Contents

1 Developmental Aspects of Pediatric Psychopharmacology......................... 1
Benedetto Vitiello, M.D.

2 Attention-Deficit/Hyperactivity Disorder 31
Jonathan Posner, M.D., and Laurence Greenhill, M.D.

7 Autism and Other Pervasive Developmental Disorders

List of Tables and Figures

Contributors

Boris Birmaher, M.D.
Professor of Psychiatry, Endowed Chair in Early Onset Bipolar Disease, Department of Psychiatry, Western Psychiatric Institute and Clinic, University of Pittsburgh Medical Center, Pittsburgh, Pennsylvania

Natoshia Raishevich Cunningham, Ph.D.
Postdoctoral Fellow, Cincinnati Children's Hospital, Cincinnati, Ohio

Christopher N. David, B.A.
Child Psychiatry Branch, National Institute of Mental Health, Bethesda, Maryland

Craig A. Erickson, M.D.
Child and Adolescent Psychiatry Fellow, Department of Psychiatry, Indiana University School of Medicine; Christian Sarkine Autism Treatment Center at the James Whitcomb Riley Hospital for Children, Indianapolis, Indiana

Robert L. Findling, M.D., M.B.A.
Professor of Psychiatry and Pediatrics and Director, Division of Child and Adolescent Psychiatry, University Hospitals Case Medical Center, Discovery and Wellness Center for Children, Case Western Reserve University School of Medicine, Cleveland, Ohio

Nitin Gogtay, M.D.
Staff Clinician, Child Psychiatry Branch, National Institute of Mental Health, Bethesda, Maryland

Pablo H. Goldberg, M.D.
Assistant Professor of Clinical Psychiatry and Medical Director of Children's Day Unit, Columbia University/New York State Psychiatric Institute, New York, New York

Laurence Greenhill, M.D.
Ruane Professor of Clinical Psychiatry, Division of Child and Adolescent Psychiatry, Columbia College of Physicians and Surgeons, Columbia University; Research Psychiatrist II, New York State Psychiatric Institute, New York, New York; Principal Investigator, New York State Research Units on Pediatric Psychopharmacology

Aysegul Selcen Guler, M.D.
Department of Child and Adolescent Psychiatry, Marmara University Faculty of Medicine, Istanbul, Turkey

Olga Jablonka, B.A.
Project Manager, Children's Day Unit, Columbia University/New York State Psychiatric Institute, New York, New York

Peter S. Jensen, M.D.
Director, The REACH Institute, New York, New York

Kevin W. Kuich, M.D.
Clinical Lecturer, Child and Adolescent Inpatient Faculty; Director, Marketing and Program Development for Inpatient Programs, Section of Child and Adolescent Psychiatry, University of Michigan, Ann Arbor, Michigan

Christopher J. McDougle, M.D.
Albert E. Sterne Professor and Chairman, Department of Psychiatry, Indiana University School of Medicine; Christian Sarkine Autism Treatment Center at the James Whitcomb Riley Hospital for Children, Indianapolis, Indiana

Molly McVoy, M.D.
Assistant Professor of Psychiatry and Assistant Training Director, Division of Child and Adolescent Psychiatry, University Hospitals Case Medical Center, Discovery and Wellness Center for Children, Case Western Reserve University School of Medicine, Cleveland, Ohio

Lourival Baptista Neto, M.D.
Assistant Clinical Professor of Psychiatry, Columbia University/New York State Psychiatric Institute, New York, New York

Elizabeth Pappadopulos, Ph.D.
Assistant Director, Center for the Advancement of Children's Mental Health at Columbia University; Assistant Professor, Clinical Psychology (in Psychiatry), Columbia University, New York, New York

Jonathan Posner, M.D.
Assistant Professor of Clinical Psychiatry, Columbia College of Physicians and Surgeons and New York State Psychiatric Institute, New York, New York

Judith L. Rapoport, M.D.
Chief, Child Psychiatry Branch, National Institute of Mental Health, Bethesda, Maryland

Moira A. Rynn, M.D.
Deputy Director of Research Psychiatry, Associate Professor of Clinical Psychiatry, Division of Child and Adolescent Psychiatry, Department of Psychiatry, Columbia University/New York State Psychiatric Institute, New York, New York

Lawrence Scahill, M.S.N., Ph.D.
Professor of Nursing and Child Psychiatry, Yale Child Study Center, New Haven, Connecticut

Kimberly A. Stigler, M.D.
Assistant Professor of Psychiatry, Department of Psychiatry, Indiana University School of Medicine; Christian Sarkine Autism Treatment Center at the James Whitcomb Riley Hospital for Children, Indianapolis, Indiana

Tiffany Thomas, M.D.
Assistant Training Director, Post-Pediatric Portal Program, Child and Adolescent Psychiatry Faculty, University Hospitals of Cleveland, Case Western Reserve University School of Medicine, Cleveland, Ohio

Benedetto Vitiello, M.D.
Chief, Child and Adolescent Treatment and Preventive Intervention Research Branch, National Institute of Mental Health, Bethesda, Maryland

Solomon G. Zaraa, D.O.
Senior Instructor, Division of Child and Adolescent Psychiatry, University Hospitals Case Medical Center, Case Western Reserve University School of Medicine, Cleveland, Ohio

Disclosure of Competing Interests

The following contributors to this book have indicated a financial interest in or other affiliation with a commercial supporter, a manufacturer of a commercial product, a provider of a commercial service, a nongovernmental organization, and/or a government agency, as listed below:

Boris Birmaher, M.D.   *Employer:* University of Pittsburgh, University of Pittsburgh Medical Center/Western Psychiatric Institute and Clinic; *Grant Support:* National Institute of Mental Health. *Consultant:* Schering-Plough; *Royalties:* Lippincott Williams & Wilkins, Random House.

Craig A. Erickson, M.D.   *Chief Medical Advisor:* Confluence Pharmaceuticals; *Consultant:* F. Hoffmann LaRoche (past), Novartis (past), Seaside Therapeutics (past); *Research Grant Support:* Bristol Myers-Squibb (past), F. Hoffmann LaRoche (past), Novartis (current), Seaside Therapeutics (current).

Robert L. Findling, M.D.   *Grant/Research Support:* AstraZeneca, Bristol-Myers Squibb, Eli Lilly, Forest, GlaxoSmithKline, Johnson & Johnson, Merck, National Institutes of Health, Novartis, Otsuka, Pfizer, Rhodes, Shionogi, Shire, Stanley Medical Research Institute, Supernus; *Consultant:* Alexza, Bristol-Myers Squibb, Dainippon Sumitomo Pharma, GlaxoSmithKline, Guilford Press, KemPharm, Lundbeck, Merck, Novartis, Otsuka, Pfizer, Physicians Postgraduate Press, Roche, Shire, Sunovion, Supernus, Transcept, WebMD; *Speakers' Bureau:* Shire; *Royalties:* American Psychiatric Publishing, Johns Hopkins University Press, Sage Publications.

Pablo H. Goldberg, M.D.   *Consultant:* ProPhase.

Laurence Greenhill, M.D.   Dr. Greenhill entered into a research contract with Rhodes Pharmaceuticals to conduct a study of Biphentin in children with ADHD. The study was completed in September 2011, and no patents were recorded or requested.

Peter S. Jensen, M.D.   *Honoraria:* Janssen-Cilag, Shire; *Grant Support:* J.W. Marriott & Alice Marriott Foundation, Shire; *Royalties:* Ballantine Books, Civic Research Institute, Guilford Press, Oxford University Press; *Part-Owner:* CATCH Services, Inc.

Elizabeth Pappadopulos, Ph.D.   *Honoraria:* Bristol-Myers Squibb.

Jonathan Posner, M.D.   *Research Support:* Shire Pharmaceuticals (investigator-initiated research agreement to study emotional processing in ADHD with fMRI).

Moira A. Rynn, M.D.   *Research Support:* Boehringer Ingelheim, Eli Lilly, Merck, National Institute of Child Health & Human Development, National Institute of Mental Health, Neuropharm, Pfizer; *Royalties:* American Psychiatric Publishing; *Honoraria:* AACAP National Conference Presentation, NSLIJ Grand Rounds.

Lawrence Scahill, M.S.N., Ph.D.   *Research Support:* Pfizer, Roche, Shire; *Consultant:* Biomarin, F. Hoffmann LaRoche, Pfizer.

Kimberly A. Stigler, M.D.   *Research Support:* Bristol-Myers Squibb, Curemark, Eli Lilly, Forest, Janssen, Seaside Therapeutics.

The following authors have no competing interests to report:
Natoshia Raishevich Cunningham, Ph.D.
Christopher N. David, B.A.
Nitin Gogtay, M.D.
Aysegul Selcen Guler, M.D.
Olga Jablonka, B.A.
Kevin W. Kuich, M.D.
Christopher J. McDougle, M.D.
Molly McVoy, M.D.
Lourival Baptista Neto, M.D.
Judith L. Rapoport, M.D.
Tiffany Thomas, M.D.
Benedetto Vitiello, M.D.
Solomon G. Zaraa, D.O.

Foreword

The use of medication to address emotional and behavioral symptoms in children and adolescents is the most rapidly changing area of pediatric mental health care and also the most controversial. Epidemiological studies show that the use of these medications overall is increasingly common, despite decreases in prescriptions for some specific drugs and classes of drugs (e.g., the decline in use of antidepressants following the U.S. Food and Drug Administration "black box" warning). The good news is that there is a growing body of research to guide our use of these interventions, which are potentially powerful in both benefits and risks. The bad news is twofold—we have far less research than we need to provide truly evidence-based treatment for each patient, and the various media are overflowing with strongly held non-research-based opinions regarding these treatments. What is a clinician to do?

The first edition (2008) of this handy clinical manual began to assist with applying both research and clinical wisdom from experience to the pharmacological treatment of youth with psychiatric symptoms and disorders. The evidence base has continued to develop, making this new edition essential. The second edition maintains the diagnosis-based chapter structure and the introductory chapter on developmental aspects of pediatric psychopharmacology. The senior author(s) of each chapter have remained. Each of these authors is a highly respected expert on the disorder covered by his or her chapter, based on extensive research and clinical experience. The final chapter in the first edition, "Disorders Primarily Seen in General Medical Settings," has not been retained. Unfortunately, there is little new research on this topic that would inform an updated chapter.

The structure of each chapter, including a concise review of research, efficient tables, and Clinical Pearls, makes this a highly useful book for child and adolescent psychiatrists as well as for pediatricians, family physicians, advanced practice nurses, and adult psychiatrists who treat children and adolescents with psychotropic medications. Medication indications, benefits, risks, and principles of use are embedded in the context of careful diagnosis and consideration of alternative or simultaneous psychosocial treatments. Rather than lists of studies with results, the authors put the body of research into perspective, noting the strengths and limitations and how the evidence is applicable to a clinical situation. Treatment of common comorbidities is included.

This book also offers an unbiased and evidence-based resource for those who do not prescribe medications, but who work with the youth who receive these treatments. Social workers, psychologists, special education professionals, and those who direct programs in child welfare or juvenile justice will find important information here.

In short, this is a book that I shall recommend to child and adolescent psychiatry fellows and the full range of child mental health professionals. No matter how small the bookshelf, this book should be on it.

Mina K. Dulcan, M.D.
Ann & Robert H. Lurie Children's Hospital of Chicago,
Northwestern University Feinberg School of Medicine,
Chicago, Illinois

Preface

The topic of pediatric psychopharmacology is compelling and often controversial. In addition, what is known about the psychopharmacological treatment of children and adolescents is rapidly changing. This book, *Clinical Manual of Child and Adolescent Psychopharmacology*, Second Edition, was designed to help clinicians provide state-of-the-art care to their patients, and to keep up to date with the most recent research available. Because the knowledge base grows so rapidly in this field, the authors have updated the first edition of this book to provide clinicians with the latest information available about the psychopharmacological treatment of children.

As in the previous edition, leading clinician-scientists were chosen to be authors so they could provide their perspectives on key aspects of the newest research in pediatric psychopharmacology. The authors have also been asked to give commentary regarding the clinical implications of the available scientific literature so that readers might have insights into how to incorporate research results into superb clinical practice. Each chapter has been revised and updated in detail, emphasizing what has been learned since the last edition of this book. New authors have been added to many of the chapters to provide the broadest perspectives on the available literature.

Since the first edition of this book, substantive research has been done in nearly every area of pediatric psychopharmacology, and major steps have been made toward improving the evidence-based practice of treating youth with psychiatric illness. Multiple studies have expanded our understanding of ways to treat youth with disruptive behavior disorders, mood disorders, anxiety disorders, pervasive developmental disorders, and psychotic illnesses. In particular, advances have been made in understanding the long-term treatment effects of medications in pediatric populations. More head-to-head studies have been completed, comparing multiple active comparators. Research designs have included a broader base of patient populations in an attempt to make the data more applicable to everyday clinical practice. More studies looking into combination therapies have been completed, helping clinicians better understand how to treat the complicated patients that present every day to a prescribing clinician's office.

The bottom line is that child and adolescent psychiatry in general, and psychopharmacology in particular, is a rapidly progressing field that is advancing in multiple directions at any given time. In order to provide the best clinical care for patients, it is important for clinicians to remain up to date with the available research. To provide a foundation for that care, much thought, energy, and consideration have been given to ensure that this Second Edition of the *Clinical Manual of Child and Adolescent Psychopharmacology* is a book that is both scientifically sound and clinically rich.

Molly McVoy, M.D.
Robert L. Findling, M.D., M.B.A.

Acknowledgments

As with any endeavor of this magnitude, this book was a truly collaborative effort. The chapter authors are extraordinarily busy, engaged experts in their field who generously volunteered their time to contribute to this book. The editorial staff at American Psychiatric Publishing (APPI) is exceptionally easy to work with, and have been generous with their time, energy, expertise and patience. In particular, many thanks go to Robert E. Hales, M.D., Editor-in-Chief of Books; John McDuffie, Editorial Director of the Books Division; Tina Coltri-Marshall, Publications Coordinator; Greg Kuny, Managing Editor; and Rebecca Richters, Senior Editor.

Finally, and most importantly, thanks to the patients we have the privilege to serve. Thanks also go to the generous support of all of our families as we work to serve our patients using the highest standards of psychiatric medicine.

1

Developmental Aspects of Pediatric Psychopharmacology

Benedetto Vitiello, M.D.

Pediatric psychopharmacology is the science behind the use of psychotropic agents to improve the mental health of children and adolescents. This discipline has four defining elements: the developing organism (in particular, the developing brain), psychopathology, chemical compounds that act on the brain, and the therapeutic intent. The interplay among these elements determines the benefits and toxicity of a particular treatment.

Many medications are prescribed to children based mainly on research conducted in adults; however, extrapolation from adult data is insufficient to in-

Disclaimer: The opinions and assertions contained in this chapter are the private views of the author and are not to be construed as official or as reflecting the views of the National Institute of Mental Health, the National Institutes of Health, or the Department of Health and Human Services.

form rational pediatric pharmacotherapy. Differences in how the developing organism treats the drug (pharmacokinetics), how the developing brain reacts to the drug (pharmacodynamics), and how psychopathology manifests itself during development have implications for both efficacy and safety, and therefore direct research is needed in children. The considerable expansion of pediatric psychopharmacology research in recent years has provided a foundation on which evidence-based pharmacotherapy can be built. In addition to the biological implications of development, special ethical and legal considerations apply when treating children for purposes of either personal care or research.

The purpose of this chapter is to describe the aspects that are specific to pediatric psychopharmacology and that make it a distinct discipline at the crossroads of child and adolescent psychiatry, pediatrics, and pharmacology.

Pharmacokinetics

Pharmacokinetics determines the availability of a drug at the site of action and thus directly influences the intensity and duration of the pharmacological activity. The basic pharmacokinetic processes of absorption, distribution, metabolism (biotransformation), and excretion are all influenced by development, as summarized in Tables 1–1 and 1–2. Because knowledge of the pharmacokinetics of a drug is critical for identifying the therapeutic dose range and frequency of administration, pediatric pharmacokinetics studies should precede and inform clinical trials aimed at testing efficacy in children (Findling et al. 2006).

Children have smaller body size than adults but a greater proportion of liver and kidney parenchyma when adjusted for body weight. Compared with adults, children also have relatively more body water, less fat, and less plasma albumin to which drugs can bind. These structural characteristics can result in a smaller volume of distribution for drugs, greater drug extraction during the first pass through the liver after oral administration, lower bioavailability, and faster metabolism and elimination (see Table 1–2). These differences mean that simply decreasing adult doses based on child weight may result in undertreatment. Adjusting by body surface area would control for both weight and height, but this approach is usually reserved for drugs with a narrow therapeutic index, such as antineoplastics, and is seldom used in pediatric psychopharmacology.

Table 1–1. Essential pharmacokinetics terminology

Term	Definition
Absorption	Process by which a drug is absorbed from the site of administration into the systemic circulation
Liver first-pass extraction	Drug metabolism that occurs when a drug goes through the liver soon after intestinal absorption, before reaching the systemic circulation
Bioavailability	Proportion of administered drug that reaches the systemic circulation
Area under the curve (AUC)	Total area under the curve that describes the drug plasma as a function of time
Metabolism (biotransformation)	Phase I: cytochrome P450 (CYP)–mediated oxidation; hydroxylation Phase II: conjugation reactions (glucuronidation, sulfation, acetylation)
Volume of distribution (V_d)	Apparent volume in which the drug is distributed after absorption (V_d = dose absorbed /C_p)
Concentration in plasma (C_p)	Drug quantity for unit of plasma (C_p = dose absorbed/V_d)
Peak plasma concentration (C_{max})	Highest plasma concentration
Time to C_{max} (T_{max})	Time that it takes from drug administration to reach C_{max}
Clearance (plasma clearance: CL)	Volume of plasma completely cleared of the drug in a unit of time; the cumulative result of drug removal that occurs in the liver, kidney, and other parts of the body (e.g., lungs, skin, bile); CL = dose absorbed/AUC
Elimination half-life ($t_{1/2}$)	Time that it takes, after full drug absorption and distribution in the body, for C_p to be reduced by 50%; a function of CL and V_d ($t_{1/2}$ = 0.693 · V_d/CL)
Steady-state plasma concentration	Stable C_p between doses that is achieved when the rate of elimination equals the rate of absorption; usually achieved after about four half-lives during constant drug administration

Table 1–2.   Developmental pharmacokinetics and its implications

Compared with adults, children have	Pharmacokinetics implications	Examples
Smaller body size	Smaller volume of distribution → higher peak plasma concentration	After 20 mg oral fluoxetine, plasma levels are twofold higher in children than in adolescents (Wilens et al. 2002)
More liver parenchyma relative to body size	Relatively greater metabolic capacity → greater first-pass liver drug extraction → reduced bioavailability → faster drug metabolism → greater metabolite/parent drug levels ratio → shorter half-life ($t_{1/2}$)	Ratio of metabolites to bupropion in plasma is 19%–80% greater in youth than in adults; mean bupropion $t_{1/2}$ is 12 hours in youth vs. 21 hours in adults (Daviss et al. 2005)
Relatively more body water and less adipose tissue	Less accumulation of drug → faster elimination	
More kidney parenchyma relative to body size	Relatively greater clearance capacity → faster drug elimination → shorter time to plasma peak → shorter $t_{1/2}$	Lithium $t_{1/2}$: 18 ± 7 hours in children vs. 22 ± 8 hours in adults (Vitiello et al. 1988)

Adolescence is characterized by marked growth in body size and redistribution of body compartments. Differences between sexes become more pronounced. In males, the percentage of total body water increases and that of body fat decreases, whereas the opposite occurs in females. These changes can produce gender differences in pharmacokinetics. Specific studies into the gender differences in adolescents have yet to be completed and may be warranted given this difference.

Drug metabolism consists in biotransformations that turn the drug into derivative products (metabolites) that are more polar and therefore more easily eliminated. (Not all drugs undergo metabolism, however. Lithium, for instance, is excreted unchanged through the kidneys.) Drug metabolism typically includes a Phase I, during which medications undergo enzymatic oxidative or hydrolytic transformations, and a Phase II, during which conjugates are formed between the drug, or its metabolites, and glucuronic acid, sulfate, glutathione, or acetate. The Phase I oxidative processes are mediated by cytochrome P450 (CYP) microsomal enzymes, which are concentrated in the liver but present in small quantity in other tissues as well.

The CYP system matures rapidly after birth. For instance, liver microsomes have only 1% of the adult CYP2D6 activity in the fetus, but this rate increases to about 20% of the adult activity by 1 month after birth. The immaturity of the CYP2D6 system at birth is one of the possible explanations for the syndrome of irritability, tachypnea, tremors, and increased muscle tone that has been observed in newborns of mothers taking selective serotonin reuptake inhibitors (SSRIs) (Chambers et al. 1996). An alternative explanation is that the syndrome represents a withdrawal reaction from the SSRI (Sanz et al. 2005). In any case, the CYP metabolizing capacity is well developed by age 3 years (DeWildt et al. 1999). Because children have proportionally greater liver parenchyma than adults, the weight-adjusted metabolic capacity is greater in childhood.

The two most important CYP enzymes in pediatric psychopharmacology are CYP3A4 and CYP2D6, which are involved in the metabolism of most psychotropics, as summarized in Table 1–3. Genetic polymorphism has been identified for CYP2D6. About 7%–10% of whites, 1%–8% of blacks, and 1%–3% of East Asians are poor metabolizers. Poor metabolizers have higher drug concentrations in plasma and other body tissues. For example, the mean elimination half-life of atomoxetine is about 5 hours in children or adults who are extensive metabolizers, but 22 hours in poor metabolizers (Sauer et al. 2005). Being a poor metabolizer can have safety implications. One case of death in a 9-year-old child with a CYP2D6 genetic deficiency was associated with unusually high plasma levels of fluoxetine (Sallee et al. 2000). Assaying for genetic polymorphism is currently not considered a routine procedure in pediatric psychopharmacology, but it may be considered for individual patients in the case of long-term treatment with drugs metabolized by CYP enzymes with genetic polymorphism (e.g., 2D6 and 2C19), drugs with a low therapeutic index (e.g., tricyclics), polypharmacy, or drugs with history of toxicity.

Possible drug-drug and drug-food interactions must be taken into account because drugs or food can inhibit, induce, or compete with specific CYP enzymes (see Table 1–3). Especially important are those genetic polymorphisms and drug interactions that involve drugs with potential toxicities at high plasma concentration. Poor metabolizer status or the concomitant administration of another drug that competes with or inhibits the metabolism of the first drug would result in increased plasma concentrations. For instance, poor metabolizers of CYP2D6 could develop toxic levels of tricyclic antidepressants. In addition, concomitant administration of fluvoxamine (an inhibitor of CYP3A4) and pimozide (metabolized by 3A4) could lead to high levels of pimozide and prolongation of the QTc interval. Finally, in sexually active female adolescents, use of oral contraceptives can induce CYP enzymes and thus increase drug metabolism and elimination.

The main route of drug elimination is through the kidneys, whereas bile, lungs, and skin account for a much smaller portion of elimination. Absolute clearance is usually lower in children than in adults, but weight-adjusted clearance is greater in children than in adults (see Table 1–2). Because of the faster elimination, the drug plasma half-life can be shorter in children than in adults (Daviss et al. 2005). A shorter elimination half-life means that plasma steady state is reached sooner during repeated administration, and that elimination is faster so that withdrawal symptoms upon discontinuation are more likely. More frequent dosing may be needed to maintain steady state and prevent withdrawal symptoms between doses.

Pharmacokinetics can also be influenced by the dose of medication and the duration of treatment, as shown in studies of sertraline in adolescents (Axelson et al. 2002). After a single dose of sertraline 50 mg in adolescents, the mean half-life was about 27 hours, but at steady state, after repeated administrations, the mean half-life decreased to about 15 hours. In addition, the steady-state half-life was found to be longer (about 20 hours) after administration of higher doses (100–150 mg). The clinical implication is that lower doses (50 mg/day) should be given twice a day to ensure consistent treatment and prevent withdrawal, whereas higher doses can be given once a day.

In pharmacokinetics studies of a number of commonly prescribed medications in pediatric populations, researchers found the pharmacokinetics of many compounds, such as escitalopram, aripiprazole, quetiapine, risperidone, and lithium, to be similar to that in adults (Findling et al. 2008, 2010a; Rao 2007; Thyssen et al. 2010). However, considerable intersubject variability was observed, suggesting that major individual differences in the time course of pharmacological effects may occur clinically.

In the case of medications such as methylphenidate and amphetamines, whose short half-lives result in short duration of action with consequent need for multiple daily doses, a variety of extended-release formulations have been developed. The first generation of extended-release formulations of methylphenidate consists of tablets of immediate- and slower-release medication, indicated with different-colored coatings. Due to considerable intersubject variability in absorption, however, the onset of action may be delayed in the morning and/or the therapeutic effect may attenuate in the afternoon. More recently, a second generation of biphasic extended-release formulations has been introduced. These formulations allow an initial bolus of medication to be absorbed immediately, followed by a second, more gradual release. The plasma pharmacokinetics curve thus shows an acute initial peak at about 1.5 hours after dosing, followed by a second peak about 3 hours later. The rationale for these biphasic release formulations rests in the observation that optimal clinical effect occurs at increasing plasma levels of methylphenidate (Swanson et al. 2003). These extended-release preparations can be administered once a day in the morning, because they allow adequate control of attention-deficit/hyperactivity disorder (ADHD) for 8–10 hours (Swanson et al. 2004).

Plasma levels are used as an indication ("surrogate marker") of drug concentration at the site of action, which, in the case of psychotropics, is not easily accessible. In fact, plasma drug levels are a rather incomplete reflection of the drug concentration in the brain, as also suggested by the rather low correlation between plasma level and clinical effects that is observed for most but not all drugs. Proton mag-

Table 1–3. Selected compounds relevant to pediatric pharmacotherapy metabolized by cytochrome P450 (CYP) enzymes

CYP enzyme	Genetic polymorphism	Substrates	Inhibitors	Inducers
3A4	None	Alprazolam	Clarithromycin	Carbamazepine
		Aripiprazole	Erythromycin	Dexamethasone
		Bupropion	Fluoxetine	Oxcarbazepine
		Buspirone	Fluvoxamine	Phenobarbital
		Citalopram	Grapefruit juice	Phenytoin
		Erythromycin	Indinavir	Primidone
		Escitalopram	Ketoconazole	Rifampin
		Ethinyl estradiol	Nefazodone	St. John's wort[†]
		Indinavir	Ritonavir	Topiramate
		Mirtazapine		
		Nefazodone		
		Pimozide		
		Quetiapine		
		Ritonavir		
		Saquinavir		
		Sertraline		
		Ziprasidone		
		Zolpidem		
2D6	Yes[a]	Amitriptyline	Amitriptyline	
		Aripiprazole	Clomipramine	
		Atomoxetine	Desipramine	
		Desipramine	Fluoxetine	
		Dextromethorphan	Haloperidol	
		Fluoxetine	Imipramine	
		Haloperidol	Nortriptyline	
		Imipramine	Paroxetine	
		Nortriptyline		
		Olanzapine		
		Paroxetine		

Table 1–3. Selected compounds relevant to pediatric pharmacotherapy metabolized by cytochrome P450 (CYP) enzymes *(continued)*

CYP enzyme	Genetic polymorphism	Substrates	Inhibitors	Inducers
2D6 *(continued)*		Perphenazine		
		Risperidone		
		Venlafaxine		
1A2	None	Amitriptyline	Ciprofloxacin	Carbamazepine
		Caffeine	Erythromycin	Modafinil
		Clozapine	Fluvoxamine	Tobacco smoke
		Fluvoxamine		
		Olanzapine		
		Theophylline		
2C9	Yes[b]	Fluoxetine	Fluoxetine	Carbamazepine
		Fluvoxamine	Fluvoxamine	Rifampin
		Ibuprofen	Modafinil	
		Naproxen	Sertraline	
2C19	Yes[c]	Amitriptyline	Fluoxetine	
		Citalopram	Fluvoxamine	
		Clomipramine	Modafinil	
		Diazepam		
		Escitalopram		
		Imipramine		
2B6	Yes[d]	Bupropion		Diazepam
				Clonazepam

[†]*Hypericum perforatum.*

[a]Poor metabolizers: 7%–10% of whites, 1%–8% of Africans, and 1%–3% of East Asians. Ultrafast metabolizers: 1%–3% of whites.

[b]Poor metabolizers: 6%–12% of whites, 4% of Africans, and 3% of East Asians.

[c]Poor metabolizers: 1%–3% of whites, 1%–3% of Africans, and 20% of East Asians.

[d]Reported in white and Japanese populations.

netic resonance spectroscopy has allowed the brain level of several drugs, such as lithium and fluoxetine, to be directly measured. For instance, a direct correlation between serum and brain lithium levels was reported in both children and adults; younger subjects, however, had a lower brain-to-serum ratio, thus suggesting that they may need higher maintenance serum lithium concentrations than adults to achieve therapeutic lithium concentrations in the brain (Moore et al. 2002).

Pharmacodynamics

Although the exact mechanism of action responsible for the therapeutic effects of many psychotropics remains unknown, the basic biochemical activity of these medications is generally considered to be similar across ages. For instance, SSRIs block the reuptake of serotonin in both children and adults, and their antidepressant effect has been found to be associated with the degree of inhibition of the serotonin transporter in platelets (Axelson et al. 2005). However, the possible effects of development on the intensity and specificity of this pharmacological activity have not been systematically evaluated.

Most psychotropics act through neurotransmitters, such as dopamine, serotonin, and norepinephrine, whose receptors undergo major changes during development (Rho and Storey 2001). Receptor density tends to peak in preschool years and then gradually declines toward adult levels in late adolescence (Chugani et al. 2001). The impact of these developmental changes on drug activity and possible clinical implications have not been fully elucidated, but the observation that there are differences between children and adults in the efficacy and safety of a number of psychotropics supports the notion that development has a significant influence on the effects of psychotropic medications. For example, amphetamine-like stimulants are more likely to induce euphoria in adults than in children, and antipsychotics are more likely to induce metabolic effects in youth than in adults (Correll et al. 2009).

Although not yet applicable to clinical care, brain imaging technology and genetics are currently used to research, respectively, specific brain targets of psychotropics and possible associations between genetic polymorphisms and pharmacological effects (Stein and McGough 2008). The practical appeal of this line of research is that it may eventually lead to a more targeted and individualized treatment approach.

Efficacy

Evidence of treatment efficacy in children is established primarily through controlled clinical trials. The theoretical framework of this methodology is the same as in adult psychopharmacology, but there are important differences when it is applied to pediatric samples. A distinctive characteristic is that collection of clinical information about both therapeutic and adverse effects of treatment often relies more on reports from adults, such as parents and teachers, than from the child. This is especially the case in the treatment of young children who have cognitive disabilities or disruptive behavior disorders. This particular feature of pediatric pharmacology makes drug evaluations in both research and practice settings more complex and time-consuming than in adults. Clinicians must integrate information from a variety of sources and arrive at a coherent conclusion about treatment effects.

A number of rating instruments have been developed and validated for assessing treatment effects on psychiatric symptoms and level of functioning in children. In the absence of biological markers of disease and treatment effects, the pharmacotherapist must rely on changes in clinical symptoms to gauge response. Although symptom rating scales have been introduced primarily for research purposes, with the goal of quantifying psychopathology at different points in time, they can and should be applied to usual clinical practice, because they help the clinician measure and document the patient's condition prospectively. Population norms have been developed for many scales for rating ADHD, depression, and anxiety symptoms in children.

For children with ADHD, parent and teacher questionnaires are typically used, such as the Conners Parent Rating Scale—Revised, the Conners Teacher Rating Scale—Revised, the Iowa Conners Teacher Rating Scale, or the Swanson, Nolan, and Pelham Version IV (SNAP-IV) rating scale. Some of these scales are available from commercial sources (e.g., the Conners scales are available from Multi-Health Systems), in the scientific literature (Conners et al. 1998a, 1998b), or at Internet sites (e.g., SNAP-IV is available at www.adhd.net). To assess treatment effects in anxiety disorders, both rating instruments completed by the child or parent, such as the Screen for Child Anxiety Related Emotional Disorders (SCARED) (Birmaher et al. 1997) or the Multidimensional Anxiety Scale for Children (MASC) (March et al. 1997), and rating scales completed by clinicians, such as the Pediatric Anxiety

Rating Scale (Research Units on Pediatric Psychopharmacology Anxiety Study Group 2002), are available. In the assessment of antidepressant treatment effects, clinician-rated scales are generally used, in particular the Children's Depression Rating Scale—Revised (Poznanski and Mokros 1996), which has been used in most placebo-controlled trials of antidepressants in children and adolescents (March et al. 2004). A number of self-administered scales, such as the Children's Depression Inventory (Kovacs 1985), the Beck Depression Inventory (Beck and Steer 1984), and the Reynolds Adolescent Depression Scale, 2nd Edition (Reynolds 2002), are commonly used in practice settings and especially with adolescents. A fairly recently developed scale to rate adolescent depression is the Quick Inventory of Depressive Symptomatology, which is available in both clinician-rated and adolescent-rated versions, and is in the public domain (Bernstein et al. 2010). Scales for rating behavior in children with cognitive disabilities are also available and have been found to be sensitive to treatment effects in autism clinical trials (Marshburn and Aman 1992; McCracken et al. 2002). Finally, scales of global functioning, such as the Children's Global Assessment Scale (Shaffer et al. 1983) and its adaptation to children with autism and other pervasive developmental disorders (Wagner et al. 2007), are used in clinical studies.

For some medications, continuity of efficacy has been consistently demonstrated between children and adults (e.g., serotonin reuptake inhibitors are effective in the treatment of obsessive-compulsive disorder, and stimulants in ADHD). For other medications, remarkable differences have been observed. Most notably, none of the placebo-controlled trials of tricyclic antidepressants have been able to show superiority of the active medication in children (Hazell et al. 1995) and, among the SSRIs, only fluoxetine and escitalopram have been found better than placebo in more than one study. It is difficult to determine whether the inability to consistently demonstrate antidepressant efficacy for the other SSRIs was mainly due to intrinsic differences in pharmacological activity among these compounds (a difference that does seem to exist in adults) or, more likely, to variability in methods and implementation across studies (Kratochvil et al. 2006).

An increasing body of research in child and adolescent psychiatry has allowed evidence-based treatment algorithms to be developed. Treatment algorithms consist of step-by-step instructions on how to treat individual patients based on their symptoms and history of previous treatment. Algorithms are therefore more detailed and specific than general treatment guidelines or practice parameters. Pediatric pharmacological algorithms have been developed for ADHD, depression, and other disorders (Birmaher and Brent 2007; McClellan et al. 2007; Pliszka and AACAP Work Group on Quality Issues 2007). The magnitude of the treatment effect relative to a control is often expressed in standard deviation units using the effect size. Among the most commonly used ways of computing an effect size is Cohen's *d* or Hedge's *g*, either of which is the difference in outcome measure between the study groups divided by the pooled standard deviation at the end of treatment (Rosenthal et al. 2000). Compared with placebo, stimulants usually have a large effect size (0.8 and above) in decreasing symptoms of ADHD (Greenhill et al. 2001). In the trials that have detected a separation between SSRI and placebo, the SSRI had a moderate effect size (0.5–0.7) when used in the treatment of major depression (March et al. 2004) or obsessive-compulsive disorder (Pediatric OCD Treatment Study 2004). However, meta-analysis of all available databases of clinical trials in pediatric depression indicates that the effect size of antidepressant medication versus placebo is small (0.25; 95% confidence interval [CI], 0.16–0.34) (Bridge at al. 2007), which is consistent with adult data (Bech et al. 2000).

It should be pointed out that the effect size is a purely mathematical computation to express a difference between means. As such, it is at times used to quantify the difference from pretreatment to posttreatment within the same treatment group. When this is done, a large effect size often emerges, because it includes the time effect. In the absence of a control condition and due to the consequent inability to distinguish treatment effect from time effect, the pretreatment to posttreatment effect size has limited meaning and cannot be taken as an index of treatment effect.

In addition to the effect size, a useful calculation is the strength of the therapeutic benefit using the number needed to treat (NNT), which is the number of patients who need to be given the treatment in order to add one more improved patient to the number of those who are expected to improve with the control condition. For example, in the Treatment for Adolescents With Depression Study (TADS), 61% of fluoxetine-treated patients improved at the end of the 12-week treatment, compared with 35% of the placebo patients (March et al. 2004). The NNT is 4 (i.e., $1/[0.61 - 0.35]$), which indicates that, on average, one needs to treat four patients in order to improve one patient more than the placebo condition. The smaller the NNT, the greater is the relative efficacy of the treatment. Clinical trials have shown that the NNTs of psychotropic medications, although variable across studies, are often quite favorable and compare well with other nonpsychiatric drugs used in pediatrics.

Because most psychiatric conditions are chronic or recurrent in nature and symptoms tend to reemerge when treatment is discontinued, pharmacological treatment of child disorders is often prolonged in time. A few studies have addressed the long-term effectiveness of pharmacotherapy in child psychiatry (Emslie et al. 2004; March et al. 2007; MTA Cooperative Group 2004; Vitiello et al. 2011). More research, however, is needed to test whether successful control of symptoms in the short term translates into better prognosis in the long term. This type of research poses many challenges from a methodological and implementation point of view because, on the one hand, conducting long-term randomized controlled trials is difficult, and, on the other hand, observational studies are usually insufficient for inferring causality.

Safety

Safety issues are paramount, especially when treating children. Pharmacological treatment during a period when the organism undergoes marked developmental changes may result in toxicities that are not seen in adults. For example, prolonged administration of phenobarbital to young children to prevent recurrence of febrile seizures impairs their cognitive development (Farwell et al. 1990). In addition, the risk of valproic acid–induced hepatotoxicity is highest for children under age 2 years and decreases with age (Bryant and Dreifuss 1996). Hepatotoxicity may be caused by a toxic metabolite, 4-ene-valproic acid, which is produced by CYP2C9 and CYP2A6 enzymes (Sadeque et al. 1997). Also, children are at higher risk than adults of developing serious rash during treatment with lamotrigine, possibly due to a higher efficiency of the CYP metabolism in children, which may result in higher levels of potentially toxic metabolites (Anderson 2002).

A general concern is that the administration of agents acting on neurotransmitter systems during rapid development may interfere with normal processes and result in unwanted long-lasting changes. The distal effects of early exposure to psychotropics have been investigated in animals. For example, administration of fluoxetine to newborn mice caused a transient inhibition of the serotonin transporter during early development and was associated with abnormal emotional behaviors when they were adults, such as reduced exploratory behavior and slower adaptation to novel environments or stimuli, which could be interpreted as signs of anxiety or depression (Ansorge et al. 2004). In another study, chronic administration of fluoxetine to young rats impaired dendritic growth and spine density in the hippocampus (Norrholm and Ouimet 2000). The relevance of these findings in animals to pediatric psychopharmacology remains unclear, but these findings raise the possibility that early exposure to psychotropics may have enduring effects on the brain.

A high level of suspicion is therefore warranted when treating children with medications and especially when the treatment is prolonged in time. Different types of adverse effects can occur (Vitiello et al. 2003). Some, such as rash or dystonias, may emerge acutely after brief drug exposure, whereas others, such as tardive dyskinesia or metabolic syndrome, may develop with chronic treatment. Some toxicities, such as lithium-induced tremor, are related to drug dose and/or plasma concentrations; others, such as withdrawal dyskinesias, emerge after drug discontinuation. Some adverse effects may be anticipated based on the mechanism of action of the medication, but others are completely unexpected and even paradoxical, such as the increased suicidality with antidepressant treatment.

As in assessing efficacy, the assessment of safety in pediatric psychopharmacology depends in large part on adult monitoring and reporting. From the perspective of the clinician, identification of treatment adverse effects is contingent on the level of detail with which the relevant information is elicited and classified. A very general and open-ended inquiry by the clinician to the child and parent during a medication management visit, such as "Any health problems since the last visit?" has been found to yield substantially less information about adverse effects than a detailed, body-system inquiry, such as "Any problems with your eyes? Ears? Throat? Breathing?…" (Greenhill et al. 2004). Obviously, the latter method of eliciting adverse effects is much more time and labor intensive than the former, and its feasibility in a busy clinical practice is therefore questionable. Research is ongoing to develop sensitive instruments to assess adverse events that can be easily administered in practice settings, such as the Pediatric Adverse Event Rating Scale (PAERS) (Wehmeier et al. 2008).

Over the years, more information has become available on the long-term safety of psychotropic medications in children. Although limited by the fact that most of the studies have been observational in nature (i.e., without an internal control group), the available data provide some guidance to clinicians. In the following paragraphs, I describe some selected safety issues that pertain to commonly used psychotropics.

Amphetamine-like stimulants can cause a dose-related delay in physical growth, in both weight and height. After 14 months of treatment, children treated with stimulant medication for ADHD grew on average 1.4 cm less in height than peers treated with behavior therapy (MTA Cooperative Group 2004). A growth deficit was found to persist in future years in continuously medicated children (Swanson et al. 2007). The mechanism underlying the interference of stimulants with skeletal growth is still being debated. Recent data suggest that chronic treatment with methylphenidate leads to transient inhibition of testosterone levels and delay in puberty (Mattison et al. 2011).

Stimulants have adrenergic effects, and concern about unwanted cardiovascular outcomes, including sudden death, has been raised (Gould et al. 2009). Recently, prospective analyses of children treated for up to 10 years did not find an increased risk for hypertension, although stimulants have a detectable effect on heart rate even with long-term use (Vitiello et al. 2012).

Because stimulant medications are drugs of potential abuse, concerns have been raised about the possibility that treatment in childhood may sensitize the brain and thus make substance abuse and dependence more likely in adolescence and adulthood. The feasibility of mounting randomized, well-controlled studies to address this issue is questionable, and researchers have relied on naturalistically treated samples. Most of these studies have not found an increased risk of substance abuse after treatment with stimulants (Biederman et al. 2008; Wilens et al. 2008).

Interesting differences in tolerability have been observed across age and type of development. Preschoolers with ADHD have lower tolerability to methylphenidate than older children (Greenhill et al. 2006; Wigal et al. 2006). Children with autism or other pervasive developmental disorders with ADHD symptoms are more sensitive to methylphenidate, as indicated by an 18% treatment discontinuation rate due to intolerable adverse events (most commonly irritability) (Research Units on Pediatric Psychopharmacology Autism Network 2005). Youth exposed to second-generation antipsychotics are more prone to gaining weight than adults (Correll et al. 2009).

Antidepressant treatment in children and adolescents has been found to be associated with increased risk for certain suicide-related events, such as thoughts about suicide and suicidal attempts, but not completed suicide (Hammad et al. 2006). In a meta-analysis including 13 placebo-controlled trials in youth with major depression, the suicidality rate was 3% for those taking antidepressant and 2% for those given placebo (Bridge et al. 2007). Similar meta-analyses of clinical trials in adults have shown a strong association between age and risk of suicidality associated with antidepressant, with an increase in risk for young adults under age 25, a neutral effect for those ages 25–64, and a protective effect for older patients (Stone et al. 2009). These data provide an example of interaction between development and pharmacological effect, even though the biological underpinning of this interaction remains unknown. In fact, the mechanisms through which antidepressants may trigger suicidality remain a matter of speculation. Some youth may become abnormally activated by the antidepressant, with display of akathisia, agitation, anxiety, insomnia, and impulsivity. For the moment, this remains a theory based on anecdotal reports, and systematic analyses of treated youth have not supported it (Vitiello et al. 2009).

Safety is a relative concept, and possible risks of pharmacotherapy must be weighed against possible risks of untreated psychopathology. Decisions about prescribing medications must also take into account the availability of effective nonpharmacological interventions. Although generally found somewhat less effective at decreasing symptoms of ADHD or depression in children and adolescents, psychotherapy can be considered in lieu of medication for mild depression, or in combination with medications for more severe cases. Psychotherapy, used either sequentially (i.e., starting first with psychotherapy, then adding medication if insufficient) or in combination (i.e., starting both psychotherapy and medication concurrently), may be able to reduce the medication dosage needed to control symptoms. Especially when treating young children, consideration should be given to using psychosocial interventions as first-step treatment. In any case, the importance of carefully monitoring children receiving psychotropics and of documenting both positive and negative outcomes has emerged as a critically important component of rational pharmacotherapy.

Ethical Aspects

Children should be given as much explanation as they can reasonably understand about their condition and the choice of possible treatments, but they cannot give legal permission for treatment, which is the responsibility of the parents. Parents are also instrumental in implementing pharmacotherapy by ensuring appropriate administration of prescribed medication and by reporting possible treatment-emergent adverse effects. Parental permission is required for child participation in research, which is subject to special regulations over and above those required for adult research participation (U.S. Department of Health and Human Services 2009; U.S. Food and Drug Administration 2001).

Only scientifically sound research investigations that use valid methodology and are posited to add new knowledge about important health issues may be ethically acceptable (Vitiello 2003). Pediatric research can be divided into two broad categories based on whether it does or does not present the prospect of direct benefit to the individual participant. *Prospect of direct benefit* refers to the fact that each participant has the potential of deriving a health benefit from participation. General acquisition of knowledge relevant to the child's condition does not satisfy the requirement of direct benefit. For being ethically acceptable, research with prospect of direct benefit must have a favorable balance between anticipated benefits and foreseeable harms. A study that tests the efficacy of a treatment intervention usually has potential for direct benefit to the research participants. In this case, the main criterion for determining whether the study is ethically acceptable is the risk-benefit ratio. The presence of a placebo arm in a randomized clinical trial is usually considered acceptable in child psychiatry conditions. Placebo does not equal absence of treatment and has been associated with substantial improvement, especially in the case of mood and anxiety disorders.

Pharmacological research that does not offer a prospect of direct benefit includes pharmacokinetics and pharmacodynamics studies. To examine the acceptability of a study in this category, one must determine whether such a study does or does not have the potential for generating essential knowledge relevant to the disorder or condition of the research participant. If the information that the study will acquire is not relevant to the child's disorder or condition (e.g., a pharmacokinetics study in healthy children who are at no increased risk for the condition being targeted by the treatment), then the research can be conducted only if it entails no more than minimal risk. *Minimal risk* is defined as "risk for harm not greater than ordinarily encountered in daily life, or during routine physical or psychological examinations or tests" [U.S. Department of Health and Human Services 2009, section 46.102(i)]. The prevailing interpretation is that the daily life, examinations, and tests of a normal child are to be used as reference, but a precise quantification of risk in ordinary daily life is not easy and remains a matter of discussion (Wendler et al. 2005).

If the study aims to acquire information relevant to the child's condition (e.g., pharmacokinetics of a medication for ADHD being studied in children with ADHD), then the research risk cannot be greater than a minor increase over minimal risk. A *minor increase over minimal risk* can be considered acceptable only if 1) it presents "experiences to the subjects that are commensurate with those inherent in their actual or expected medical, dental, psychological, social, or educational situations" [U.S. Department of Health and Human Services 2009, 45 C.F.R. 46.406(b)] and 2) the study has the potential to generate new knowledge considered of "vital importance" for understanding or treating the child's disorder or condition.

Research that is not otherwise approvable based on these criteria, but that presents an opportunity to understand, prevent, or alleviate a serious problem affecting the health or welfare of children, can be referred to the U.S. Secretary of Health and Human Services for further review under regulations at 45 C.F.R. 46.407 (U.S. Department of Health and Human Services 2009) and 21 C.F.R. 50.56 (U.S. Food and Drug Administration 2001). Studies in which psychotropic medications are given to children who are physically and mentally healthy with the goal of better understanding the drugs' mechanisms of action on the brain usually fall into this category, because nontherapeutic administration of a psychotropic drug would generally be considered to pose more than minimal risk. For example, a protocol for a brain magnetic resonance imaging study of healthy children ages 9 and older receiving a single oral dose of dextroamphetamine was referred in 2004 by the institutional review board of the National Institute of Mental Health under 45 C.F.R. 46.407 (Couzin 2004). This study was reviewed and approved by the Pediatric Ethics Subcommittee of the U.S. Food and Drug Administration's (FDA's) Pediatric Advisory Committee in September 2004. The reviewers determined that a single administration of dextroamphetamine 10 mg to a child age 9 years or older entails more than minimal risk, because the potential adverse effects are more than those expected in a routine visit to a doctor, but is limited to a minor increase over minimal risk. That being the case, and because the study had the potential to generate critically important information on the brain effects of a commonly used medication in children, the research was approved.

The process of informing parents and children about the aims, procedures, potential risks and benefits of research participation, presence of alternative treatments, and rights of research participants is critical for obtaining their informed permission and assent. In general, children ages 7 and older are able to provide assent, and this is often documented in writing with an appropriate assent form. With proper communication and explanation by researchers, parents can achieve a good understanding of both research procedures and participant rights. By age 16, youths have a level of understanding similar to that of their parents (Vitiello et al. 2009).

A number of public and private Web sites provide detailed information about child participation in research and the process of determining whether a particular project is ethically acceptable (Children's Hospital Boston 2012; Office for Human Research Protections 2012).

Regulatory Aspects

A number of psychotropic medications have received approved pediatric indications by the FDA, whereas others are used for off-label indications (Table 1–4). Off-label use of a drug is not in itself an inappropriate practice because such use is often supported by considerable empirical evidence and is consistent with treatment guidelines. However, parents need to be advised that an off-label use of a medication is going to be prescribed so they can make fully informed decisions about the treatment of their child.

Consequent to the recognition in the mid-1990s of the widespread and increasing off-label use of medications in children, major initiatives were started to increase pediatric research and thus acquire the necessary information for appropriate drug use in children. In 1997, the U.S. Congress passed the Food and Drug Administration Modernization Act of 1997 (P.L. 105-

115), which provided financial incentives to pharmaceutical companies in re-turn for conducting pediatric research. This legislation was then further ex-panded and extended by the U.S. Congress under the Best Pharmaceuticals for Children Act of 2002 (P.L. 107-109) and its later updates. The incentive (i.e., a 6-month extension in the drug patent exclusivity) has substantially changed the approach of industry to pediatric pharmacology, including also pediatric psychopharmacology. Both pharmacokinetics and clinical trials have been conducted in children under the additional exclusivity program.

For medications for which pediatric data are needed but which are already off patent, the incentive of additional patent exclusivity cannot apply. In these cases, the Best Pharmaceuticals for Children Act established a program that arranges for the necessary studies to be conducted with funding by the Na-tional Institutes of Health. For example, a contract to study lithium carbonate in children has been funded under this initiative (Findling et al. 2010b).

In addition, legislation to prevent the pediatric off-label use of future medications was enacted with the Pediatric Research Equity Act of 2003 (P.L. 108-155). This act provides the FDA with the authority to request industry to conduct pediatric studies of a drug, even before its approval for adult use, when there is indication that the drug is likely to be prescribed to children.

Conclusions

Pediatric psychopharmacology is a field in rapid expansion due to intense re-search activities. It is also the object of frequent debate and, at times, contro-versy in the media and the general public. The therapeutic value of a number of psychotropics is now well documented for both the short term and inter-mediate term. Knowledge gaps remain in the understanding of the long-term impact of pharmacotherapy with respect to both efficacy and safety. Practic-ing rational pharmacotherapy requires integration of knowledge at different levels, including developmental psychopathology, pharmacology, and drug regulation and bioethics, and a considerable investment of time on the part of the treating clinician and the child's parents.

Table 1–4. Pediatric indications approved by the U.S. Food and Drug Administration (FDA) and off-label use of selected psychotropic medications

Medication	FDA-approved indication(s)	Relative child age	Off-label use
Methylphenidate	ADHD	≥6 years	ADHD: <6 years
Dexmethylphenidate	ADHD	≥6 years	ADHD: <6 years
Amphetamines	ADHD	≥3 years	
Atomoxetine	ADHD	≥6 years	ADHD: <6 years
Clonidine	ADHD	≥6 years	Tourette's disorder
Guanfacine	ADHD	≥6 years	Tourette's disorder
Fluoxetine	MDD	≥8 years	MDD: <8 years
	OCD	≥7 years	Other anxiety disorders: ≥6 years
Sertraline	OCD	≥6 years	OCD, anxiety disorders: ≥6 years
			MDD: ≥6 years
Citalopram	None		OCD, other anxiety disorders: ≥6 years
			MDD: ≥6 years
Escitalopram	MDD	≥12 years	MDD: 6–11 years
Paroxetine	None		OCD, other anxiety disorders: ≥6 years
			MDD: ≥6 years
Fluvoxamine	OCD	≥7 years	Other anxiety disorders: ≥6 years
Venlafaxine	None		MDD: ≥6 years
Bupropion	None		MDD: ≥6 years
			ADHD: ≥6 years
Clomipramine	OCD	≥10 years	
Haloperidol	Psychosis, Tourette's disorder, hyperactivity, severe behavioral problems, explosive hyperexcitability	≥3 years	

Table 1–4. Pediatric indications approved by the U.S. Food and Drug Administration (FDA) and off-label use of selected psychotropic medications *(continued)*

Medication	FDA-approved indication(s)	Relative child age	Off-label use
Pimozide	Tourette's disorder	≥12 years	
Risperidone	Schizophrenia	≥13 years	Aggression
	Bipolar disorder	≥10 years	Tourette's disorder
	"Irritability" in autism	5–16 years	
Quetiapine	Schizophrenia	≥13 years	Aggression
	Bipolar disorder	≥10 years	Tourette's disorder
Aripiprazole	Schizophrenia	≥13 years	Aggression
	Bipolar disorder	≥10 years	Tourette's disorder
	"Irritability" in autism	5–16 years	
Olanzapine	Schizophrenia	≥13 years	Aggression
	Bipolar disorder	≥10 years	Tourette's disorder
Lithium	Bipolar disorder	≥12 years	Bipolar disorder: <12 years Aggression
Valproate	Epilepsy	From infancy	Mania, aggression
Carbamazepine	Epilepsy	From infancy	Mania, aggression
Oxcarbazepine	Epilepsy	≥4 years	Mania, aggression
Lamotrigine	Epilepsy	≥2 years	Depression in bipolar disorder

Note. ADHD=attention-deficit/hyperactivity disorder; MDD=major depressive disorder; OCD=obsessive-compulsive disorder.

Clinical Pearls

- Simply decreasing adult medication doses on the basis of child weight can result in undertreatment because of faster drug elimination in children.
- Assessing treatment effects and safety requires collection and integration of data from different sources (i.e., child, parent, teacher).

- Safety is paramount, and a high level of suspicion is warranted when treating children with medication, especially at the beginning of treatment and when multiple medications are used.
- Younger children tend to be more sensitive to adverse effects of medications.
- Children should have their condition explained to the extent that they can understand and, whenever possible, asked for their assent to treatment.

References

Anderson GD: Children versus adults: pharmacokinetics and adverse-effects differences. Epilepsia 43 (suppl 3):53–59, 2002

Ansorge MS, Zhou M, Lira A, et al: Early life blockade of the 5-HT transporter alters emotional behavior in adult mice. Science 306:879–881, 2004

Axelson DA, Perel JM, Birmaher B, et al: Sertraline pharmacokinetics and dynamics in adolescents. J Am Acad Child Adolesc Psychiatry 41:1037–1044, 2002

Axelson DA, Perel JM, Birmaher B, et al: Platelet serotonin reuptake inhibition and response to SSRIs in depressed adolescents. Am J Psychiatry 162:802–804, 2005

Bech P, Cialdella P, Haugh MC, et al: Meta-analysis of randomized controlled trials of fluoxetine vs. placebo and tricyclic antidepressants in the short-term treatment of major depression. Br J Psychiatry 176:421–428, 2000

Beck AT, Steer RA: Internal consistencies of the original and revised Beck Depression Inventory. J Clin Psychol 140:1365–1367, 1984

Bernstein IH, Rush AJ, Trivedi MH, et al: Psychometric properties of the Quick Inventory of Depressive Symptomatology in adolescents. Int J Methods Psychiatr Res 19:185–194, 2010

Best Pharmaceuticals for Children Act of 2002, Pub. L. No. 107-109, 115 Stat. 1408.

Biederman J, Monuteaux MC, Spencer T, et al: Stimulant therapy and risk for subsequent substance use disorders in male adults with ADHD: a naturalistic controlled 10-year follow-up study. Am J Psychiatry 165:597–603, 2008

Birmaher B, Brent DA, Chiappetta L, et al: The Screen for Child Anxiety Related Emotional Disorders (SCARED): scale construction and psychometric characteristics. J Am Acad Child Adolesc Psychiatry 38:1230–1236, 1997

Birmaher B, Brent DA: Practice parameter for the assessment and treatment of children and adolescents with depressive disorders. J Am Acad Child Adolesc Psychiatry 46:1503–1526, 2007

Bridge JA, Iyengar S, Salary CB, et al: Clinical response and risk for reported suicidal ideation and suicide attempts in pediatric antidepressant treatment: a meta-analysis of randomized controlled trials. JAMA 297:1683–1696, 2007

Bryant AE, Dreifuss FE: Valproic acid hepatic fatalities. III: I.S. experience since 1986. Neurology 46:465–469, 1996

Chambers CD, Johnson KA, Dick LM, et al: Birth outcomes in pregnant women taking fluoxetine. N Engl J Med 335:1010–1015, 1996

Children's Hospital Boston (Harvard Medical School): The Children's Hospital Boston's interactive parents' guide to medical research. Available at: www.bostonchild.vitalconsent.com/bstnchld/index.html. Accessed May 9, 2012.

Chugani DC, Muzik O, Juhasz C, et al: Postnatal maturation of human GABAA receptors measured with positron emission tomography. Ann Neurol 49:618–626, 2001

Conners CK, Sitarenios G, Parker JD, et al: The revised Conners' Parent Rating Scale (CPRS-R): factor structure, reliability, and criterion validity. J Abnorm Child Psychol 26:257–268, 1998a

Conners CK, Sitarenios G, Parker JD, et al: Revision and restandardization of the Conners' Teacher Rating Scale (CTRS-R): factor structure, reliability, and criterion validity. J Abnorm Child Psychol 26:279–291, 1998b

Correll CU, Manu P, Olshanskiy V, et al: Cardiometabolic risk of second-generation antipsychotic medications during first-time use in children and adolescents. JAMA 302:1765–1773, 2009

Couzin J: Pediatric study of ADHD drug draws high-level public review. Science 305:1088–1089, 2004

Daviss WB, Perel JM, Rudolph GR, et al: Steady-state pharmacokinetics of bupropion SR in juvenile patients. J Am Acad Child Adolesc Psychiatry 44:349–357, 2005

DeWildt SN, Kearns GL, Leader JS, et al: Cytochrome P450 3A: ontogeny and drug disposition. Clin Pharmacokinet 37:485–505, 1999

Emslie GJ, Heiligenstein JH, Hoog SL, et al: Fluoxetine treatment for prevention of relapse of depression in children and adolescents: a double-blind, placebo-controlled study. J Am Acad Child Adolesc Psychiatry 43:1397–1405, 2004

Farwell JR, Lee YJ, Hirtz DG, et al: Phenobarbital for febrile seizures—effects on intelligence and on seizure recurrence. N Engl J Med 322:364–369, 1990

Findling RL, McNamara NK, Stansbrey RJ, et al: The relevance of pharmacokinetic studies in designing efficacy trials in juvenile major depression. J Child Adolesc Psychopharmacol 16:131–145, 2006

Findling RL, Kauffman RE, Sallee FR, et al: Tolerability and pharmacokinetics of aripiprazole in children and adolescents with psychiatric disorders: an open-label, dose-escalation study. J Clin Psychopharmacol 28:441–446, 2008

Findling RL, Johnson JL, McClellan J, et al: Double-blind maintenance safety and effectiveness findings from the Treatment of Early Onset Schizophrenia Spectrum (TEOSS) study. J Am Acad Child Adolesc Psychiatry 49:583–594, 2010a

Findling RL, Landersdorfer CB, Kafantaris V, et al: First-dose pharmacokinetics of lithium carbonate in children and adolescents. J Clin Psychopharmacol 30:404–10, 2010b

Food and Drug Administration Modernization Act of 1997, Pub. L. No. 105-115, 111Stat. 2296.

Gould M, Walsh BT, Munfakh JL: Sudden death and use of stimulant medications in children. Am J Psychiatry 166:992–1001, 2009

Greenhill LL, Swanson JM, Vitiello B, et al: Impairment and deportment responses to different methylphenidate doses in children with ADHD: the MTA titration trial. J Am Acad Child Adolesc Psychiatry 40:180–187, 2001

Greenhill LL, Vitiello B, Fisher P, et al: Comparison of increasingly detailed elicitation methods for the assessment of adverse events in pediatric psychopharmacology. J Am Acad Child Adolesc Psychiatry 43:1488–1496, 2004

Greenhill LL, Abikoff H, Chuang S, et al: Efficacy and safety of immediate-release methylphenidate treatment for preschoolers with ADHD. J Am Acad Child Adolesc Psychiatry 45:1284–1293, 2006

Hammad TA, Laughren T, Racoosin J: Suicidality in pediatric patients treated with antidepressant drugs. Arch Gen Psychiatry 63:332–339, 2006

Hazell P, O'Connell D, Heathcote D, et al: Efficacy of tricyclic drugs in treating child and adolescent depression: a meta-analysis. BMJ 310:897–901, 1995

Kovacs M: The Children's Depression Inventory (CDI). Psychopharmacol Bull 21:995–998, 1985

Kratochvil CJ, Vitiello B, Walkup J, et al: SSRIs in pediatric depression: is the balance between benefits and risks favorable? J Child Adolesc Psychopharmacol 16:11–24, 2006

March JS, Parker JD, Sullivan K, et al: The Multidimensional Anxiety Scale for Children (MASC): factor structure, reliability, and validity. J Am Acad Child Adolesc Psychiatry 36:554–565, 1997

March J, Silva S, Petrycki S, et al: Fluoxetine, cognitive-behavioral therapy, and their combination for adolescents with depression: Treatment for Adolescents With Depression Study (TADS) randomized controlled trial. JAMA 292:807–820, 2004

March JS, Silva S, Petrycki S, et al: The Treatment for Adolescents With Depression Study (TADS): long-term effectiveness and safety outcomes. Arch Gen Psychiatry 64:1132–1143, 2007

Marshburn EC, Aman MG: Factor validity and norms for the Aberrant Behavior Checklist in a community sample of children with mental retardation. J Autism Dev Disord 22:357–373, 1992

Mattison DR, Plant TM, Lin HM, et al: Pubertal delay in male nonhuman primates (Macaca mulatta) treated with methylphenidate. Proc Natl Acad Sci USA 108:16301–16306, 2011

McClellan J, Kowatch R, Findling RL, et al: Practice parameter for the assessment and treatment of children and adolescents with bipolar disorder. J Am Acad Child Adolesc Psychiatry 46:107–125, 2007

McCracken JT, McGough J, Shah B, et al; Research Units on Pediatric Psychopharmacology Autism Network: Risperidone in children with autism and serious behavioral problems. N Engl J Med 347:314–321, 2002

Moore CM, Demopulos CM, Henry ME, et al: Brain-to-serum lithium ratio and age: an in vivo magnetic resonance spectroscopy study. Am J Psychiatry 159:1240–1242, 2002

MTA Cooperative Group: National Institute of Mental Health Multimodal Treatment Study of ADHD follow-up: changes in effectiveness and growth after the end of treatment. Pediatrics 113:762–769, 2004

Norrholm SD, Ouimet CC: Chronic fluoxetine administration to juvenile rats prevents age-associated dendritic spine proliferation in hippocampus. Brain Res 883:205–215, 2000

Office for Human Research Protections: Special Protections for Children as Research Subjects. Available at: www.hhs.gov/ohrp/policy/populations/children.html. Accessed May 9, 2012.

Pediatric OCD Treatment Study: Cognitive-behavior therapy, sertraline, and their combination for children and adolescents with obsessive-compulsive disorder: the Pediatric OCD Treatment Study (POTS) randomized controlled trial. JAMA 292:1969–1976, 2004

Pediatric Research Equity Act of 2003, Pub. L. No. 108-155, 117 Stat. 1936–1943.

Pliszka S; AACAP Work Group on Quality Issues: Practice parameter for the assessment and treatment of children and adolescents with attention-deficit/hyperactivity disorder. J Am Acad Child Adolesc Psychiatry 46:894–921, 2007

Poznanski EO, Mokros HB: Manual for the Children's Depression Rating Scale—Revised. Los Angeles, CA, Western Psychological Services, 1996

Rao N: The clinical pharmacokinetics of escitalopram. Clin Pharmacokinet 46:281–290, 2007

Research Units on Pediatric Psychopharmacology Anxiety Study Group: The Pediatric Anxiety Rating Scale (PARS): development and psychometric properties. J Am Acad Child Adolesc Psychiatry 41:1061–1069, 2002

Research Units on Pediatric Psychopharmacology Autism Network: Randomized, controlled, crossover trial of methylphenidate in pervasive developmental disorders with hyperactivity. Arch Gen Psychiatry 62:1266–1274, 2005

Reynolds WM: Professional Manual for the Reynolds Adolescents Depression Scale, 2nd Edition. Lutz, FL, Psychological Assessment Resources, 2002

Rho JM, Storey TW: Molecular ontogeny of major neurotransmitter receptor systems in the mammalian central nervous system: norepinephrine, dopamine, serotonin, acetylcholine, and glycine. J Child Neurol 16:271–279, 2001

Rosenthal R, Rosnow R, Rubin DB: Contrasts and Effect Sizes in Behavioral Research. Cambridge, UK, Cambridge University Press, 2000

Sadeque AJ, Fisher MB, Korzekwa KR, et al: Human CYP2C9 and CYP2A6 mediate formation of the hepatotoxin 4-ene-valproic acid. J Pharmacol Exp Ther 283:698–703, 1997

Sallee FR, DeVane CL, Ferrell RE: Fluoxetine-related death in a child with cytochrome P-450 2D6 genetic deficiency. J Child Adolesc Psychopharmacol 10:27–34, 2000

Sanz EJ, De-las-Cuevas C, Kiuru A, et al: Selective serotonin reuptake inhibitors in pregnant women and neonatal withdrawal syndrome: a database analysis. Lancet 365:482–487, 2005

Sauer JM, Ring BJ, Witcher JM: Clinical pharmacokinetics of atomoxetine. Clin Pharmacokinet 44:571–590, 2005

Shaffer D, Gould M, Brasic J, et al: A children's global assessment scale (CGAS). Arch Gen Psychiatry 40:1228–1231, 1983

Stein MA, McGough JJ: The pharmacogenomic era: promise for personalizing attention deficit hyperactivity disorder therapy. Child Adolesc Psychiatr Clin N Am 17:475–490, 2008

Stone M, Laughren T, Jones ML, et al: Risk of suicidality in clinical trials of antidepressants in adults: analysis of proprietary data submitted to US Food and Drug Administration. BMJ 339:b2880, 2009

Swanson JM, Gupta S, Lam A, et al: Development of a new once-a-day formulation of methylphenidate for the treatment of attention-deficit/hyperactivity disorder: proof-of-concept and proof-of-product studies. Arch Gen Psychiatry 60:204–211, 2003

Swanson JM, Wigal SB, Wigal T, et al: A comparison of once-daily extended-release methylphenidate formulations in children with attention-deficit/hyperactivity disorder in the laboratory school (the Comacs Study). Pediatrics 113:E206–E216, 2004

Swanson JM, Elliott GR, Greenhill LL, et al: Effects of stimulant medication on growth rates across 3 years in the MTA follow-up. J Am Acad Child Adolesc Psychiatry 46:1014–1026, 2007

Thyssen A, Vermeulen A, Fuseau E, et al: Population pharmacokinetics of oral risperidone in children, adolescents and adults with psychiatric disorders. Clin Pharmacokinet 49:465–478, 2010

U.S. Department of Health and Human Services: Protection of human subjects. 45 C.F.R. 46 (Subparts A–D): Protections of Human Subjects. 2009. Available at: www.hhs.gov/ohrp/humansubjects/guidance/45cfr46.html. Accessed May 9, 2012.

U.S. Food and Drug Administration: Additional safeguards for children in clinical investigations of FDA-regulated products. Fed Regist 66:20589–20600, 2001

Vitiello B: Ethical considerations in psychopharmacological research involving children and adolescents. Psychopharmacol 171:86–91, 2003

Vitiello B, Behar D, Malone R, et al: Pharmacokinetics of lithium carbonate in children. J Clin Psychopharmacol 8:355–539, 1988

Vitiello B, Riddle MA, Greenhill LL, et al: How can we improve the assessment of safety in child and adolescent psychopharmacology? J Am Acad Child Adolesc Psychiatry 42:634–641, 2003

Vitiello B, Silva S, Rohde P, et al: Suicidal events in the Treatment for Adolescents With Depression Study (TADS). J Clin Psychiatry 70:741–747, 2009

Vitiello B, Emslie G, Clarke G, et al: Long-term outcome of adolescent depression initially resistant to selective serotonin reuptake inhibitor treatment: a follow-up study of the TORDIA sample. J Clin Psychiatry 72:388–396, 2011

Vitiello B, Elliott GR, Swanson JM, et al: Blood pressure and heart rate in the Multimodal Treatment of Attention Deficit/Hyperactivity Disorder Study over 10 years. Am J Psychiatry 169:167–177, 2012

Wagner A, Lecavalier L, Arnold LE, et al: Developmental Disabilities Modification of Children's Global Assessment Scale (DD-CGAS). Biol Psychiatry 19:629–635, 2007

Wehmeier PM, Schacht A, Lehmann M, et al: Emotional well-being in children and adolescents treated with atomoxetine for attention-deficit/hyperactivity disorder: findings from a patient, parent and physician perspective using items from the Pediatric Adverse Event Rating Scale (PAERS). Child Adolesc Psychiatry Ment Health 28:11, 2008

Wendler D, Belsky L, Thompson KM, et al: Quantifying the federal minimal risk standard: implications for pediatric research without a prospect of direct benefit. JAMA 294:826–832, 2005

Wigal T, Greenhill LL, Chuang S, et al: Safety and tolerability of methylphenidate in preschool children with ADHD. J Am Acad Child Adolesc Psychiatry 45:1294–1303, 2006

Wilens TE, Cohen L, Biederman J, et al: Fluoxetine pharmacokinetics in pediatric patients. J Clin Psychopharmacol 22:568–575, 2002

Wilens TE, Adamson J, Monuteaux MC, et al: Effect of prior stimulant treatment for attention-deficit/hyperactivity disorder on subsequent risk for cigarette smoking and alcohol and drug use disorders in adolescents. Arch Pediatr Adolesc Med 162:916–921, 2008

2

Attention-Deficit/Hyperactivity Disorder

Jonathan Posner, M.D.
Laurence Greenhill, M.D.

Attention-deficit/hyperactivity disorder (ADHD) is a frequently diagnosed behavioral condition (American Psychiatric Association 2000). The prevalence of ADHD has been estimated, in the U.S. National Health Interview Survey, to be 6.7% of all school-age children (Woodruff et al. 2004). The Centers for Disease Control and Prevention (CDC) reported a point prevalence of 9% for school-age children ages 6–17 (Pastor and Reuben 2008). This rate is close to the estimate of 7.5% found in an epidemiological survey of elementary and secondary school children in Minnesota (Barbaresi et al. 2002).

ADHD is a chronic disorder. Follow-up studies of school-age children diagnosed early with ADHD suggest that 60%–80% will continue to meet the full DSM-IV-TR criteria (American Psychiatric Association 2000) for the disorder throughout their teenage years (Barkley et al. 1990; Biederman et al.

1996). These data indicate that the condition does not resolve with the onset of puberty. Estimates are that 2%–27% (Barkley et al. 2002; Mannuzza et al. 1993) will continue to meet the criteria for the disorder into adult life. Epidemiological studies using a two-stage probability sample screen of 3,199 individuals ages 19–44 estimated the point prevalence of adult ADHD to be 4.4% (Kessler et al. 2006).

The prevalence of ADHD in school-age children may be gleaned from comprehensive reviews (Bauermeister et al. 1994; Bird et al. 1988; Szatmari 1992) and from epidemiological surveys conducted in the United States (Visser and Lesesne 2006), such as in Pittsburgh, Pennsylvania (Costello 1989); Puerto Rico (Bird et al. 1988); and the Great Smoky Mountain area of rural North Carolina (Costello et al. 2003). Similar research was conducted in other countries, such as Australia (Connell et al. 1982), Norway (Vikan 1985), England (Taylor et al. 1991), the Netherlands (Verhulst et al. 1992), Canada (Szatmari et al. 1989), Germany (Esser et al. 1996), and New Zealand (Anderson et al. 1987). Rates for ADHD range from 2.0% to 6.3% (Szatmari et al. 1989), but the predominantly inattentive subtype of ADHD (attention-deficit disorder) shows a wider range, between 2.2% and 12.6% (Velez et al. 1989). A meta-analysis has shown a worldwide prevalence of ADHD of 5.29%, with significant variability caused by diagnostic criteria, source of information, requirement of impairment for diagnosis, and geographic origin of the studies (Polanczyk et al. 2007).

Diagnosis of ADHD

ADHD is a heterogeneous condition characterized by a persistent, developmentally inappropriate pattern of gross motor overactivity, inattention, and impulsivity that impairs academic, social, and family function. The condition was first described in the nineteenth century. The most recent definition of the disorder appears in DSM-IV-TR, which subdivides it into three subtypes: predominantly hyperactive-impulsive, predominantly inattentive, and combined. More recent studies suggest that these ADHD subtypes may not be stable over time if preschool children with ADHD are followed until they are early adolescents (Lahey and Willcutt 2010). Two-thirds of young children with ADHD also meet criteria for other childhood psychiatric disorders, including anxiety, depressive, oppositional defiant, conduct, and mood disorders. These comorbid psychiatric conditions are thought to increase the impairment associated with ADHD.

By adulthood, children who were diagnosed with ADHD may no longer meet full symptom criteria necessary for the diagnosis, yet their symptoms often continue to cause significant impairment. For this reason, the DSM-5 work group for ADHD is considering reducing the threshold of symptoms required for adults with ADHD (American Psychiatric Association, DSM-5 Development 2012). DSM-IV-TR requires the persistence of six or more symptoms of inattentiveness or hyperactivity/impulsivity for at least 6 months at a level that is maladaptive and exceeds the norm for the subject's age group. In addition, there is an age-at-onset criterion (before 7 years), a duration criterion (symptoms must have persisted more than 6 months), a pervasiveness criterion (the symptoms must cause impairment in more than one setting), and a differential diagnosis criterion (symptoms cannot be better explained by a different disorder).

Diagnostic Procedures

Guidelines for diagnosing ADHD in an office practice have been published by the American Academy of Pediatrics (2011) and the American Academy of Child and Adolescent Psychiatry (AACAP) (Pliszka 2007). Because ADHD is so prevalent, the AACAP recommends that screening for ADHD should be part of any patient's mental health assessment. The practitioner can accomplish such screening by asking questions about inattention, impulsivity, and hyperactivity, and then asking whether such symptoms cause impairment. Parents and teachers can help by filling out rating scales containing DSM-IV-TR symptoms of ADHD before the practitioner starts the first interview. A positive screen on a rating scale, however, does not constitute a definitive ADHD diagnosis.

A medical history should be carried out by a child psychiatrist during the diagnostic evaluation; if a decision is made to treat the child with medication, then the family can be referred to a pediatrician to obtain a physical examination. If the patient's medical examination and history are unremarkable, no additional laboratory or neurological testing is required (Pliszka 2007). Likewise, neuropsychological testing has limited sensitivity and/or specificity for ADHD and is not indicated in a diagnostic evaluation of the disorder. When a comorbid learning disorder is suspected, neuropsychological testing may be helpful (Pliszka 2007).

The next diagnostic procedure includes an interview with the child or adolescent to determine whether other psychiatric disorders are present that would better explain the symptoms causing impairment. Although it is helpful to interview a preschool- or school-age child with the parent present, older children and adolescents should be interviewed alone, because they are more likely to discuss symptoms of substance use, suicidal ideation or behavior, or depression without a parent listening.

Because a majority of children with ADHD also have at least one other Axis I psychiatric disorder (Biederman et al. 1991), the clinician should make inquiries about symptoms of oppositional defiant disorder, conduct disorder, depression, anxiety disorders, tic disorders, substance use disorders, and mania. Symptoms of these conditions can be captured by parent symptom checklists (e.g., the Child Behavior Checklist [Achenbach and Ruffle 2000]) and rating scales (e.g., the Swanson, Nolan, and Pelham Version IV [SNAP-IV] rating scale]; Collett et al. 2003). In addition, the clinician should obtain information about the family history, patient's prenatal history, developmental milestones, and medical history.

Diagnostic Controversy

ADHD diagnosis has been controversial because no confirmatory laboratory tests are available to corroborate that the diagnosis is accurate and because the condition is treated with psychostimulants, medications deemed to be abusable by the U.S. Drug Enforcement Administration (DEA) (Parens and Johnston 2009). The diagnosis of ADHD is further complicated because the criteria have been revised four times since 1970. The most recent criteria, from DSM-IV-TR, are listed in Table 2–1. The DSM-IV-TR criteria for ADHD will be replaced by the DSM-5 criteria, which are under development.

The American Psychiatric Association's DSM-5 ADHD work group reviewed the diagnostic criteria established for DSM-IV (American Psychiatric Association 1994). The panel reported a number of areas of weakness (American Psychiatric Association, DSM-5 Development 2012). Some of these criticisms are listed on the APA's DSM-5 Web site (www.dsm5.org) and include the following:

- The DSM-IV subtypes have been shown to be unstable over time (Lahey and Willcutt 2010).
- The DSM-IV criteria underrepresent impulsivity (only three symptoms of impulsivity are provided in the diagnostic criteria).
- The adult criteria for ADHD do not allow for a decline in the number of symptoms with age without a reduction in impairment.
- The age at onset of 7 years is not borne out in the literature as a critical age, because children with onsets between 7 and 12 years do not show a difference in outcomes (Keiling et al. 2010).
- DSM-IV requires a large number of symptom criteria for ADHD, and clinicians may have difficulty remembering all of them.

These criticisms are being addressed with modifications to the criteria for ADHD diagnosis, which will be finalized before the scheduled DSM-5 publication date of May 2013.

Because no laboratory test can confirm ADHD, the diagnosis must be established by history taken from multiple informants, including the child, the parents, and the teacher. The clinician should consider each of the major components of the DSM-IV-TR criteria: age at onset (before 7 years), requirement for impairment in a minimum of two settings, 6-month duration of symptoms, and a differential diagnosis that rules out other diagnostic conditions that can cause inattention, overactivity, or impulsivity. Confirmation depends on specific ADHD symptom criteria that encompass the type, duration, severity, and frequency of ADHD problems present. The clinician must confirm that the patient has at least six of nine ADHD symptoms in either or both the inattention and hyperactivity-impulsivity symptom lists, counting a symptom as present only if it occurs often (at least half the time). The symptoms must start in childhood and follow a chronic course.

The other area of controversy involving ADHD is the use of psychostimulants to treat the disorder. The controversy is related to their classification as drugs of abuse. At the 1998 Consensus Development Conference on ADHD sponsored by the National Institutes of Health (Kupfer et al. 2000), a panel concluded that stimulants are effective in reducing the defining ADHD symptoms in the short term, but that the controversy about their long-term use demands serious consideration. The panel noted a lack of evidence for their long-term benefits and/or safety; the known risks of treatment; wide

Table 2–1. DSM-IV-TR diagnostic criteria for attention-deficit/ hyperactivity disorder

A. Either (1) or (2):

(1) six (or more) of the following symptoms of **inattention** have persisted for at least 6 months to a degree that is maladaptive and inconsistent with developmental level:

Inattention

(a) often fails to give close attention to details or makes careless mistakes in schoolwork, work, or other activities

(b) often has difficulty sustaining attention in tasks or play activities

(c) often does not seem to listen when spoken to directly

(d) often does not follow through on instructions and fails to finish schoolwork, chores, or duties in the workplace (not due to oppositional behavior or failure to understand instructions)

(e) often has difficulty organizing tasks and activities

(f) often avoids, dislikes, or is reluctant to engage in tasks that require sustained mental effort (such as schoolwork or homework)

(g) often loses things necessary for tasks or activities (e.g., toys, school assignments, pencils, books, or tools)

(h) is often easily distracted by extraneous stimuli

(i) is often forgetful in daily activities

(2) six (or more) of the following symptoms of **hyperactivity-impulsivity** have persisted for at least 6 months to a degree that is maladaptive and inconsistent with developmental level:

Hyperactivity

(a) often fidgets with hands or feet or squirms in seat

(b) often leaves seat in classroom or in other situations in which remaining seated is expected

(c) often runs about or climbs excessively in situations in which it is inappropriate (in adolescents or adults, may be limited to subjective feelings of restlessness)

(d) often has difficulty playing or engaging in leisure activities quietly

(e) is often "on the go" or often acts as if "driven by a motor"

(f) often talks excessively

Impulsivity

(g) often blurts out answers before questions have been completed

(h) often has difficulty awaiting turn

(i) often interrupts or intrudes on others (e.g., butts into conversations or games)

Table 2–1. DSM-IV-TR diagnostic criteria for attention-deficit/ hyperactivity disorder *(continued)*

B. Some hyperactive-impulsive or inattentive symptoms that caused impairment were present before age 7 years.

C. Some impairment from the symptoms is present in two or more settings (e.g., at school [or work] and at home).

D. There must be clear evidence of clinically significant impairment in social, academic, or occupational functioning.

E. The symptoms do not occur exclusively during the course of a pervasive developmental disorder, schizophrenia, or other psychotic disorder and are not better accounted for by another mental disorder (e.g., mood disorder, anxiety disorder, dissociative disorder, or a personality disorder).

Code based on type:

314.01 **Attention-Deficit/Hyperactivity Disorder, Combined Type:** if both Criteria A1 and A2 are met for the past 6 months

314.00 **Attention-Deficit/Hyperactivity Disorder, Predominantly Inattentive Type:** if Criterion A1 is met but Criterion A2 is not met for the past 6 months

314.01 **Attention-Deficit/Hyperactivity Disorder, Predominantly Hyperactive-Impulsive Type:** if Criterion A2 is met but Criterion A1 is not met for the past 6 months

Coding note: For individuals (especially adolescents and adults) who currently have symptoms that no longer meet full criteria, "In Partial Remission" should be specified.

Source. Reprinted from *Diagnostic and Statistical Manual of Mental Disorders,* 4th Edition, Text Revision. Washington, DC, American Psychiatric Association, 2000. Copyright © 2000 American Psychiatric Association. Used with permission.

variation in prescribing practices among practitioners; and an absence of evidence regarding the appropriate ADHD diagnostic threshold above which the benefits of psychostimulant therapy outweigh the risks.

The conclusions drawn at the 1998 Consensus Development Conference were not as positive as those reached by the Council on Scientific Affairs of the American Medical Association. After reviewing hundreds of trials involving thousands of patients, the council concluded that "the risk-benefit ratio of stimulant treatment in ADHD must be evaluated and monitored on an ongoing basis in each case, but in general is highly favorable" (Goldman et al. 1998, p. 1106).

Treatment of ADHD

Fortunately, ADHD responds to both psychosocial and psychopharmacological treatments (Richters et al. 1995). Recent reports suggest that 3.6% of children in the United States received treatment with stimulants in 2008, up from 2.4% in 1996, with the greatest growth among adolescents (6%) (Zuvekas and Vitello 2012). If all ADHD medication treatments are included, over 4 million people—2.5 million age 18 and younger and 1.5 million older than age 18—in the United States take pills every day to alleviate ADHD symptoms. Earlier estimates (Swanson et al. 1995b) suggested that from 1990 to 1993, the number of outpatient visits for ADHD increased from 1.6 million to 4.2 million per year, and the amount of methylphenidate manufactured increased from 1,784 to 5,110 kg per year.

Medications of choice for ADHD are the psychostimulants (Greenhill et al. 2002a, 2002b), which include various preparations of methylphenidate and amphetamines. Long-duration oral stimulant preparations (Biederman et al. 2002), the stimulant transdermal patch (McGough et al. 2006), atomoxetine (Michelson et al. 2003), and the daytime alertness drug modafinil (Greenhill et al. 2006a) have been introduced within the last decade and a half. These agents have been tested for efficacy in multisite double-blind, randomized, parallel-design, placebo-controlled trials, and their safety has been monitored in longer-term open-label studies.

Psychostimulants produce a robust response, reducing core ADHD symptoms within 30 minutes of administration when the proper dose is given to a patient. This rapid and robust response explains, to some degree, why published drug research in the past four decades has focused mainly on studying stimulants (Vitiello and Jensen 1995). Rather than explore novel compounds, academic researchers have relied on either methylphenidate or amphetamines to study response patterns, adverse events, determination of "normalization" during drug treatment, and characteristics among nonresponders.

Using Stimulants to Treat ADHD

Psychopharmacological treatment of ADHD should begin with medications approved by the U.S. Food and Drug Administration (FDA) (Table 2–2). These medications have been tested for short-term efficacy and safety in at least two different randomized controlled trials (RCTs). Stimulants are highly effective in reducing ADHD symptoms. Meta-analyses of 62 methylphenidate treatment RCTs, lasting 3 months or less, revealed large effect sizes (standard deviation [SD] = 0.8) when ratings were made by teachers and moderate effect sizes (SD = 0.5) when ratings were made by parents (Schachter et al. 2001). Six methylphenidate treatment RCTs involving adults with ADHD (N = 140) revealed large effect sizes (0.9) when patients were rated by their physicians (Faraone et al. 2004).

The FDA currently approves two groups of stimulants for treatment of ADHD in the pediatric population. These medications are available in both brand and generic formulations: amphetamines (Adderall, Dexedrine, Vyvanse) and methylphenidates (Concerta, Focalin, Metadate ER, Metadate CD, methylphenidate, Methylin, Ritalin, Ritalin-SR, Ritalin LA, transdermal methylphenidate). The individual characteristics of these medications are described in Table 2–2. Dextroamphetamine and methylphenidate are structurally related to the catecholamines (dopamine and norepinephrine) (McCracken 1991). The term *psychostimulant* used for these compounds refers to their ability to increase central nervous system (CNS) activity in some but not all brain regions.

Compared with placebo, psychostimulants have a significantly greater ability to reduce ADHD symptoms, such as overactivity (e.g., fidgetiness and off-task behavior during direct observation), and to eliminate behavior that disrupts the classroom (e.g., constant requests of the teacher during direct observation) (Jacobvitz et al. 1990). In experimental settings, stimulants have been shown to improve child behavior during parent-child interactions (Barkley and Cunningham 1979) and problem-solving activities with peers (Whalen et al. 1989). The behavior of children with ADHD has a tendency to elicit negative, directive, and controlling behavior from parents and peers (Campbell 1973). When these children begin taking stimulants, their mothers' rates of disapproval, commands, and control diminishes to the extent seen between mothers and their children who do not have ADHD (Barkley and

Table 2–2. Medications used in the treatment of attention-deficit/hyperactivity disorder

Medication	Duration of action	Pediatric		Adult	
		Starting dose	Typical dose	Starting dose	Typical dose
Dexmethylphenidate					
Focalin (Novartis)	6 hours[a]	2.5 mg A.M.	5 mg bid	2.5 mg bid	10 mg bid
Focalin XR (Novartis)	8–12 hours; dual pulse	5 mg A.M.	10 mg A.M.	5 mg A.M.	20 mg A.M.
D,L-Methylphenidate					
Short-acting (immediate release)	3–5 hours				
Methylin Oral Solution (Shionogi)		5 mg tid	10 mg tid	10 mg bid	20 mg tid
Methylin Chewable Tablets (Shionogi)		5 mg tid	10 mg tid	10 mg bid	20 mg tid
Intermediate-acting	3–8 hours				
Metadate ER (Celltech)	Single pulse	10 mg bid	30 mg A.M.	10 mg bid	80 mg A.M.
Ritalin-SR (Novartis)	Single pulse	20 mg A.M.	40 mg	20 mg A.M.	80 mg A.M.
Long-acting	8–12 hours				
Metadate CD (Celltech)	8–10 hours; dual pulse	10 mg A.M.	30 mg A.M.	20 mg A.M.	80 mg A.M.
Concerta (McNeil)	8–12 hours; ascending single pulse	18 mg A.M.	36 mg A.M.	18 mg A.M.	72 mg A.M.
Ritalin LA (Novartis)	8–10 hours; dual pulse	10 mg A.M.	30 mg A.M.	10 mg A.M.	80 mg A.M.
Daytrana (Noven)	10–12 hours; transdermal single pulse	10 mg patch qd × 9 hours, off 15 hours	30 mg patch qd × 9 hours, off 15 hours	10 mg patch qd × 9 hours, off 15 hours	60 mg patch qd × 9 hours, off 15 hours

Table 2–2. Medications used in the treatment of attention-deficit/hyperactivity disorder *(continued)*

Medication	Duration of action	Pediatric		Adult	
		Starting dose	Typical dose	Starting dose	Typical dose
Dextroamphetamine					
Short-acting					
Generic	4–6 hours	5 mg bid	10 mg bid	5 mg bid	15 mg bid
Long-duration	6–8 hours				
Generic		5 mg A.M.	15 mg A.M.	5 mg A.M.	30 mg A.M.
Dexedrine Spansule (Amedra)		5 mg A.M.	15 mg A.M.	5 mg A.M.	30 mg A.M.
Amphetamine mixed salts					
Generic	4–6 hours	5 mg bid	10 mg bid	5 mg bid	15 mg bid
Adderall (Shire)		5 mg bid	10 mg bid	5 mg bid	10 mg bid
Adderall XR (Shire)	8–10 hours; dual pulse	5 mg A.M.	30 mg A.M.	5 mg A.M.	60 mg A.M.
Lisdexamfetamine					
Vyvanse (Shire)	10–12 hours	30 mg A.M.	50 mg A.M.	30 mg A.M.	70 mg A.M.

Table 2–2. Medications used in the treatment of attention-deficit/hyperactivity disorder *(continued)*

Medication	Duration of action	Pediatric		Adult	
		Starting dose	Typical dose	Starting dose	Typical dose
Nonstimulants					
Atomoxetine (Strattera; Eli Lilly)	24 hours	0.5 mg/kg/ day in divided doses (bid)	1.2 mg/kg/day in divided doses (bid)	40 mg/day in divided doses (bid)	100 mg/day in divided doses (bid)
Clonidine extended release (Kapvay; Shionogi)					
Guanfacine extended release (Intuniv; Shire)	24 hours	1 mg A.M.; 0.05–0.08 mg/kg/day	0.12 mg/kg/ day up to 4 mg/day	1 mg/day	Up to 4 mg/ day

aLimited data.

Cunningham 1979; Barkley et al. 1984; Humphries et al. 1978). In the laboratory, stimulant-treated children with ADHD demonstrate major improvements during experimenter-paced continuous performance tests (Halperin et al. 1992), paired-associate learning, cued and free recall, auditory and reading comprehension, spelling recall, and arithmetic computation (Pelham and Bender 1982; Stephens et al. 1984). Some studies show correlations between methylphenidate plasma levels and performance on a laboratory task, but plasma levels rarely correlate with clinical response. Likewise, hyperactive conduct-disordered children and preadolescents show reductions in aggressive behavior when treated with stimulants, as observed in structured and unstructured school settings (Hinshaw 1991). Stimulants also can reduce the display of covert antisocial behaviors, such as stealing and property destruction (Hinshaw et al. 1992).

No single theory explains the psychostimulant mechanism of action on the CNS that ameliorates ADHD symptoms. The theory that the drug's effect is based on a single neurotransmitter has been discounted (Zametkin and Rapoport 1987), as has the belief in the drug's ability to correct the under- or overaroused CNS in the child with ADHD (Solanto 1984). A two-part theory of stimulant action has been postulated (McCracken 1991), in which stimulants increase dopamine release, producing enhanced autoreceptor-mediated inhibition of ascending dopamine neurons, while simultaneously increasing adrenergic-mediated inhibition of the noradrenergic locus coeruleus via epinephrine activity. This theory awaits confirmation from basic research in animals and imaging studies in humans.

Brain imaging has reported few consistent psychostimulant effects on glucose metabolism. Although some studies using positron emission tomography (PET) and ^{18}F-labeled fluorodeoxyglucose in adults with ADHD have shown that stimulants lead to increased brain glucose metabolism in the striatal and frontal regions (Ernst and Zametkin 1995), other studies (Matochik et al. 1993, 1994) have been unable to find a change in glucose metabolism during acute and chronic stimulant treatment.

Psychostimulants are thought to release catecholamines and block their reuptake. Methylphenidate, like cocaine, has affinity for the dopamine transporter (DAT), and DAT blockade is now regarded as the putative mechanism for psychostimulant action in the human CNS. PET scan data show that ^{11}C-labeled methylphenidate concentration in brain is maximal in the striatum, an area rich in dopamine terminals where DAT resides (Volkow et al. 1995). These PET scans reveal a significant difference in the pharmacokinetics of [^{11}C]methylphenidate and [^{11}C]cocaine. Although both drugs display rapid uptake into striatum, methylphenidate is cleared more slowly from brain. The authors speculated that this slow reversal of binding to the DAT means that methylphenidate is not as reinforcing as cocaine and, therefore, does not lead to as much self-administration as does cocaine. More recently, the same authors (Volkow et al. 2001) were able to show that therapeutic doses of oral methylphenidate significantly increase extracellular dopamine in the human brain: "DA decreases the background firing rates and increases signal-to-noise in target neurons[;] we postulate that the amplification of weak DA signals in subjects with ADHD by methylphenidate would enhance task-specific signaling, improving attention and decreasing distractibility" (p. 1). Results from a functional MRI (fMRI) study suggest that psychostimulants may be effective in suppressing activation in the so-called "default mode" or task-negative neural circuit (Peterson et al. 2009). This neural circuit becomes increasingly deactivated as attentional demands increase. Failure to suppress, or deactivate, this circuit is associated with attentional lapses (Weissman et al. 2006). Children with ADHD show impaired suppression of the task-negative circuit during attentionally demanding tasks; psychostimulants seem to normalize this suppression and improve task performance. Additional fMRI studies suggest that psychostimulants may have direct effects on affective circuits, offering a potential explanation for the palliative effect that psychostimulants can have on emotional impulsivity in hyperactive children (Posner et al. 2011a, 2011b).

One of the most important findings in the stimulant treatment literature is the high degree of short-term efficacy results for *behavioral* targets, with weaker effects shown for *cognition and learning*. Conners (personal communication, 1993) noted that 0.8, 1.0, and 0.9 effect sizes were reported for behavioral improvements in the Type 4 meta-analytic reviews of stimulant drug actions (Kavale 1982; Ottenbacher and Cooper 1983; Thurber and Walker 1983). These behavioral responses to stimulant treatment, when compared with placebo, resembled the treatment efficacy of antibiotics. Less powerful effects were found for laboratory measures of cognitive changes, in particular on the continuous performance task, for which the effect size was 0.6 and 0.5 for omissions and commissions, respectively, in a within-subject design (Milich et al. 1989) and 0.6 and 1.8, respectively, in a between-subject study (Steinhausen and Kreuzer 1981).

Psychostimulants continue to show behavioral efficacy in the Type 1 RCTs published since 1985 (Table 2–3). These modern-day controlled trials have matured along with the field and now utilize multiple-dose conditions with multiple stimulants (Elia et al. 1991), parallel designs (Spencer et al. 1995), and a common definition of response as normalization (Abikoff and Gittelman 1985a; Rapport et al. 1994). These studies test psychostimulants in special ADHD populations, including adolescents (Klorman et al. 1990; Wilens et al. 2006), adults (Spencer et al. 1995), subjects with mental retardation (Horn et al. 1991), and subjects with comorbid anxiety disorders, internalizing disorders, and tic disorders (Gadow et al. 1995). As shown in Table 2–3, 70% of ADHD subjects respond to stimulants, whereas less than 13% respond to placebo (Greenhill et al. 2001).

Studies have also been conducted that attempt to evaluate stimulant nonresponders. Some drug trials (e.g., Douglas et al. 1988) report a 100% response rate in small samples in which multiple methylphenidate doses are used. Other results indicate that a trial involving two stimulants separately at different times harvests the most responders, with those not responding to one medication showing a response to the other. Elia et al. (1991) reduced the 32% nonresponse rate of a single psychostimulant to less than 4% when two stimulants, dextroamphetamine and methylphenidate, were titrated one at a time sequentially in the same subject. However, if the sample includes children with comorbidity, the rate of medication nonresponse might be higher.

Finally, few studies have used the placebo discontinuation model, double-blind or single-blind, to determine whether the child continues to respond to stimulants after 1 or more years of treatment. One study revealed that 80% of children with ADHD relapsed when switched, in a single-blind fashion, from methylphenidate to placebo after 8 months of treatment (H. Abikoff, personal communication, 1994). Even so, these observations about the rare nonresponder do not address the rate of placebo response. More of the current industry-sponsored RCTs are parallel designs—an approach that can assess whether the placebo response emerges at some point over the entire drug trial. However, few treatment studies prescreen for placebo responders, so the percentage of actual medication responders in any sample of children with ADHD might be closer to 55%, not the 75%–96% often quoted. Fur-

Table 2–3.   Controlled studies showing stimulant efficacy in attention-deficit/hyperactivity disorder drug treatments (N = 3,125)

Study	N	Age range (years)	Design	Drug (dose)	Duration	Response	Comment
Abikoff and Gittelman 1985b	28	6–12	ADHD, controls	MPH (41 mg); PB	8 weeks	80.9%	Normalization in children with ADHD.
Taylor et al. 1987	38	6–10	Crossover	MPH (0.2–1.4); PB	6 weeks	58%	Better response in children with severe ADHD symptoms.
Douglas et al. 1988	19	7–13	Crossover	MPH (0.15, 0.3, 0.6); PB	2 weeks	100%	Linear dose-response relationships.
Rapport et al. 1988	22	6–10	Crossover	MPH (5, 10, 15 mg); PB	5 weeks	72%	MPH response same in home and at school.
Barkley et al. 1989	74	6–13	Crossover (37 aggressive, 37 nonaggressive)	MPH (0.3, 0.5); PB	4 weeks	80%	Aggression responsive to MPH.
Whalen et al. 1989	25	6.3–12	Crossover	MPH (0.3, 0.5); PB	5 weeks	48%–72%	MPH helps, but does not normalize, peer status.
Klorman et al. 1990	48	12–18	Crossover	MPH (0.26 tid); PB bid	6 weeks	MPH 60%	Less medical benefits for adolescents.

Table 2–3. Controlled studies showing stimulant efficacy in attention-deficit/hyperactivity disorder drug treatments (N = 3,125) *(continued)*

Study	N	Age range (years)	Design	Drug (dose)	Duration	Response	Comment
Pelham et al. 1990	22	8–13	Crossover	MPH (10 mg bid); PB bid; DEX Spansule (10 mg); PEM (56.25 mg qd)	24 days	Stimulant: 68%	DEX Spansule, PEM best for behavior; 27% did best with DEX, 18% with SR, 18% with PEM, and 5% with MPH bid.
Barkley et al. 1991	40	6–12	Crossover (23 ADHD, 17 ADHD-W)	MPH (5, 10, 15 mg bid); PB bid	6 weeks	ADHD, 95% ADHD-W, 76%	Few children with ADHD-W responded; need low dose.
Elia et al. 1991	48	6–12	Crossover	MPH (0.5, 0.8, 1.5); PB bid; DEX (0.25, 0.5, 0.75)	6 weeks	MPH: 79% DEX: 86%	Response rate for two stimulants: 96%.
DuPaul and Rapport 1993	31	6–12	Crossover (31 ADHD, 25 controls)	MPH (20 mg); PB bid	6 weeks	78% (behavior) 61% (attention)	MPH can normalize classroom behavior; academics did not normalize in 25% of subjects with ADHD.

Table 2–3.   Controlled studies showing stimulant efficacy in attention-deficit/hyperactivity disorder drug treatments (*N* = 3,125) (*continued*)

Study	*N*	Age range (years)	Design	Drug (dose)	Duration	Response	Comment
DuPaul et al. 1994	40	6–12	Crossover (12 high ANX, 17 moderate ANX, 11 low ANX)	MPH (5, 10, 15 mg); PB single dose	6 weeks	High: 68% nortriptyline Moderate: 70% nortriptyline Low: 82% nortriptyline	25% of children with comorbid internalizing disorders deteriorated while taking medications; ADHD subjects with comorbid internalizing disorders were less likely to experience normalization of behavior or to respond to MPH.
Rapport et al. 1994	76	6–12	Crossover	MPH (5, 10, 15, 20 mg); PB	5 weeks	94% (behavioral) 53% (attention)	MPH normalizes behavior more than it does academic performance; higher doses better; linear dose-response curve.
Douglas et al. 1995	17	6–11	Crossover	MPH (0.3, 0.6, 0.9); PB	4 weeks	70% (behavior)	No cognitive toxicity at high doses; linear dose-response curves.
Gadow et al. 1995	34	6–12	Crossover (ADHD+tic)	MPH (0.1, 0.3, 0.5); PB	8 weeks	MPH: 100%	No nonresponders in terms of behavior; physicians' motor tic ratings showed two minimal increases while subjects were taking drug; only effects over 8 weeks of treatment studied.

Table 2–3. Controlled studies showing stimulant efficacy in attention-deficit/hyperactivity disorder drug treatments (*N* = 3,125) (*continued*)

Study	*N*	Age range (years)	Design	Drug (dose)	Duration	Response	Comment
Pelham et al. 1995	28	5–12	Crossover	PEM (18.75, 37.5, 75, 112.5 mg); PB od	7 weeks	PEM: 89% PB: 0%	PEM dosage of ≥37.5 mg/day lasts 2–7 hours; efficacy and time course equal to those of MPH.
Spencer et al. 1995	23	18–60	Crossover	MPH (1 mg/kg/day)	7 weeks	MPH: 78% PB: 4%	MPH at 1 mg/kg/day led to improvement in adults equivalent to that seen in children.
Tannock et al. 1995a	40	6–12	Crossover (22 ADHD, 18 ADHD-ANX)	MPH (0.3, 0.6)	2 weeks	70%	Activity level better in both groups; working memory not improved in anxious children.
Tannock et al. 1995b	28	6–12	Crossover	MPH (0.3, 0.6, 0.9); PB	2 weeks	70%	Effects on behavior: dose-response curve linear, but effects on response inhibition U-shaped; suggests adjustment of dose on objective measures.
Castellanos et al. 1997	20	6–13	Crossover	MPH (45 mg); DEX (22.5 mg)	9 weeks	ADHD + TS	Dose-related tics at high doses.
Gillberg et al. 1997	62	6–12	Parallel	MAS (17 mg); PB	60 weeks	70%; 27%–40% improved	No dropouts, but only 25% placebo group at 15-month assessment.

Table 2–3. Controlled studies showing stimulant efficacy in attention-deficit/hyperactivity disorder drug treatments (N = 3,125) (continued)

Study	N	Age range (years)	Design	Drug (dose)	Duration	Response	Comment
McGough et al. 2006	97	6–17	Crossover	MTS on 9 hours/day (12.5, 18.75, 25, 37.5 cm²); PB	2 weeks	79.8%	MPH transdermal system well tolerated and significantly more efficacious than PB; FDA registration trial
Klein et al. 1997	84	6–15	Parallel	MPH (1.0)	5 weeks	MPH: 59%–78% PB: 9%–29%	MPH reduced ratings of antisocial behaviors.
Musten et al. 1997	31	4–6	Crossover	MPH (0.3, 0.5); PB	3 weeks	MPH>PB	MPH improves attention in preschoolers.
Schachar et al. 1997	91	6–12	Parallel	MPH (33.5 mg); PB	52 weeks	0.7 SD effect size	15% side effects: affective, overfocusing led to dropouts.
Swanson et al. 1998	29	7–14	Crossover	MAS (5, 10, 15, 20 mg); PB; MPH	7 weeks	100%	Adderall peaks at 3 hours; MPH at 1.5 hours.
MTA Cooperative Group 1999a	579	7–9	Parallel	MPH (<0.8 tid)	14 months	MPH: 77% DEX: 10% None: 13%	Titration trial for multisite multimodal study; full study data for 288 subjects taking 38.7 mg MPH.
Greenhill et al. 2001	277	6–12	Parallel	Long-acting MPH; PB	3 weeks	70%	Mean total daily dose = 40 mg; FDA registration.

Table 2–3. Controlled studies showing stimulant efficacy in attention-deficit/hyperactivity disorder drug treatments (N = 3,125) (continued)

Study	N	Age range (years)	Design	Drug (dose)	Duration	Response	Comment
Wolraich et al. 2001	282	6–12	Parallel	OROS-MPH (36 mg); immediate-release MPH tid; PB	4 weeks	62%	Concerta rated effective by teachers and parents; FDA registration trial.
Greenhill et al. 2002a	321	6–16	Parallel	MPH-MR (Metadate ER) (20, 60 mg qd); PB tid	3 weeks	MPH-MR: 64% PB: 27%	Mean MPH-MR ER daily dose = 40.7 mg (1.28 mg/kg/day).
Wigal et al. 2004	132	6–17	Parallel	D-MPH; DL-MPH; PB bid	4 weeks	D-MPH: 67% DL-MPH: 49%	Average D-MPH dose (18.25 mg) was as safe and effective as half of the average DL-MPH dose (32.14 mg).
Greenhill et al. 2006a	165	3–5.5	Crossover	Immediate-release MPH (1.25, 2.5, 5, 7.5 mg tid); PB tid	70 weeks	88%	Optimal immediate-release MPH dosage = 14.22±8.1 mg/day (0.7±0.4 mg/kg/day); treatment effect sizes less than those in school-age children.

Table 2–3.   Controlled studies showing stimulant efficacy in attention-deficit/hyperactivity disorder drug treatments (N = 3,125) (continued)

Study	N	Age range (years)	Design	Drug (dose)	Duration	Response	Comment
Greenhill et al. 2006b	97	6–17	Parallel	D-MPH-ER (Focalin LA) (5–30 mg qd); PB	7 weeks	D-MPH-ER: 67.3% PB: 13.3%	Mean D-MPH-ER daily dose = 24 mg.
Wilens et al. 2006	177	13–18	Parallel	OROS-MPH (18, 36, 54, 72 mg qd); PB	2 weeks	OROS-MPH: 52% PB: 31%	OROS-MPH well tolerated and effective in adolescents at total daily dose of up to 72 mg; FDA trial evidence for adolescents 72 mg.

Note.   Doses listed as mg/kg/dose, and medication is given twice daily, unless otherwise stated.
ADHD = attention-deficit/hyperactivity disorder; ADHD-W = attention-deficit disorder without hyperactivity; ANX = anxiety; DEX = dextroamphetamine; ER = extended release; FDA = U.S. Food and Drug Administration; MAS = mixed amphetamine salts (Adderall); MPH = methylphenidate; MTS = methylphenidate transdermal system; OROS-MPH = osmotic-release oral system formulation of methylphenidate; MR = modified release; PB = placebo; PEM = pemoline; TS = Tourette syndrome.

thermore, these estimates apply to group effects and do not inform the clinician about the individual patient.

Methylphenidate: Short-Acting Preparations

Pharmacokinetics. Methylphenidate forms the active ingredient of the majority of stimulant medications prescribed in the United States. With the exception of the two dexmethylphenidate products (Focalin and Focalin XR; methyl α-phenyl-2-piperidineacetate hydrochloride), methylphenidate is a racemic mixture composed of the *d*- and *l-threo* enantiomers. The *d-threo* enantiomer is more pharmacologically active than the *l-threo* enantiomer. Methylphenidate is thought to block the reuptake of dopamine into the presynaptic neuron in the CNS and increase the concentration of these neurotransmitters in the synaptic cleft.

Methylphenidate absorption into the systemic circulation is rapid after the immediate-release tablet is swallowed, so that effects on behavior can be seen within 30 minutes. Plasma concentration reaches a peak by 90 minutes, with a mean half-life of about 3 hours and a 3- to 5-hour duration of action. Although children take one immediate-release dose just after breakfast, most will require a second dose at lunch (which for young children must be given by the school nurse) and a third dose just after school in the afternoon to prevent loss of effectiveness as well as rebound crankiness and tearfulness. Long-duration preparations now are used to overcome the need for multiple daily doses of methylphenidate, and these preparations are currently the mainstay of practice.

Metabolism and excretion. In humans, methylphenidate is metabolized extrahepatically via de-esterification to α-phenylpiperidine acetic acid (PPA, ritalinic acid), an inactive metabolite. About 90% of radiolabeled methylphenidate is recovered from the urine.

Dosage and administration. Immediate-release methylphenidate tablets may be used to augment long-duration forms, such as OROS (osmotic-release oral system) methylphenidate, in clinical practice to provide a boost in the morning or to smooth withdrawal in the late afternoon. When used as the main ADHD treatment, immediate-release methylphenidate should be initiated at low morning doses, 5 mg for children and 10 mg for adults. The dose should be increased every 3–5 days by adding noontime and afternoon doses until the three-times-daily schedule is achieved. The dosage should be increased through the recommended range up to 20 mg three times daily, which is equivalent to a total daily dose (TDD) of 60 mg.

Efficacy: clinical trials. Myriad RCTs (see Schachter et al. 2001 for meta-analysis), in addition to a half century of the drug's use in the community, have supported methylphenidate's safety and efficacy for ADHD treatment in youth (Greenhill et al. 2002b; Pliszka 2007). Investigators for the National Institute of Mental Health (NIMH) Multimodal Treatment of ADHD (MTA) study identified immediate-release methylphenidate to be the most effective initial treatment strategy for their trial, in which 579 children, ages 7–10 years, with combined-type ADHD were randomly assigned to receive methylphenidate alone, behavior therapy alone, methylphenidate plus behavior therapy, or community care (MTA Cooperative Group 1999a). A double-blind, placebo-controlled titration protocol was used to titrate each MTA subject to his or her *best* immediate-release dose, which was given according to a three-times-per-day dosing schedule (Greenhill et al. 1996, 2001). Similar methods were used in the NIMH Preschool ADHD Treatment Study. This study employed a randomized clinical trial of immediate-release methylphenidate in 165 preschool children with ADHD, ages 3–5.5 years (Greenhill 2001). Both studies showed a response rate of more than 75% among children exposed to methylphenidate. However, the mean *best* immediate-release methylphenidate TDD varied by age, with preschoolers doing best at a dosage of 14.4 ± 0.75 mg/day (0.75 mg/kg/day) and school-age children in the MTA doing best at 31.2 ± 0.55 mg/day (0.95 mg/kg/day). Immediate-release effect sizes were greater in school-age children (1.2 per teacher rating scales, and 0.8 per child self-report at 30 mg/day) than in preschoolers (0.8 per teacher rating scales, and 0.5 per parent rating scales at 14 mg/day), but optimal TDDs were higher in the former.

Adverse effects specifically associated with methylphenidate. Short- and long-duration methylphenidate preparations demonstrate the same adverse-effect profile during placebo-controlled randomized clinical trials. Adverse effects include appetite loss, weight decrease, headache, abdominal pain, delay in sleep onset, and new-onset tics. Other adverse effects reported as infrequent are nausea, abdominal pain, dryness of the throat, dizziness, palpitations, headache, akathisia, dyskinesia, and drowsiness. Rare but serious adverse effects include angina, tachycardia, urticaria, fever, arthralgia, exfoliative dermatitis, erythema multiforme, and thrombocytopenic purpura. Also rare are tactile hallucinations (including formication), phobias of insects, leukopenia, anemia, eosinophilia, transient depression, sudden unexpected death, and hair loss. Neuroleptic malignant syndrome (NMS) has been reported very rarely and only when methylphenidate is used in combination with other drugs that are by themselves associated with NMS.

Drug-drug interactions. Methylphenidate interacts with few medications. These include monoamine oxidase inhibitors (isocarboxazid, phenelzine, selegiline, and tranylcypromine), as well as antibiotics with monoamine oxidase–inhibiting activity (linezolid), leading to blood pressure elevations and an increase in methylphenidate serum concentrations. In addition, phenytoin, phenobarbital, tricyclic antidepressants, and warfarin increase the serum concentrations of methylphenidate. The effects of centrally acting antihypertensives (guanadrel, methyldopa, and clonidine) can be reduced by methylphenidate. NMS has been reported in one patient treated with both venlafaxine and methylphenidate.

Methylphenidate: Long-Duration Preparations

Long-duration methylphenidate preparations address the problems of short-acting methylphenidate with a once-daily dosing format and have become a mainstay of clinical practice in the United States (Biederman et al. 2002, 2007c; Greenhill et al. 2002a, 2006c; McCracken et al. 2003; Pelham et al. 1999; Swanson et al. 2004; Wolraich et al. 2001; Zuvekas and Vitiello 2012). A meta-analysis comparing atomoxetine to immediate-release methylphenidate and OROS methylphenidate indicates that the longer-duration OROS formulation shows significantly greater effect size than atomoxetine, but the immediate-release methylphenidate shows no difference in efficacy compared with atomoxetine (Hanwella et al. 2011). Although most medications use methylphenidate as the active ingredient, the formulations differ in the number and shape of methylphenidate pulses that they release into the blood circulation. The range of medications includes the older, single-pulse methylphenidate drugs such as Ritalin-SR; newer dual-pulse beaded methylphenidate products such as Metadate CD, Ritalin LA, and Focalin XR; and complex-release formulations such as OROS methylphenidate (Concerta).

Methylphenidate, single-pulse, sustained-release.   Single-pulse, sustained-release methylphenidate formulations (Ritalin-SR and Metadate ER) are formulated in a wax-matrix preparation to prolong release. They display a slower onset of action than immediate-release methylphenidate, produce lower serum concentrations, and have a 6- to 8-hour duration of action (Birmaher et al. 1989). Clinicians regard these products as less effective in practice than immediate-release or dual-pulse beaded methylphenidate or OROS methylphenidate preparations. To compensate for the reduced effectiveness of single-pulse, sustained-release methylphenidate, clinicians administer them twice daily or give them with an immediate-release tablet in the morning to compensate for the slow onset of action.

Methylphenidate, beaded.   Beaded methylphenidate products are an extended-release formulation with a bimodal release profile. In Ritalin LA, this profile is created by using a proprietary SODAS (spheroidal oral drug absorption system) technology involving a mixture of immediate-release and delayed-release beads. These preparations help young children who have difficulty swallowing pills because the capsule can be opened, and the tiny medication spheres can be sprinkled into applesauce.

Each Ritalin LA capsule contains half the dose as immediate-release methylphenidate beads and half as enteric-coated delayed-release beads, thus providing a two-pulse release system that mimics the use of immediate-release methylphenidate given in two doses 4 hours apart. In a single dose, Ritalin LA 10-, 20-, 30-, and 40-mg capsules provide the same amount of methylphenidate as twice-daily doses of 5, 10, 15, and 20 mg, respectively, of the immediate-release preparation. Given once daily, Ritalin LA exhibits a lower second-peak concentration ($C_{max}2$), higher interpeak minimum concentrations, and less peak-to-peak trough fluctuations in serum concentration of methylphenidate than immediate-release methylphenidate tablets given 4 hours apart. This effect may be due to the earlier onset and more prolonged absorption of the delayed-release beads. The efficacy of Ritalin LA in ADHD treatment was established in one controlled trial involving 132 children, ages 6–12, who met DSM-IV criteria for ADHD (Wigal et al. 2004).

Dexmethylphenidate

Pharmacokinetics.   Dexmethylphenidate hydrochloride (Focalin) is the *d-threo* enantiomer of racemic methylphenidate. The drug's plasma concentration increases rapidly after ingestion, reaching a maximum in the fasted state at about 1–1.5 hours postdose (Quinn et al. 2004; Wigal et al. 2004). Plasma levels of dexmethylphenidate are comparable to those achieved following immediate-release methylphenidate doses given as capsules in twice the total milligram amount.

Focalin XR is an extended-release formulation of dexmethylphenidate with a bimodal release that includes proprietary SODAS technology similar to that of Ritalin LA. Each Focalin XR capsule contains half the dose as immediate-release beads and half as enteric-coated, delayed-release beads. In a single dose, Focalin XR 5-, 10-, and 20-mg capsules provide the same amount of dexmethylphenidate as Focalin at dosages of 2.5, 5, and 10 mg, respectively, given twice daily.

Efficacy: clinical trials. The immediate-release dexmethylphenidate (5-, 10-, or 20-mg/day total dose) preparation, *d,l-threo*-methylphenidate hydrochloride (10-, 20-, or 40-mg/day total dose), or placebo was given twice daily to 132 patients in a multicenter, 4-week, parallel-group study (Keating and Figgitt 2002). Patients treated with dexmethylphenidate showed a statistically significant improvement in SNAP-ADHD teacher-rated symptom scores from baseline compared with patients who received placebo.

The long-duration preparation, Focalin XR, was shown to be effective in a randomized, double-blind, placebo-controlled, parallel-group study of 103 pediatric patients, ages 6–17. Using mean change from baseline scores on the teacher-rated Conners ADHD/DSM-IV Scales (CADS-T), the study authors reported significantly greater decrease in ADHD scores for youth taking the active Focalin XR than for youth receiving placebo (Greenhill et al. 2006c). The drug's effectiveness for adult ADHD was reported in a 5-week, randomized, double-blind, parallel-group, placebo-controlled study of 221 adults, ages 18–60, who met DSM-IV criteria for ADHD on the DSM-IV Attention-Deficit/Hyperactivity Disorder Rating Scale (DSM-IV ADHD-RS). Signs and symptoms of ADHD were far fewer for adults taking 20-, 30-, and 40-mg daily doses than for those randomly assigned to receive placebo (Spencer et al. 2007a).

OROS Methylphenidate

Pharmacokinetics. The OROS methylphenidate caplet (Concerta) uses an osmotic delivery system to produce ADHD symptom reduction for up to

12 hours (Swanson et al. 2004; Wolraich et al. 2001). Immediate-release methylphenidate is applied to the outside of the OROS caplet to provide immediate drug benefits in the first 2 hours after it is swallowed. The long-duration component is delivered by an osmotic pump (OROS) that gradually releases the drug over a 10-hour period, producing a slightly ascending methylphenidate serum concentration curve. Taken once daily, it mimics the serum concentrations produced by taking immediate-release methylphenidate three times daily, but with less variation (Modi et al. 2000). Long-duration preparations containing the dual-pulse beaded technology have claimed greater efficacy than OROS methylphenidate for controlling ADHD symptoms in the early morning hours (Swanson et al. 2004).

Efficacy: clinical trials. Two double-blind, placebo-controlled, randomized clinical trials have tested the efficacy and safety of OROS methylphenidate compared with immediate-release methylphenidate for children with ADHD (Swanson et al. 2003; Wolraich et al. 2001). The results show that once-daily dosing with OROS methylphenidate matches the robust reduction of ADHD symptoms for the active preparation and low placebo-response rates reported in the MTA study for methylphenidate. In addition, compared with immediate-release methylphenidate given three times daily, OROS methylphenidate has been demonstrated in a small study ($N = 6$) to have a longer duration of effect in reducing ADHD-induced driving impairments in the evening (Cox et al. 2004).

Special Oral Methylphenidate Preparations

Methylin chewable tablets and Methylin oral solution are two forms of a short-duration branded methylphenidate generic that has been formulated for young children who have difficulty swallowing pills or capsules. Methylin chewable tablets show peak plasma methylphenidate concentrations in 1–2 hours (T_{max}), with a mean peak concentration (C_{max}) of 10 ng/mL after a 20-mg chewable tablet is taken. High-fat meals delay the peak by 1 hour (1.5 and 2.4 hours for fasted and fed states, respectively), which is similar to what is seen with an immediate-release methylphenidate tablet. Methylin chewable tablets are available in 2.5-, 5-, and 10-mg doses. Methylin oral solution is available in 5 mg/5 cc and 10 mg/5 cc strengths. No large-scale clinical trials have been published in which Methylin chewable tablets or oral solution was used.

Transdermal Methylphenidate Preparations

Transdermal methylphenidate (Daytrana) is steadily absorbed after application of the patch, but the levels do not reach peak until 7–9 hours later, with no noticeable reduction of ADHD symptoms for the first 2 hours. Interestingly, this delivery method bypasses the first-pass effect, so that blood levels of L-methylphenidate are higher than obtained from the oral route. Steady dosing with the patch results in higher peak methylphenidate levels than does equivalent dosing with OROS methylphenidate, suggesting increased absorption. Duration of action for a 9-hour wear period is about 11.5 hours. A double-blind, placebo-controlled, crossover study conducted in a laboratory classroom showed that children wearing active versus placebo patch had significantly lower ADHD symptom scores and higher math test scores for postdose hours 2 through 9 (McGough et al. 2006). Transdermal methylphenidate appears to be as effective as other long-duration preparations, but adverse effects, including anorexia, insomnia, and tics, occur more frequently with the patch, and mild skin reactions are common.

Amphetamines

Pharmacokinetics.   As with methylphenidate, amphetamines are manufactured in the dextro isomer, as in dextroamphetamine (Dexedrine, lisdexamfetamine) or in racemic forms, with mixtures of D-amphetamine and L-amphetamine (Adderall or Adderall XR). Efficacy of these amphetamine products resembles the efficacy of the methylphenidate products in controlling overactivity, inattention, and impulsivity in patients with ADHD. Some children who experience severe adverse effects associated with taking methylphenidate may respond without such problems when taking amphetamine products. Absorption of this preparation is rapid, and the plasma levels of the drug peak 3 hours after oral administration. All the amphetamines are metabolized hepatically. Acidification of the urine increases urinary output of amphetamines (Greenhill et al. 2002b). Taking the medication with ascorbic acid or fruit juice decreases absorption, whereas taking it with alkalinizing agents such as sodium bicarbonate increases it (Vitiello 2006).

Effects of dextroamphetamine can be seen within 1 hour of ingestion, and the duration of action lasts up to 5 hours, which is somewhat longer than with methylphenidate. Nevertheless, twice-daily administration is needed to extend the immediate-release preparation treatment throughout the school day.

Racemic Adderall and Adderall XR.   Adderall and Adderall XR are amphetamine salt mixtures. Adderall XR is a dual-pulse capsule preparation that includes both immediate- and extended-release beads. There is no evidence that these mixed amphetamine salts offer any advantage over methylphenidate or dextroamphetamine, but some patients may respond better to one than another.

Lisdexamfetamine dimesylate (Vyvanse) is the first formulation of amphetamine available for the treatment of ADHD in a prodrug formulation intended for a single, long-duration, daily-dose regimen. The preparation is inactive parenterally because the D-amphetamine molecule is covalently bonded to L-lysine, an essential amino acid. After ingestion, the pharmacologically active D-amphetamine is released when the covalent bond is cleaved. This bond is an amide bond, which means that a digestive proteolytic enzyme or enzymes in the digestive tract are the agents of release. Only minimal amounts of D-amphetamine are released when the drug is administered parenterally (Mickel et al. 2006). The lisdexamfetamine prodrug was designed to have much reduced potential for abuse, diversion, or overdose toxicity (Jasinski and Krishnan 2009).

In two double-blind, placebo-controlled, randomized clinical trials in a total of 342 children with ADHD, the children taking lisdexamfetamine, in doses of 30–50 mg for 3 or 4 weeks, improved more on ADHD rating scales than those taking placebo. The first study, a Phase II, double-blind, placebo-controlled, randomized, crossover design in children ($N=52$) with ADHD, showed significant reductions for lisdexamfetamine dimesylate and mixed amphetamine salts in trained but blind observer ratings of ADHD behavior differences across 8 hourly sessions of a 12-hour day when compared with placebo (Biederman et al. 2007a). The second study, a multisite, Phase III, randomized controlled clinical trial of 290 children with ADHD, ages 6–12, with a parallel design, showed significant decreases in ADHD behaviors, as reported by parents for morning, afternoon, and early evening on the Conners Parent Rating Scale (Biederman et al. 2007b).

Adverse Effects Reported With Stimulants

Adverse effects frequently reported during stimulant use include delay of sleep onset, headache, appetite decrease, and weight loss. Infrequently observed adverse effects include emotional lability and tics.

Standard Warnings

All stimulant products carry a warning on the package insert that the product should be used with care in patients with a history of drug dependence or alcoholism. In addition, there is a warning about sudden death that may be associated with preexisting cardiac abnormalities or other serious heart problems. For adults, the warning includes sudden death but also extends to stroke and myocardial infarction. Adults are also warned that they should be cautious about taking stimulants if they have preexisting hypertension, heart failure, recent myocardial infarction, or ventricular arrhythmia. Patients with preexisting psychotic and bipolar psychiatric illness are cautioned against taking stimulants because of their psychotomimetic properties at high dosages. Additionally, there is a warning about stimulants' ability to slow growth rates and lower the convulsive threshold in children.

Basis of Warnings About Serious, Unexpected Adverse Events
Associated With Stimulant Use

Stimulant benefits have had to be weighed against reports of serious, unexpected adverse events in populations taking stimulants for ADHD treatment. These concerns arose from the FDA review of cardiovascular and psychiatric adverse events associated with approved stimulant medications. On June 30, 2005, the agency began this review by examining the passive surveillance reports associated with OROS methylphenidate (Concerta) (www.fda.gov/ohrms/dockets/ac/05/transcripts/2005-4152t2_Transcript.pdf). The review uncovered 135 adverse events, including 36 psychiatric adverse events and 20 cardiovascular events. In particular, the reports included 12 instances of tactile and visual hallucinations (classified under "psychosis") during OROS methylphenidate use—the same clinical phenomena seen in cases of alcoholic delirium. These OROS methylphenidate adverse-event reports represent 135 of 1.3 million cases, and thus these events are rare and unexpected.

More worrisome were reports of 20 cases of sudden unexpected death (14 children and 6 adults) and 12 cases of stroke in patients taking mixed amphetamine salts (Adderall XR). This led Health Canada to temporarily suspend the sales of Adderall XR in 2005 (www.hc-sc.gc.ca/ahc-asc/media/advisories-avis/_2005/2005_01-eng.php). Five patients had preexisting structural heart defects. The rest of the victims had "family histories of ventricular tachycardia, association of death with heat exhaustion, fatty liver, heart attack, and type 1 diabetes." The rate of sudden, unexpected death is estimated to be 0.5 per 100,000 patient-years in patients taking mixed amphetamine salts and 0.19 per 100,000 patient-years in patients taking methylphenidate, whereas the rate of sudden, unexpected death in the general population has been estimated at 1.3–1.6 per 100,000 patient-years (Liberthson 1996). Patients with preexisting heart disease should be referred to a cardiologist before initiating stimulant treatment. More recent studies (Cooper et al. 2011; Olson et al. 2012; Vitiello et al. 2012) have shown no significant differences in risks of vascular events or symptoms with stimulant use.

In summary, serious unexpected cardiac or psychiatric adverse events associated with taking stimulants are extremely rare. These rates are too low to prove a causal association with stimulants in patients with no history of previous heart disease. Routine electrocardiograms and echocardiograms are not indicated prior to starting stimulant treatment in patients with unremarkable medical histories and physical examinations.

Recommendations Concerning Cardiac Contraindications to Stimulant Use

Before prescribing stimulants, the physician should first ask whether the patient or his or her family has a history of structural heart disease and whether they have previously consulted with a cardiologist. Known cardiac problems that raise a caution about using stimulants include tetralogy of Fallot, cardiac artery abnormalities, and obstructive subaortic stenosis. Clinicians should be alert if the patient has hypertension or complains of syncope, arrhythmias, or chest pain, because these may be indicators of hypertrophic cardiomyopathy. This condition has been associated with sudden, unexpected death in patients taking stimulants.

Growth Slowdown

Growth slowdown is another infrequent adverse reaction to psychostimulants. Reduction in growth velocity has been the most consistently researched long-term side effect for stimulants (Greenhill 1984). Even with the plethora of studies done in this area (Greenhill 1981), myriad methodological difficulties prevent an easy interpretation. Few studies employ the optimal controls, which include untreated children with ADHD, a psychiatric control group, and an ADHD group receiving treatment with a class of medications other than stimulants. However, even these studies differ in the quality of compliance measures used and in whether the children were taking stimulants on weekends or used the stimulants throughout the summer. One large controlled study (Gittelman-Klein et al. 1988) reported growth rate reductions among a subgroup of children, but growth may resume immediately when stimulant treatment is discontinued (Safer et al. 1975).

In the MTA Cooperative Group (2004) study, growth slowdown for height and weight was reported for children with ADHD, ages 7–10, who were treated with methylphenidate at a mean dosage of 30 mg/day. School-age children grew 1.0 cm less and gained 2.5 kg less than predicted from CDC growth charts. Similar effects were observed for preschool children (Swanson et al. 2007), who grew 1.5 cm less in height and gained 2.5 kg less in weight than predicted while being treated with methylphenidate at a mean dosage of 14 mg/day.

Safer and Allen (1973; Safer et al. 1972, 1975) first reported that treatment for 2 or more years with methylphenidate and dextroamphetamine could produce decrements in the rate of weight gain on age-adjusted growth rate charts. Dextroamphetamine, with a half-life of two to three times that of methylphenidate, produces more sustained effects on the rate of weight gain than methylphenidate, as well as suppressing mean sleep-related prolactin concentrations (Greenhill 1981). In methylphenidate-treated children with ADHD who were followed for 2–4 years, dose-related decreases in weight velocity were seen (Gittelman-Klein et al. 1988; Satterfield et al. 1979), with some tolerance of the suppressive effect developing in the second year (Satterfield et al. 1979). Hechtman et al. (1984) reported growth slowdown in untreated children with ADHD, suggesting that differential growth in such children may be associated with the ADHD disorder itself. Spencer et al. (1996) detected similar differential growth for children with ADHD that could be associated with the disorder itself and not only with stimulant treatment.

The psychostimulant mechanism for any growth slowdown is unknown. Primate studies with exposure to oral methylphenidate in clinical dosages in young monkeys led to a 6-month delay in the onset of puberty but no loss of weight or height (Mattison et al. 2011). Early theories blamed the drug's putative growth-suppressant action on its effects on growth hormone or prolactin, but research studies involving 13 children treated for 18 months with 0.8 mg/day of dextroamphetamine (Greenhill et al. 1981) and 9 children treated for 12 months with 1.2 mg/kg/day of methylphenidate (Greenhill et al. 1984) failed to demonstrate a consistent change in growth hormone release. The most parsimonious explanation for this drug effect is the medication's suppression of appetite, leading to reduced caloric intake. No study, however, has collected the standardized diet diaries necessary to track calories consumed by children with ADHD who are taking psychostimulants (Greenhill et al. 1981).

In any case, the growth effects of methylphenidate appear to be minimal. Satterfield et al. (1979) followed 110 children and found decreases in the rate of height growth during the first year of psychostimulant treatment, but this effect reversed during the second year of treatment. An initial growth loss during treatment was seen in 65 children followed to age 18, but these children caught up during adolescence and reached heights predicted from their parents' heights (Gittelman and Mannuzza 1988). These results confirm the observations by Roche et al. (1979) that psychostimulants have mild and transitory effects on weight and only rarely interfere with height acquisition. Height and weight should be measured at 6-month intervals during stimulant treatment and recorded on age-adjusted growth forms to determine the presence of a drug-related reduction in height or weight velocity. If such a decrement is discovered during maintenance therapy with psychostimulants, a reduction in dosage or change to another class of medication can be carried out, as shown in reports of growth changes in the NIMH MTA and the NIMH Preschool ADHD Treatment Study (Biederman et al. 2010; Faraone et al. 2008; Swanson et al. 2007). In addition, evidence indicates that treatment of children with ADHD using the nonstimulant atomoxetine is similarly associated with a transient growth suppression (Spencer et al. 2007b).

Motor or vocal tics have been reported in up to 1% of children taking methylphenidate (Ickowicz et al. 1992). A controlled trial of children with ADHD and chronic tic disorder who were taking methylphenidate (Gadow et al. 1995) reported significant improvement in ADHD symptoms without consistent worsening or increase in tic frequency for all subjects. However, the TDD of methylphenidate used never exceeded 20 mg. These low dosages and the short length of the 8-week study do not resemble the higher dosages and longer treatment duration found in clinical practice, where tics may appear after several months of drug administration.

Clinical literature has held that methylphenidate lowers the seizure threshold, although the treatment of patients with ADHD and seizures shows no change in seizure frequency (Klein 1995).

Adverse Effects Associated With Discontinuation
of Treatment With Stimulants

The most common adverse effects associated with discontinuation of stimulant treatment in controlled trials are twitching (motor or vocal tics), anorexia, insomnia, and tachycardia, with reported incident rates of approximately 1%.

Contraindications to Stimulant Treatment

Several clinical conditions have been worsened by stimulant treatment. Florid psychosis, mania, concurrent substance abuse, Tourette's disorder, and eating disorders are common contraindications to stimulant use. Structural cardiac lesions and hypertensive states are additional contraindications to the use of stimulants to treat ADHD.

Stimulant Medications in Practice

In the mid-1990s, over 85% of psychostimulant prescriptions written in the United States were for methylphenidate (Safer et al. 1996; L. Williams and J. Swanson, unpublished paper, 1996). The rate of methylphenidate prescription writing increased fourfold from 1990 to 1995. The drug's indications, pharmacology, adverse-effect profile, and usage directions are frequently highlighted in reviews (e.g., Dulcan 1990; Wilens and Biederman 1992). Methylphenidate has become the first-line psychostimulant for ADHD, followed by dextroamphetamine and atomoxetine (Richters et al. 1995). As the longer-acting amphetamine preparations (lisdexamfetamine, mixed amphetamine salts extended release) have been increasingly marketed from 2000 to 2011, these two major groups now are prescribed equally often. Dextroamphetamine has identical efficacy to methylphenidate (Arnold et al. 1978; Elia et al. 1991; Pelham et al. 1990; Vyborova et al. 1984; Winsberg et al. 1974). Arnold (2000) noted that of the 141 subjects in these studies, 50 responded better to dextroamphetamine, and only 37 responded better to methylphenidate.

Outpatient visits devoted to ADHD increased from 1.6 million per year in 1990 to 4.2 million visits (and 6 million stimulant drug prescriptions) in 1993 (Swanson et al. 1995b). During those visits, 90% of the children were given prescriptions, 71% of which were for methylphenidate. Methylphenidate production in the United States increased from 1,784 to 5,110 kg per year during the same time period (Vitiello and Jensen 1997). It has been estimated that 3.6% of U.S. youth ages 6–17 were given prescriptions for stimulants in 2008 (Zuvekas and Vitiello 2012). However, specific epidemiological surveys suggest that 12-month prescription rates for the school-age group, ages 6–12, may be higher, ranging from 6% in urban settings (Safer et al. 1996) to 7% in rural settings (Angold et al. 2000) and extending up to 10% in some communities (LeFever et al. 1999).

Psychostimulant use has increased fivefold since 1989, and this increase has raised concerns at the DEA—which regulates production of these drugs—about the risks of abuse and diversion. Increased psychostimulant use could be attributed to increases in ADHD prevalence, a change in the ADHD diagnosis, improved recognition of ADHD by physicians, broadened indications for use, or an increase in drug diversion and prescription for profit or abuse (Goldman et al. 1998). Analyses of managed-care data sets reveal a 2.5-fold increase in prescribing from 1990 to 1995 that can be accounted for by longer durations of treatment, inclusion of girls and patients with predominantly inattentive ADHD subtype, and treatment of high school students (Safer et al. 1996). A more recent study by IMS Health reported that physicians wrote 51.5 million prescriptions for ADHD medications in 2010, with a total value of $7.42 billion, an increase of 83% from the $4.05 billion sold in 2006; this increase partially accounts for shortages of mixed amphetamine salts (Harris 2012). An epidemiologically based survey conducted in four communities found that only one-eighth of children diagnosed with ADHD received adequate stimulant treatment (Jensen et al. 1999); another survey, conducted in rural North Carolina, found that many school-age children taking stimulants did not meet DSM-IV criteria for ADHD (Angold et al. 2000; Copeland et al. 2011; Merikangas et al. 2010).

Because of reports of hepatotoxicity during postmarketing surveillance by the FDA from 1975 to 1990, pemoline is no longer available in the United States. However, pemoline is effective. A randomized clinical trial by Pelham et al. (1995) comparing four doses of once-daily pemoline with placebo showed a 72% rate of response for pemoline at a dosage of 37.5 mg/day.

Stimulant responsiveness or rates of side effects were originally thought to be affected by the presence of comorbid anxiety symptoms. Pliszka (1989) gave 43 subjects with ADHD either methylphenidate (0.25–0.4 mg/kg or 0.45–0.70 mg/kg) or placebo for 4 weeks. For the 22 subjects with comorbid anxiety symptoms, the active stimulant treatment showed less efficacy when compared with placebo, as judged by teachers' global ratings, with no increase in side effects. This result might be explained by the strong placebo response in the group. Tannock et al. (1995a) reported findings from a treatment study involving 40 children with ADHD, some with (n = 18) and some without (n = 22) comorbid anxiety symptoms, in a double-blind, randomized, crossover design with three methylphenidate doses (0.3, 0.6, and 0.9 mg/kg). The two groups showed equal decreases in motor activity, but the group with comorbid anxiety did more poorly on a serial addition task and had a differential heart-rate response to methylphenidate. DuPaul et al. (1994) found that compared with children with ADHD and no comorbid anxiety, 40 children with ADHD and comorbid anxiety were less likely to respond to methylphenidate and showed more side effects for three methylphenidate doses (5, 10, and 15 mg) and placebo. However, the study did not collect ratings for anxiety symptoms, so the direct effect of methylphenidate on such symptoms was not recorded.

Subsequent data do not support these early impressions. One controlled study (Gadow et al. 1995) that tested the methylphenidate effects in children with comorbid anxiety symptoms found equally good responses in those with and those without the anxiety disorder. These divergent data leave open the question of whether comorbid anxiety symptoms predict poor response to stimulant treatment.

Predicting drug response in an individual child with ADHD is difficult. Although pretreatment patient characteristics (young age, low rates of anxiety, low severity of disorder, and high IQ) may moderate a good response to methylphenidate on global rating scales (Buitelaar et al. 1995), most research shows that neurological, physiological, or psychological measures of functioning are not reliable predictors of response to psychostimulants (Pelham and Milich 1991; Zametkin and Rapoport 1987). In the NIMH MTA study, participants with comorbid anxiety disorders responded to behavioral treatments better than to stimulant medication; for families receiving public assistance, medication management decreased closeness in parent-child interactions; and regular attendance at physician visits mediated the benefits of stimulant treatment (MTA Cooperative Group 1999b).

There has been no universally agreed-upon criterion for how much the symptoms must change, once a child responds, before the clinician stops increasing the dosage. Furthermore, there is no standard for the outcome measure. For example, should global ratings alone be used, or should they be combined with more "objective" academic measures, such as percentage of correct answers on completed lists of math problems? Some have advocated a 25% reduction of ADHD symptoms as a threshold, whereas others suggest continuing to adjust the dosage until the child's behavior and classroom performance are normalized.

The concept of *normalization* has helped standardize the definition of a categorical responder across domains and studies. Studies now use normal classroom controls instead of just statistical significance to determine whether a child's improvement from treatment is clinically meaningful. Treatment was noted to remove differences between children with ADHD and nonreferred classmates on measures of activity and attention (Abikoff and Gittelman 1985a), but not for positive peer nominations (Whalen et al. 1989). Further advances occurred when investigators used statistically derived definitions of clinically meaningful change during psychotherapeutic treatment (Jacobson and Truax 1991). Rapport et al. (1994) used this technique to calculate reliable change and normalization on the Conners Abbreviated Teacher Rating Scale (ATRS) using national norms. They determined that a child's behavior would be considered normalized when his or her ATRS score fell closer to the mean of the normal population than to the mean of the ADHD population. Using this technique in a controlled trial of four methylphenidate doses in children with ADHD, Rapport et al. found that methylphenidate normalized behavior and, to a lesser extent, academic performance (94% and 53%, respectively). Similarly, DuPaul and Rapport (1993) found that methylphenidate normalized behavior for all children with ADHD who were treated, but normalized academic performance for only 75% of the children. In another study, DuPaul et al. (1994) reported that normalization in behavior and academic performance occurred less often when subjects with ADHD had high levels of comorbid internalizing disorders. Swanson et al. (2001), applying this approach to the cumulative distribution curves on the SNAP parent and teacher behavior ratings at the end of the MTA study, found that 88% of children without ADHD, 68% of children with ADHD treated with medication plus behavior therapy, and 56% of children with ADHD treated with medication alone achieved symptom scores of 1 or less, which represent a *normal* response on those scales.

Limitations of Stimulant Treatment for ADHD

Although 3- to 7-month treatment studies carried out in groups of children with ADHD show impressive reductions in symptoms (for a review, see Schachar and Tannock 1993), clinicians must manage individual children with ADHD over years. When examined over periods greater than 6 months, children taking these medications fail to maintain academic improvement (Gadow 1983) or to improve the social problem–solving deficits that accompany ADHD. However, most long-term stimulant studies reporting lack of academic improvement have been uncontrolled, and many of the children followed were not taking stimulants consistently, so it is not possible to draw conclusions about whether stimulant treatment reverses academic failure over time. In an authoritative review, Schachar and Tannock (1993) found that of the more than 100 controlled studies of stimulant efficacy in the literature, only 18 studies lasted as long as 3 months. Because the duration of ADHD treatment extends from first grade through college, there is growing interest in showing that stimulant treatment is effective over the long run.

In a dual-site multimodal treatment study (Abikoff et al. 2004) in which children were treated for more than 2 years, medication-alone treatment was as effective as combination treatment involving medication plus psychosocial interventions. However, this study did not include a no-medication group. Concern about drawing long-term conclusions from short-term benefits in the psychostimulant literature became one of the driving forces behind the implementation of the 14-month NIMH MTA study (MTA Cooperative Group 1999a; Richters et al. 1995). The study attempted to address long-term stimulant use by including a no-medication psychosocial treatment–only arm in a sample of 576 children with ADHD.

Other caveats have been expressed about psychostimulant use for ADHD treatment in children. First, even with the relatively low rate of nonresponse (Elia et al. 1991), a small number of patients experience unmanageable side effects. Approximately 25% of children with ADHD are not helped by the first psychostimulant given or experience side effects so bothersome that meaningful dose adjustments cannot be made (DuPaul and Barkley 1990). Second, indications for choosing a particular psychostimulant and the best methods for adjusting the dose remain unclear, and these factors may prove confusing to the clinician and family. Although methylphenidate is regarded as the drug of choice for ADHD treatment, controlled treatment studies show no particular advantage of this medication over dextroamphetamine. Third, the credibility of many treatment studies is limited by methodological problems, including failure to control for prior medication treatment and inappropriately short washout periods.

In addition to the widely accepted short-term side effects of stimulants, more theoretical but still controversial concerns have been expressed. A few studies have reported problems with dissociation of cognitive and behavioral responses to methylphenidate (Sprague and Sleator 1977). Concerns have also been raised about children treated with stimulants who may develop negative self-attributions, coming to believe that they are incapable of functioning without the medication. In addition, investigators have sometimes found that stimulant effects may be influenced by the patient's IQ or age (Buitelaar et al. 1995; Pliszka 1989). Some authors have speculated that dose-response measures of academic performance in stimulant-treated children with ADHD may be influenced by state-dependent learning (Pliszka 1989; Swanson and Kinsbourne 1976). Finally, the possibility that stimulant medication response is related to the presence of minor physical anomalies, neurological soft signs, or metabolic or nutritional status has yet to be explored.

The practitioner may find it difficult to cull specific guidelines about dosing an individual patient from the studies involving large groups of children with ADHD. There is no universally agreed-upon method for dosing with these medications; some practitioners use the child's weight as a guideline (dose-by-weight method), and others titrate each child's response through the approved dosage range until clinical response occurs or side effects limit further dosage increases (stepwise-titration method). Rapport et al. (1989) demonstrated that there is no consistent relationship between weight-adjusted methylphenidate dosages and behavioral responses, calling into question the widely accepted practice of standardizing methylphenidate dosages by weight adjustment. Dose response can be conceptualized as a simple linear function (Gittelman and Kanner 1986) in some children with ADHD and as a curvilinear pattern in others. These relationships may vary in the same child, with one type for cognitive performance and another type for the behavioral domain (Sprague and Sleator 1977).

Adverse reactions to medications show the same variability and may appear unpredictable during different phases of the medication absorption or metabolic phases. Although long-term adverse reactions, such as inhibition of linear growth in children, have been shown to resolve by adulthood, no long-term, prospective studies have been published that show results of maintaining adolescents on psychostimulants through the critical period of the long bone epiphyses fusion. Therefore, more evidence remains to be gathered showing that continuously treated adolescents will reach the final height predicted from their parents' size (Greenhill 1981).

Nonstimulant Medication Treatments

Because of the controversy surrounding the use of controlled stimulant drugs in children, clinicians and parents may prefer nonstimulant medications for the treatment of ADHD. All stimulant medications approved for use in children with ADHD are classified by the DEA as drugs of abuse and are controlled. Besides the controversy, other problems face the family with children using stimulants for ADHD. Stimulants, which cause insomnia, cannot be given too late in the day. Methylphenidate's attention-enhancing effects, which last only 3–4 hours, are often needed in the late evening to help school-age children with their homework but may result in delayed sleep onset and insomnia. Adverse effects, including severe weight loss, headaches, insomnia, and tics, can also occur.

March et al. (1994) suggested that a nonstimulant may be used when there is an unsatisfactory response to two different stimulants; this approach is supported by the results of the studies of Elia et al. (1991). Other ADHD treatment parameters, as well as the Texas Children's Medication Algorithm Project, recommend the use of nonstimulants when stimulants cannot be used because of inadequate response, unwanted side effects, or parental preference (Pliszka et al. 2000).

Atomoxetine

Atomoxetine, a selective norepinephrine reuptake inhibitor, is the first drug approved by the FDA to treat ADHD both in children and in adults because of its efficacy in RCTs (Michelson 2004; Michelson et al. 2001, 2002, 2003, 2004). Atomoxetine is neither a controlled substance nor a stimulant. It is rapidly absorbed, and peak serum concentrations occur in 1 hour without food and in 3 hours with food. The drug undergoes hepatic metabolism with the cytochrome P450 (CYP) 2D6 isozyme (CYP2D6), and is then glucuronidated and excreted in urine. Plasma elimination half-life averages 5 hours for most patients. However, 5%–10% of patients have a polymorphism for the allele that codes for CYP2D6, and for them the half-life of atomoxetine can be as long as 24 hours. The pharmacodynamics differ from the pharmacokinetics in that the duration of action in reducing symptoms of ADHD is much longer than the pharmacokinetic half-life, so ADHD symptoms can be managed with once-daily dosing. Atomoxetine also can be given in the evening, whereas stimulants cannot. It is valued as a treatment for patients who have not responded to or cannot tolerate stimulants, or for those who do not want treatment with a schedule II stimulant ("Atomoxetine [Strattera] for ADHD" 2003).

Efficacy. Atomoxetine's effect size in reducing symptoms of ADHD was calculated to be 0.7, which indicates a medium effect size. This calculation was borne out in a double-blind, placebo-controlled treatment study by significantly higher response rates in patients who were randomly assigned to immediate-release stimulants (0.91) rather than once-daily atomoxetine (0.62) (Faraone et al. 2003; Newcorn et al. 2008). In practice, some clinicians have been concerned by the low numbers of children with ADHD who respond to atomoxetine.

Dosage and administration. Atomoxetine is available in 10-, 18-, 25-, 40-, 60-, 80-, and 100-mg capsules. To limit adverse effects, youth weighing 70 kg or less should have the medication started at 0.5 mg/kg/day in divided doses, with the dosage increased after 1 week to a target of 1.2 mg/kg/day. The maximum TDD is 1.4 mg/kg or 100 mg, whichever is less. Patients with hepatic dysfunction should take half the usual dose.

Drug interactions. Atomoxetine and monoamine oxidase inhibitors should not be used together or within 2 weeks of each other. The initial dosage of atomoxetine should not be increased rapidly if the patient is also taking a potent CYP2D6 inhibitor, such as fluoxetine (Prozac).

Adverse effects. Somnolence, nausea, decreased appetite, and vomiting have occurred in children starting to take atomoxetine, particularly when the dosage is increased from the initial to top levels within 3 days. Children who are slow metabolizers displayed higher rates of decreased appetite. The FDA has added two warnings to the atomoxetine package insert instructions. The first warning, added on December 17, 2004, was based on reports of severe liver injury and jaundice in two patients (one adult and one child). The FDA warned that atomoxetine should be discontinued in patients who develop jaundice or have dark urine or who have laboratory evidence of liver injury. A second warning, added on September 29, 2005, was based on the report by Eli Lilly stating that 5 of 1,800 youth in atomoxetine trials spontaneously reported suicidal ideation, whereas none of the youth randomly assigned to placebo made such reports. The FDA required that atomoxetine's label carry a black box warning about its possible association with suicidality. It is noteworthy that both warnings are based on spontaneous reports, not systematically elicited adverse effects.

Bupropion

Bupropion, an antidepressant with noradrenergic activity, has been reported to be effective for some ADHD symptoms in placebo-controlled trials (Casat et al. 1989; Clay et al. 1988; Simeon et al. 1986). Barrickman et al. (1995) reported that bupropion was equivalent to methylphenidate in the treatment of 15 children with ADHD, who showed equal improvements from both medications on the Clinical Global Impression Scale, the Conners teacher and parent rating scales, and the Continuous Performance Test, as well as ratings of anxiety and depression. The study showed an order effect that suggested a carryover from one drug condition to the next. Also, subjects were not assigned to receive placebo in the crossover, so the study was not placebo controlled. A multisite, double-blind, placebo-controlled trial of bupropion revealed that teachers could detect a reduction of ADHD symptoms at a significant level but that parents could not (Conners et al. 1996). This finding suggests that bupropion is a second-line, off-label agent for ADHD treatment.

Clonidine and Guanfacine

Clonidine is an α_2 presynaptic receptor agonist indicated for adult hypertension. The drug has been touted as a nonstimulant treatment for aggressive children with ADHD. Previously limited by its short half-life, clonidine has been reformulated into extended-release tablets (CLON-XR; Kapvay) that can be dosed once or twice daily. Following two Phase III trials, Kapvay has received FDA approval for the treatment of ADHD in children, when used either alone or in conjunction with a psychostimulant. Jain et al. (2011) conducted an 8-week, placebo-controlled, fixed-dose trial that randomly assigned 238 hyperactive children to receive either placebo, Kapvay 0.2 mg/day, or Kapvay 0.4 mg/day. By week 5, greater reductions in ADHD symptoms were detected in both of the clonidine-treated groups than in the placebo group.

Connor et al. (2000) conducted a pilot study comparing methylphenidate, clonidine, or their combination in 24 children with ADHD and comorbid aggression and either oppositional defiant disorder or conduct disorder. Although all groups showed improvement, the group taking clonidine showed a decrease in fine motor speed. Connor et al. (1999), in reviewing this clonidine study and others in a meta-analysis, concluded that clonidine has a moderate effect size of 0.56 on ADHD symptoms in children and adolescents with comorbid conduct disorder, developmental delay, and tic disorders.

Although Connor et al. (1999) concluded that clonidine may be an effective second-tier treatment for ADHD symptoms, its clinical use is associated with many side effects. Reports coming into the FDA's MedWatch postmarketing surveillance system indicated that 23 children treated simultaneously with clonidine and methylphenidate experienced drug reactions, including heart rate and blood pressure abnormalities. Among that group, four experienced severe adverse events, including death (Swanson et al. 1995a).

Guanfacine, another α_2 presynaptic agonist, has also been reformulated into extended-release tablets (Intuniv). Biederman et al. (2008) completed an 8-week, double-blind, placebo-controlled, fixed-dosage escalation study that randomly assigned 345 children with ADHD to receive either placebo or extended-release guanfacine 2 mg/day, 3 mg/day, or 4 mg/day. ADHD symptom scores were significantly reduced in all of the groups given guanfacine instead of placebo. Many clinicians feel that side effects such as sedation and hypotension are less common in patients taking guanfacine than in those taking clonidine, although head-to-head trials of these medications in hyperactive children are absent. The FDA has granted a new indication for long-duration guanfacine (Intuniv), which allows the medication to be given with a stimulant in cases in which the ADHD does not respond to a stimulant alone. It was proven effective as an add-on medication in a controlled clinical trial (Spencer et al. 2009).

Modafinil

Modafinil is a nonstimulant with no cardiovascular effects that is used for narcolepsy treatment. It also has been used off-label for ADHD treatment. Its mechanism of action has not been determined. Some claim it may inhibit sleep-promoting neurons by blocking norepinephrine uptake ("New Indications for Modafinil [Provigil]" 2004). Modafinil was found to be equivalent to 600 mg of caffeine (approximately six cups of coffee) in maintaining alertness and performance in sleep-deprived healthy adults (Wesensten et al. 2002). A report of Stevens-Johnson syndrome in a child and reports of visual hallucinations emerged from large sponsor-supported registration trials, after which the manufacturer withdrew its application to the FDA for a new indication for use of modafinil in treating ADHD.

Selective Serotonin Reuptake Inhibitors

Selective serotonin reuptake inhibitors (SSRIs) enjoy a reputation for high efficacy and low adverse effects reported in adults with major depressive disorder. Castellanos found no signs of efficacy for SSRIs in the treatment of ADHD in children in the seven studies (68 children) he reviewed (X. Castellanos, unpublished paper, 1996).

Monitoring Treatment

The AACAP practice parameter for ADHD (Pliszka 2007) recommends that during a psychopharmacological intervention for ADHD, the patient should be monitored for treatment-emergent side effects. The effectiveness of regular monthly visits and dosage adjustments based on tolerability and lingering ADHD symptoms was shown in the MTA study (MTA Cooperative Group 1999a). Those subjects assigned the medication management by NIMH protocol had significantly lower ADHD symptom scores than those followed by the providers in the community. When compared, the children in the MTA study had five times the rate of appointments, increased feedback from the teacher to the provider, and higher mean methylphenidate TDDs.

Monitoring can be done through direct visits between patient and provider, by phone calls with the patient and family, or even by e-mail contact. Teacher input should be sought at least once in the fall and once in the spring for patients with ADHD who are attending primary, middle, or high school.

Monitoring should follow a predetermined plan that is worked out with the patient and, if the patient is a child, with the parents. Generally, monitoring visits are scheduled weekly during the initial dosage adjustment phase, then monthly for the first few months of maintenance. After that, the visits can be regularly scheduled but less frequent. During the monitoring visit, the clinician should collect information on the exact dosage used and the schedule according to which the stimulants were administered, including time(s) of day. The clinician should ask about skipped doses. The clinician should raise questions about the common and less common side effects, both acute and long term. The family and clinician should then consider whether the patient should continue taking the stimulant at the same dosage or whether the dosage should be changed. A new prescription should be written and a new appointment scheduled. The patient should leave the visit with a prescription, a plan for administration, possibly a schedule for intervisit phone contact, and the next appointment date.

The practitioner and family should agree on the pattern of stimulant treatment. They may decide on continuous daily administration of stimulant medications or may opt for treatment only on school days, with the patient not taking the drug on weekends and holidays. Those patients with more impairing ADHD symptoms will benefit from treatment with stimulants every day of the year. Patients should have their need for continued treatment with stimulant medication verified once annually through a brief period of medication discontinuation. The discontinuation period should be planned for a part of the school year when testing is not in progress.

A key monitoring component involves developing strategies for maintaining adherence to treatment. These include the option to adjust stimulant dosages to reduce treatment-emergent adverse effects. When a treatment-emergent adverse effect appears, the practitioner would do well to assess the impairment induced. Some adverse effects may not interfere with the child's health or cause significant interruption of routine. If the adverse effect worsens, then dosage reduction is indicated. If the reduction alleviates the adverse effect but leads to worsening of the ADHD symptoms, the clinician may want to consider switching the patient to another stimulant.

The AACAP practice parameter (Pliszka 2007) suggests that adjunctive pharmacotherapy can be used to deal with a troublesome adverse effect during stimulant treatment. Patients with stimulant-induced delay of sleep onset may benefit from antihistamines, clonidine, or a bedtime dose (3 mg) of melatonin (Tjon Pian Gi et al. 2003). Gadow et al. (1999) found that children with ADHD and comorbid tic disorders often show a decrease in tic frequency when they begin taking a stimulant.

Choice of Medication

An international consensus statement (Kutcher et al. 2004), the AACAP practice parameter for ADHD (Pliszka 2007), the Texas Children's Medication Algorithm Project (Pliszka et al. 2006), and the American Academy of Pediatrics (2011) all recommend stimulant medications as the first line of treatment for school-age children with ADHD. The 2011 American Academy of Pediatrics guidelines widen the age of indication down to age 4 and through adolescence. Direct comparisons of methylphenidate and atomoxetine in a double-blind, randomized, multisite trial (Buitelaar et al. 2007; Michelson et al. 2004; Newcorn et al. 2006) have shown a decided benefit for methylphenidate and confirm the meta-analysis by Faraone et al. (2003) suggesting that methylphenidate had a larger effect size (0.91) than atomoxetine (0.62). However, atomoxetine might take precedence if the family has an aversion to stimulants or if the patient has comorbid anxiety or chronic motor tics or is an adolescent or adult with a substance abuse problem.

According to the AACAP practice parameter, treatment should begin with either an amphetamine- or methylphenidate-based stimulant in long-duration formulation. The specific drug chosen can be based on its rapidity of onset, duration of action, and effectiveness for the specific patient in treatment. Short-acting stimulants can be used at first for small children and/or preschoolers if there is no long-acting preparation available in a low enough dose. Dual-pulse methylphenidate and amphetamine products (e.g., Metadate CD, Ritalin LA, Focalin XR) have strong effects in the morning and early afternoon, but the effects wear off by late afternoon. These drugs work best for children with academic problems at the beginning and middle of the school day, for those whose appetite is strongly suppressed, or for those whose sleep onset is delayed during stimulant treatment. Because transdermal stimulants are reported to have a higher-than-average number of adverse effects, orally administered stimulants should be used first. Atomoxetine should be employed only if the family does not want treatment with a controlled substance or if the patient fails full-dose-range trials of both a long-duration methylphenidate and a long-duration amphetamine formulation.

The AACAP practice parameter for ADHD (Pliszka 2007) wisely points out that none of the extant practice guidelines should be interpreted as justification for requiring that a patient experience treatment failure (or adverse effects) with one agent before allowing the trial of another.

Conclusions

In the United States, psychostimulant medications have become a mainstay in the treatment of ADHD primarily based on their proven efficacy during short-term controlled studies. In fact, the majority of children with ADHD will respond to either methylphenidate or dextroamphetamine, so nonresponders are rare (Elia et al. 1991). Although the long-term response of children with ADHD to psychostimulants has not been examined in a controlled study much longer than 24 months (Jacobvitz et al. 1990), anecdotal reports suggest that children relapse when their medication is withdrawn and respond when it is restarted. Optimal treatment involves initial titration to an optimal dosage, followed by regular appointments with a clinician who remains in regular contact with the teacher or school (Greenhill et al. 2001).

The effects of psychostimulants are rapid, dramatic, and normalizing. The risk of long-term side effects remains low, and no substantial impairments have emerged to lessen the remarkable therapeutic benefit-risk ratio of these medications. More expensive and demanding treatments, including behavior modification and cognitive-behavioral therapies, have, at best, only equaled psychostimulant treatment. The combination of behavioral and medication therapies is more effective than medication alone in reducing symptoms associated with ADHD (MTA Cooperative Group 1999b). The NIMH MTA follow-up study has shown that initial random assignment of participants to medication alone, behavioral therapy alone, the combination, or treatment as usual in the community for 14 months produced no differences in outcome after 3 years of follow-up (Molina et al. 2009). Psychostimulant treatment research has flourished, but ample opportunity exists for more studies of nonstimulant medications. Not all patients respond to psychostimulants, particularly those patients with comorbid psychiatric disorders. Another important concern involves the effects of medication on the acquisition of social skills in children with ADHD (Hinshaw 1991). The aim of the new psychopharmacological studies will be to target populations with comorbid disorders (e.g., children with ADHD and comorbid anxiety disorder) and to examine differential responses to new medications in these patients versus those without additional psychiatric diagnoses.

Clinical Pearls

- Screen for ADHD during routine mental health assessments by asking questions about inattention, impulsivity, and hyperactivity, and questioning whether such symptoms cause impairment.
- Begin medication treatment with either an amphetamine or a methylphenidate-based stimulant in a long-duration formulation. Use orally administered stimulants first because transdermal stimulants are reported to have a higher-than-average number of adverse effects.
- Remember that there is no universally agreed-upon method for dosing with stimulants; some practitioners use the dose-by-weight method, and others use the stepwise-titration method.
- Ask about the patient's and family's history of structural heart disease. Be alert if the patient has hypertension or complains of syncope, arrhythmias, or chest pain.
- Measure a child's height and weight at 6-month intervals during treatment and record the results on age-adjusted growth forms. If a decrement is present, reduce the medication's dosage or change to another class of medication.
- Use nonstimulant treatment when a patient has an unsatisfactory response to two different stimulants, or when stimulants cannot be used because of inadequate response, unwanted side effects, or parental preference.
- Remain aware that best treatment practices involve initial titration to optimize dosage, regular appointments to monitor for treatment-emergent side effects, and remaining in regular contact with the teacher or school.

References

Abikoff H, Gittelman R: Hyperactive children treated with stimulants: is cognitive training a useful adjunct? Arch Gen Psychiatry 42:953–961, 1985a

Abikoff H, Gittelman R: The normalizing effects of methylphenidate on the classroom behavior of ADDH children. J Abnorm Child Psychol 13:33–44, 1985b

Abikoff H, Hechtman L, Klein RG, et al: Symptomatic improvement in children with ADHD treated with long-term methylphenidate and multimodal psychosocial treatment. J Am Acad Child Adolesc Psychiatry 43:802–811, 2004

Achenbach TM, Ruffle TM: The Child Behavior Checklist and related forms for assessing behavioral/emotional problems and competencies. Pediatr Rev 21:265–271, 2000

American Academy of Pediatrics, Subcommittee on Attention-Deficit/Hyperactivity Disorder, Steering Committee on Quality Improvement and Management: ADHD: clinical practice guideline for the diagnosis, evaluation, and treatment of attention-deficit/hyperactivity disorder in children and adolescents. Pediatrics 128:2011–2654, 2011

American Psychiatric Association: Diagnostic and Statistical Manual of Mental Disorders, 4th Edition. Washington, DC, American Psychiatric Association, 1994

American Psychiatric Association: Diagnostic and Statistical Manual of Mental Disorders, 4th Edition, Text Revision. Washington, DC, American Psychiatric Association, 2000

American Psychiatric Association, DSM-5 Development: A 06 attention deficit/hyperactivity disorder. Proposed revision. May 1, 2012. Available at: www.dsm5.org/ProposedRevision/Pages/proposedrevision.aspx?rid=383. Accessed May, 10, 2012.

Anderson JC, Williams S, McGee R, et al: DSM-III disorders in preadolescent children: prevalence in a large sample from the general population. Arch Gen Psychiatry 44:69–76, 1987

Angold A, Erkanli A, Egger HL, et al: Stimulant treatment for children: a community perspective. J Am Acad Child Adolesc Psychiatry 39:975–984, 2000

Arnold LE: Methylphenidate vs amphetamine: comparative review. Journal of Attention Disorders 3:200–211, 2000

Arnold LE, Christopher J, Huestis R, et al: Methylphenidate vs. dextroamphetamine vs. caffeine in minimal brain dysfunction: controlled comparison by placebo washout design with Bayes' analysis. Arch Gen Psychiatry 35:463–473, 1978

Atomoxetine (Strattera) for ADHD. Med Lett Drugs Ther 45:11–12, 2003

Barbaresi W, Katusic SK, Colligan RC, et al: How common is attention-deficit/hyperactivity disorder? Incidence in a population-based birth cohort in Rochester, Minn. Arch Pediatr Adolesc Med 156:217–224, 2002

Barkley RA, Cunningham CE: The effects of methylphenidate on the mother-child interactions of hyperactive children. Arch Gen Psychiatry 36:201–208, 1979

Barkley RA, Karlsson J, Strzelecki E, et al: Effects of age and Ritalin dosage on the mother-child interactions of hyperactive children. J Consult Clin Psychol 52:750–758, 1984

Barkley RA, McMurray MB, Edelbrock CS, et al: The response of aggressive and non-aggressive ADHD children to two doses of methylphenidate. J Am Acad Child Adolescent Psychiatry 28:873–881, 1989

Barkley RA, Fischer M, Edelbrock CS, et al: The adolescent outcome of hyperactive children diagnosed by research criteria, I: an 8-year prospective follow-up study. J Am Acad Child Adolesc Psychiatry 29:546–557, 1990

Barkley RA, DuPaul GJ, McMurray MB: Attention deficit disorder with and without hyperactivity: clinical response to three dose levels of methylphenidate. Pediatrics 87:519–531, 1991

Barkley RA, Fischer M, Smallish L, et al: The persistence of attention-deficit/hyperactivity disorder into young adulthood as a function of reporting source and definition of disorder. J Abnorm Psychol 111:279–289, 2002

Barrickman LL, Perry PJ, Allen AJ, et al: Bupropion versus methylphenidate in the treatment of attention-deficit hyperactivity disorder. J Am Acad Child Adolesc Psychiatry 34:649–657, 1995

Bauermeister JJ, Canino G, Bird H: Epidemiology of disruptive behavior disorders. Child Adolesc Psychiatr Clin N Am 3:177–194, 1994

Biederman J, Newcorn J, Sprich S: Comorbidity of attention-deficit/hyperactivity disorder with conduct, depressive, anxiety, and other disorders. Am J Psychiatry 148:564–577, 1991

Biederman J, Faraone S, Milberger S, et al: A prospective 4-year follow-up study of attention-deficit hyperactivity and related disorders. Arch Gen Psychiatry 53:437–446, 1996

Biederman J, Lopez FA, Boellner SW, et al: A randomized, double-blind, placebo-controlled, parallel-group study of SLI381 (Adderall XR) in children with attention-deficit/hyperactivity disorder. Pediatrics 110:258–266, 2002

Biederman J, Boellner SW, Childress A, et al: LD and mixed amphetamine salts extended release in children with ADHD: a double-blind, placebo-controlled, crossover analog classroom study. Bio Psychiatry 62:970–976, 2007a

Biederman J, Krishnan S, Zhang Y, et al: Efficacy and tolerability of lisdexamfetamine dimesylate (NRP-104) in children with ADHD; a phase III, multicenter, randomized, double-blind, forced-dose, parallel group study. Clin Ther 29:450–463, 2007b

Biederman J, Mick EO, Surman C, et al: Comparative efficacy and tolerability of OROS and immediate release formulations of methylphenidate in the treatment of adults with attention-deficit/hyperactivity disorder. BMC Psychiatry 7:49, 2007c

Biederman J, Melmed RD, Patel A, et al: A randomized, double-blind, placebo-controlled study of guanfacine extended release in children and adolescents with attention-deficit/hyperactivity disorder. Pediatrics 121:E73–E84, 2008

Biederman J, Spencer TJ, Monuteaux MC, et al: A naturalistic ten-year prospective study of height and weight in children with attention-deficit hyperactivity disorder grown up: sex and treatment effects. J Pediatr 157:635–640, 2010

Bird HR, Canino G, Rubio-Stipec M, et al: Estimates of the prevalence of childhood maladjustment in a community survey in Puerto Rico: the use of combined measures. Arch Gen Psychiatry 45:1120–1126, 1988

Birmaher B, Greenhill LL, Cooper TB, et al: Sustained release methylphenidate: pharmacokinetic studies in ADHD males. J Am Acad Child Adolesc Psychiatry 28:768–772, 1989

Buitelaar JK, Van der Gaag RJ, Swaab-Barneveld H, et al: Prediction of clinical response to methylphenidate in children with attention-deficit hyperactivity disorder. J Am Acad Child Adolesc Psychiatry 34:1025–1032, 1995

Buitelaar JK, Michelson D, Danckaerts M, et al: A randomized, double-blind study of continuation treatment for attention-deficit/hyperactivity disorder after 1 year. Biol Psychiatry 61:694–699, 2007

Campbell S: Mother-child interaction in reflective, impulsive, and hyperactive children. Dev Psychol 8:341–349, 1973

Casat CD, Pleasants DZ, Schroeder D, et al: Bupropion in children with attention deficit disorder. Psychopharmacol Bull 25:198–201, 1989

Castellanos FX, Giedd JN, Elia J, et al: Controlled stimulant treatment of ADHD and comorbid Tourette's syndrome: effects of stimulant and dose. J Am Acad Child Adolesc Psychiatry 36:589–596, 1997

Clay T, Gualtieri C, Evans P, et al: Clinical and neurophysiological effects of the novel antidepressant bupropion. Psychol Bull 24:143–148, 1988

Collett BR, Ohan JL, Myers KM: Ten-year review of rating scales, V: scales assessing attention-deficit/hyperactivity disorder. J Am Acad Child Adolesc Psychiatry 42:1015–1037, 2003

Connell H, Irvine L, Rodney J: Psychiatric disorder in Queensland primary school children. Aust Paediatr J 18:177–180, 1982

Conners CK, Casat CD, Gualtieri CT, et al: Bupropion hydrochloride in attention deficit disorder with hyperactivity. J Am Acad Child Adolesc Psychiatry 35:1314–1321, 1996

Connor DF, Fletcher KE, Swanson JM: A meta-analysis of clonidine for symptoms of attention-deficit hyperactivity disorder. J Am Acad Child Adolesc Psychiatry 38:1551–1559, 1999

Connor DF, Barkley RA, Davis HT: A pilot study of methylphenidate, clonidine, or the combination in ADHD comorbid with aggressive oppositional defiant or conduct disorder. Clin Pediatr 39:15–25, 2000

Cooper WO, Habel LA, Sox CM, et al: ADHD drugs and serious cardiovascular events in children and young adults. N Engl J Med 365:1896–1904, 2011

Copeland W, Shanahan L, Costello E, et al: Cumulative prevalence of psychiatric disorders by young adulthood: a prospective cohort study analysis from the Great Smoky Mountains Study. J Am Acad Child Adolesc Psychiatry 50:252–261, 2011

Costello EJ: Child psychiatric disorders and their correlates: a primary care pediatric sample. J Am Acad Child Adolesc Psychiatry 28:851–855, 1989

Costello EJ, Mustillo S, Erkanli A, et al: Prevalence and development of psychiatric disorders in childhood and adolescence. Arch Gen Psychiatry 60:837–844, 2003

Cox DJ, Merkel RL, Penberthy JK, et al: Impact of methylphenidate delivery profiles on driving performance of adolescents with attention-deficit/hyperactivity disorder: a pilot study. J Am Acad Child Adolesc Psychiatry 43:269–275, 2004

Douglas VI, Barr RG, Amin K, et al: Dosage effects and individual responsivity to methylphenidate in attention deficit disorder. J Child Psychol Psychiatry 29:453–475, 1988

Douglas VI, Barr RG, Desilets J, et al: Do high doses of stimulants impair flexible thinking in attention-deficit hyperactivity disorder? J Am Acad Child Adolesc Psychiatry 34:877–885, 1995

Dulcan M: Using psychostimulants to treat behavior disorders of children and adolescents. J Child Adolesc Psychopharmacol 1:7–20, 1990

DuPaul GJ, Barkley RA: Medication therapy, in Attention-Deficit Hyperactivity Disorder: A Handbook for Diagnosis and Treatment, 2nd Edition. Edited by Barkley RA. New York, Guilford, 1990, pp 573–612

DuPaul GJ, Rapport MD: Does methylphenidate normalize the classroom performance of children with attention deficit disorder? J Am Acad Child Adolesc Psychiatry 32:190–198, 1993

DuPaul GJ, Barkley RA, McMurray MB: Response of children with ADHD to methylphenidate: interaction with internalizing symptoms. J Am Acad Child Adolesc Psychiatry 33:894–903, 1994

Elia J, Borcherding BG, Rapoport JL, et al: Methylphenidate and dextroamphetamine treatments of hyperactivity: are there true nonresponders? Psychiatry Res 36:141–155, 1991

Ernst M, Zametkin A: The interface of genetics, neuroimaging, and neurochemistry in attention-deficit hyperactivity disorder, in Psychopharmacology: The Fourth Generation of Progress, 4th Edition. Edited by Bloom F, Kupfer D. New York, Raven, 1995, pp 1643–1652

Esser G, Schmidt M, Woerner W: Epidemiology and course of psychiatric disorders in school-age children: results of a longitudinal study. J Child Psychol Psychiatry 31:243–253, 1996

Faraone SV, Spencer TJ, Aleardi M, et al: Comparing the efficacy of medications used for ADHD using meta-analysis. Presentation at the 156th annual meeting of the American Psychiatric Association, San Francisco, CA, May 17–22, 2003

Faraone SV, Spencer T, Aleardi M, et al: Meta-analysis of the efficacy of methylphenidate for treating adult attention-deficit/hyperactivity disorder. J Clin Psychopharmacol 24:24–29, 2004

Faraone SV, Biederman J, Morley CP, et al: Effect of stimulants on height and weight: a review of the literature. J Am Acad Child Adolesc Psychiatry 47:994–1009, 2008

Gadow KD: Effects of stimulant drugs on academic performance in hyperactive and learning disabled children. J Learn Disabil 16:290–299, 1983

Gadow KD, Sverd J, Sprafkin J, et al: Efficacy of methylphenidate for attention-deficit hyperactivity disorder in children with tic disorder. Arch Gen Psychiatry 52:444–455, 1995

Gadow KD, Sverd J, Sprafkin, J, et al: Long-term methylphenidate therapy in children with comorbid attention-deficit hyperactivity disorder and chronic multiple tic disorder. Arch Gen Psychiatry 56:330–336, 1999

Gillberg C, Melander H, von Knorring AL, et al: Long-term stimulant treatment of children with attention-deficit hyperactivity disorder symptoms: a randomized, double-blind, placebo-controlled trial. Arch Gen Psychiatry 54:857–864, 1997

Gittelman R, Kanner A: Psychopharmacotherapy, in Psychopathological Disorders of Childhood, 3rd Edition. Edited by Quay H, Werry J. New York, Wiley, 1986, pp 455–495

Gittelman R, Mannuzza S: Hyperactive boys almost grown up: methylphenidate effects on ultimate height. Arch Gen Psychiatry 45:1131–1134, 1988

Gittelman-Klein R, Landa B, Mattes JA, et al: Methylphenidate and growth in hyperactive children. Arch Gen Psychiatry 45:1127–1130, 1988

Goldman L, Genel M, Bazman R, et al: Diagnosis and treatment of attention-deficit/ hyperactivity disorder. JAMA 279:1100–1107, 1998

Greenhill LL: Stimulant-relation growth inhibition in children: a review, in Strategic Interventions for Hyperactive Children. Edited by Gittelman M. Armonk, NY, ME Sharpe, 1981, pp 39–63

Greenhill LL: Stimulant related growth inhibition in children: a review, in The Psychobiology of Childhood. Edited by Shopsin B. New York, SP Medical and Scientific Books, 1984, pp 135–157

Greenhill LL: Preschool ADHD Treatment Study (PATS): science and controversy. The Economics of Neuroscience 3:49–53, 2001

Greenhill LL, Puig-Antich J, Chambers W, et al: Growth hormone, prolactin, and growth responses in hyperkinetic males treated with D-amphetamine. J Am Acad Child Adolesc Psychiatry 20:84–103, 1981

Greenhill LL, Puig-Antich J, Novacenko H, et al: Prolactin, growth hormone and growth responses in boys with attention deficit disorder and hyperactivity treated with methylphenidate. J Am Acad Child Adolesc Psychiatry 23:58–67, 1984

Greenhill LL, Abikoff HB, Arnold LE, et al: Medication treatment strategies in the MTA study: relevance to clinicians and researchers. J Am Acad Child Adolesc Psychiatry 35:1304–1313, 1996

Greenhill LL, Swanson JM, Vitiello B, et al: Impairment and deportment responses to different methylphenidate doses in children with ADHD: the MTA titration trial. J Am Acad Child Adolesc Psychiatry 40:180–187, 2001

Greenhill LL, Findling RL, Swanson JM: A double-blind, placebo-controlled study of modified-release methylphenidate in children with attention-deficit/hyperactivity disorder. Pediatrics 109:E39, 2002a

Greenhill LL, Pliszka S, Dulcan MK, et al: American Academy of Child and Adolescent Psychiatry: practice parameter for the use of stimulant medications in the treatment of children, adolescents, and adults. J Am Acad Child Adolesc Psychiatry 41(suppl):26S–49S, 2002b

Greenhill LL, Biederman J, Boellner SW, et al: A randomized, double-blind, placebo-controlled study of modafinil film-coated tablets in children and adolescents with attention-deficit/hyperactivity disorder. J Am Acad Child Adolesc Psychiatry 45:503–511, 2006a

Greenhill LL, Kollins S, Abikoff H, et al: Efficacy and safety of immediate-release methylphenidate treatment for preschoolers with ADHD. J Am Acad Child Adolesc Psychiatry 45:1284–1293, 2006b

Greenhill LL, Muniz R, Ball RR, et al: Efficacy and safety of dexmethylphenidate extended-release capsules in children with attention-deficit/hyperactivity disorder. J Am Acad Child Adolesc Psychiatry 45:817–823, 2006c

Halperin JM, Matier K, Bedi G, et al: Specificity of inattention, impulsivity, and hyperactivity to the diagnosis of attention-deficit hyperactivity disorder. J Am Acad Child Adolesc Psychiatry 31:190–196, 1992

Hanwella R, Senanayake M, de Silva V: Comparative efficacy and acceptability of methylphenidate and atomoxetine in treatment of attention deficit hyperactivity disorder in children and adolescents: a meta-analysis. BMC Psychiatry 11:176, 2011

Harris G: F.D.A. finds short supply of attention deficit drugs. The New York Times, January 1, 2012, pp A1, A17

Hechtman L, Weiss G, Perlman T: Hyperactives as young adults: past and current substance abuse and antisocial behavior. Am J Orthopsychiatry 54:415–425, 1984

Hinshaw S: Effects of methylphenidate on aggressive and antisocial behavior. Proceedings of the American Academy of Child and Adolescent Psychiatry 7:31–32, 1991

Hinshaw S, Heller T, McHale JP: Covert antisocial behavior in boys with attention-deficit hyperactivity disorder: external validation and effects of methylphenidate. J Consult Clin Psychol 60:274–281, 1992

Horn WF, Ialongo NS, Pascoe JM, et al: Additive effects of psychostimulants, parent training, and self-control therapy with ADHD children. J Am Acad Child Adolesc Psychiatry 30:233–240, 1991

Humphries T, Kinsbourne M, Swanson J: Stimulant effects on cooperation and social interaction between hyperactive children and their mothers. J Child Psychol Psychiatry 19:13–22, 1978

Ickowicz A, Tannock R, Fulford P, et al: Transient tics and compulsive behaviors following methylphenidate: evidence from a placebo controlled double blind clinical trial. Presented at the 39th Annual Meeting of the American Academy of Child and Adolescent Psychiatry, Washington, DC, October 1992

Jacobson NS, Truax P: Clinical significance: a statistical approach to defining meaningful change in psychotherapy research. J Consult Clin Psychol 59:12–19, 1991

Jacobvitz D, Sroufe LA, Stewart M, et al: Treatment of attentional and hyperactivity problems in children with sympathomimetic drugs: a comprehensive review. J Am Acad Child Adolesc Psychiatry 29:677–688, 1990

Jain R, Segal S, Kollins SH, et al: Clonidine extended-release tables for pediatric patients with attention-deficit/hyperactivity disorder. J Am Acad Child Adolesc Psychiatry 50:171–179, 2011

Jasinski DR, Krishnan S: Abuse liability and safety of oral lisdexamfetamine dimesylate in individuals with a history of stimulant abuse. J Psychopharmacol 23:419–427, 2009

Jensen PS, Kettle L, Roper MT, et al: Are stimulants overprescribed? Treatment of ADHD in four U.S. communities. J Am Acad Child Adolesc Psychiatry 38:797–804, 1999

Kavale K: The efficacy of stimulant drug treatment for hyperactivity: a meta-analysis. J Learn Disabil 15:280–289, 1982

Keating GM, Figgitt DP: Dexmethylphenidate. Drugs 62:1899–1904, 2002

Keiling C, Keiling RR, Frick PJ, et al: The age at onset of ADHD. Am J Psychiatry 167:14–15, 2010

Kessler R, Adler L, Barkley R, et al: The prevalence and correlates of adult ADHD in the United States: results from the National Comorbidity Survey Replication. Am J Psychiatry 4:716–723, 2006

Klein RG: The role of methylphenidate in psychiatry. Arch Gen Psychiatry 52:429–433, 1995

Klein RG, Abikoff H, Klass E, et al: Clinical efficacy of methylphenidate in conduct disorder with and without attention deficit hyperactivity disorder. Arch Gen Psychiatry 54:1073–1080, 1997

Klorman R, Brumaghim JT, Fitzpatrick PA, et al: Clinical effects of a controlled trial of methylphenidate on adolescents with attention deficit disorder. J Am Acad Child Adolesc Psychiatry 29:702–709, 1990

Kollins SH, Jain R, Brams M, et al: Clonidine extended-release tablets as add-on therapy to psychostimulants in children and adolescents with ADHD. Pediatrics 127:E1406–E1413, 2011

Kupfer DJ, Baltimore RS, Berry DA, et al: National Institutes of Health Consensus Development Conference Statement: diagnosis and treatment of attention-deficit/hyperactivity disorder (ADHD). J Am Acad Child Adolesc Psychiatry 39:182–193, 2000

Kutcher S, Aman M, Brooks SJ, et al: International consensus statement on attention-deficit/hyperactivity disorder (ADHD) and disruptive behaviour disorders (DBDs): clinical implications and treatment practice suggestions. Eur Neuropsychopharmacol 14:11–28, 2004

Lahey BB, Willcutt EG: Predictive validity of a continuous alternative to nominal subtypes of attention-deficit/hyperactivity disorder for DSM-V. J Clin Child Adolesc Psychol 39:761–775, 2010

LeFever GB, Dawson KV, Morrow AL: The extent of drug therapy for attention deficit-hyperactivity disorder among children in public schools. Am J Public Health 89:1359–1364, 1999

Liberthson RR: Current concepts: sudden death from cardiac causes in children and young adults. N Engl J Med 334:1039–1044, 1996

Mannuzza S, Klein RG, Bessler A, et al: Adult outcome of hyperactive boys: educational achievement, occupational rank, and psychiatric status. Arch Gen Psychiatry 50:565–576, 1993

March J, Conners CK, Erhardt D, et al: Pharmacotherapy of attention-deficit hyperactivity disorder. Ann Drug Ther 2:187–213, 1994

Matochik JA, Nordahl TE, Gross M, et al: Effects of acute stimulant medication on cerebral metabolism in adults with hyperactivity. Neuropsychopharmacology 8:377–386, 1993

Matochik JA, Liebenauer LL, King AC, et al: Cerebral glucose metabolism in adults with attention deficit hyperactivity disorder after chronic stimulant treatment. Am J Psychiatry 151:658–664, 1994

Mattison DR, Plant TM, Lin HM, et al: Pubertal delay in male nonhuman primates (Macaca mulatta) treated with methylphenidate. Proc Natl Acad Sci USA 108:16301–16306, 2011

McCracken JT: A two-part model of stimulant action on attention-deficit hyperactivity disorder in children. J Neuropsychiatry Clin Neurosci 3:201–209, 1991

McCracken JT, Biederman J, Greenhill LL, et al: Analog classroom assessment of a once-daily mixed amphetamine formulation, SLI381 (Adderall XR), in children with ADHD. J Am Acad Child Adolesc Psychiatry 42:673–683, 2003

McGough JJ, Wigal SB, Abikoff H, et al: A randomized, double-blind, placebo-controlled, laboratory classroom assessment of methylphenidate transdermal system in children with ADHD. J Atten Disord 9:476–485, 2006

Merikangas KR, He J, Burstein M, et al: Lifetime prevalence of mental disorders in U.S. adolescents: results from the National Comorbidity Survey Replication—Adolescent Supplement (NCS-A). J Am Acad Child Adolesc Psychiatry 49:980–989, 2010

Michelson D: Results from a double-blind study of atomoxetine, OROS methylphenidate, and placebo. Presented at the 51st Annual Meeting of the American Academy of Child and Adolescent Psychiatry, Washington, DC, October 2004

Michelson D, Faries D, Wernicke J, et al: Atomoxetine in the treatment of children and adolescents with attention-deficit/hyperactivity disorder: a randomized, placebo-controlled, dose-response study. Pediatrics 108:E83, 2001

Michelson D, Allen AJ, Busner J, et al: Once-daily atomoxetine treatment for children and adolescents with attention deficit hyperactivity disorder: a randomized, placebo-controlled study. Am J Psychiatry 159:1896–1901, 2002

Michelson D, Adler L, Spencer T, et al: Atomoxetine in adults with ADHD: two randomized, placebo-controlled studies. Biol Psychiatry 53:112–120, 2003

Michelson D, Buitelaar JK, Danckaerts M, et al: Relapse prevention in pediatric patients with ADHD treated with atomoxetine: a randomized, double-blind, placebo-controlled study. J Am Acad Child Adolesc Psychiatry 43:896–904, 2004

Mickel T, Krishnan S, Bisho B, et al: Abuse-resistant amphetamine compounds. U.S. Patent US7 105486. September 12, 2006. Available at: www.google.com/patents/US20050054561. Accessed May 10, 2012.

Milich R, Licht BG, Murphy DA, et al: Attention-deficit hyperactivity disordered boys' evaluations of and attributions for task performance on medication versus placebo. J Abnorm Psychol 98:280–284, 1989

Modi NB, Wang B, Noveck RJ, et al: Dose-proportional and stereospecific pharmacokinetics of methylphenidate delivered using an osmotic, controlled-release oral delivery system. J Clin Pharmacol 40:1141–1149, 2000

Molina BS, Hinshaw SP, Swanson JM, et al: The MTA at 8 years: prospective follow-up of children treated for combined-type ADHD in a multisite study. J Am Acad Child Adolesc Psychiatry 48:484–500, 2009

MTA Cooperative Group: A 14-month randomized clinical trial of treatment strategies for attention-deficit/hyperactivity disorder. The MTA Cooperative Group. Multimodal Treatment Study of Children With ADHD. Arch Gen Psychiatry 56:1073–1086, 1999a

MTA Cooperative Group: Moderators and mediators of treatment response for children with attention-deficit/hyperactivity disorders. Arch Gen Psychiatry 56:1088–1096, 1999b

MTA Cooperative Group: National Institute of Mental Health Multimodal Treatment Study of ADHD follow-up: changes in effectiveness and growth after the end of treatment 37. Pediatrics 113:762–769, 2004

Musten LM, Firestone P, Pisterman S, et al: Effects of methylphenidate on preschool children with ADHD: cognitive and behavioral functions. J Am Acad Child Adolesc Psychiatry 36:1407–1415, 1997

New indications for modafinil (Provigil). Med Lett Drugs Ther 46:34–35, 2004

Newcorn J, Michelson D, Kratochvil C, et al: Low-dose atomoxetine for maintenance treatment of attention-deficit/hyperactivity disorder. Pediatrics 118:E1701–E1706, 2006

Newcorn J, Kratochvil CJ, Allen AJ, et al: Atomoxetine and osmotically released methylphenidate for the treatment of attention-deficit/hyperactivity disorder: acute comparison and differential response. Am J Psychiatry 165:721–730, 2008

Olson M, Huang C, Gerhard T, et al: Stimulants and vascular events in youth with attention-deficit/hyperactivity disorder. J Am Acad Child Adolesc Psychiatry 51:147–156, 2012

Ottenbacher KJ, Cooper HM: Drug treatment of hyperactivity in children. Dev Med Child Neurol 25:358–366, 1983

Parens E, Johnston J: Facts, values, and attention-deficit hyperactivity disorder (ADHD): an update on the controversies. Child Adolesc Psychiatry Ment Health 3:1, 2009

Pastor PN, Reuben CA: Diagnosed attention deficit hyperactivity disorder and learning disability: United States, 2004–2006. Vital Health Statistics, series 10, no 237. July 2008. Available at: www.cdc.gov/nchs/data/series/sr_10/Sr10_237.pdf. Accessed May 10, 2012.

Pelham W, Bender ME: Peer relationships in hyperactive children: description and treatment, in Advances in Learning and Behavioral Disabilities. Edited by Gadow KD, Bialer I. Greenwich, CT, JAI Press, 1982, pp 365–436

Pelham WE, Milich R: Individual differences in response to Ritalin in classwork and social behavior, in Ritalin: Theory and Patient Management. Edited by Greenhill LL, Osman B. New York, Mary Ann Liebert, 1991, pp 203–222

Pelham WE, Greenslade KE, Vodde-Hamilton M, et al: Relative efficacy of long-acting stimulants on children with attention deficit-hyperactivity disorder: comparison of standard methylphenidate, sustained-release methylphenidate, sustained-release dextroamphetamine, and pemoline. Pediatrics 86:226–237, 1990

Pelham WE, Swanson JM, Furman MB, et al: Pemoline effects on children with ADHD: a time-response by dose-response analysis on classroom measures. J Am Acad Child Adolesc Psychiatry 34:1504–1513, 1995

Pelham WE, Aronoff HR, Midlam JK, et al: A comparison of Ritalin and Adderall: efficacy and time-course in children with attention-deficit/hyperactivity disorder. Pediatrics 103:E43, 1999

Peterson BS, Potenza MN, Zang Z, et al: An fMRI study of the effects of psychostimulants on default-mode processing during Stroop task performance in youths with ADHD. Am J Psychiatry 166:1286–1294, 2009

Pliszka SR: Effect of anxiety on cognition, behavior, and stimulant response in ADHD. J Am Acad Child Adolesc Psychiatry 28:882–887, 1989

Pliszka SR; AACAP Work Group on Quality Issues: Practice parameter for the assessment and treatment of attention-deficit/hyperactivity disorder. J Am Acad Child Adolesc Psychiatry 46:894–921, 2007

Pliszka SR, Greenhill LL, Crismon ML, et al: The Texas Children's Medication Algorithm Project: report of the Texas Consensus Conference Panel on Medication Treatment of Childhood Attention-Deficit/Hyperactivity Disorder, part II: tactics. Attention-deficit/hyperactivity disorder. J Am Acad Child Adolesc Psychiatry 39:920–927, 2000

Pliszka SR, Crismon ML, Hughes CW, et al: The Texas Children's Medication Algorithm Project: revision of the algorithm for pharmacotherapy of attention-deficit/hyperactivity disorder. J Am Acad Child Adolesc Psychiatry 45:642–657, 2006

Polanczyk G, de Lima MS, Horta BL, et al: The worldwide prevalence of ADHD: a systematic review and metaregression analysis. Am J Psychiatry 164:942–948, 2007

Posner J, Maia TV, Fair D, et al: The attenuation of dysfunctional emotional processing with stimulant medication: an fMRI study of adolescents with ADHD. Psychiatry Res 30:151–160, 2011a

Posner J, Nagel BJ, Maia TV, et al: Abnormal amygdalar activation and connectivity in adolescents with attention-deficit/hyperactivity disorder. J Am Acad Child Adolesc Psychiatry 50:838–837, 2011b

Quinn D, Wigal S, Swanson J, et al: Comparative pharmacodynamics and plasma concentrations of d-threo-methylphenidate hydrochloride after single doses of d-threo-methylphenidate hydrochloride and d,l-threo-methylphenidate hydrochloride in a double-blind, placebo-controlled, crossover laboratory school study in children with attention-deficit/hyperactivity disorder. J Am Acad Child Adolesc Psychiatry 43:1422–1429, 2004

Rapport MD, Stoner G, DuPaul GJ, et al: Attention deficit disorder and methylphenidate: a multilevel analysis of dose-response effects on children's impulsivity across settings. J Am Acad Child Adolesc Psychiatry 27:60–69, 1988

Rapport MD, DuPaul GJ, Kelly KL: Attention deficit hyperactivity disorder and methylphenidate: the relationship between gross body weight and drug response in children. Psychopharmacol Bull 25:285–290, 1989

Rapport MD, Denney C, DuPaul GJ, et al: Attention deficit disorder and methylphenidate: normalization rates, clinical effectiveness, and response prediction in 76 children. J Am Acad Child Adolesc Psychiatry 33:882–893, 1994

Richters JE, Arnold LE, Jensen PS, et al: NIMH collaborative multisite Multimodal Treatment Study of Children with ADHD: background and rationale. J Am Acad Child Adolesc Psychiatry 34:987–1000, 1995

Roche AF, Lipman RS, Overall JE, et al: The effects of stimulant medication on the growth of hyperactive children. Pediatrics 63:847–849, 1979

Safer DJ, Allen RP: Factors influencing the suppressant effects of two stimulant drugs on the growth of hyperactive children. Pediatrics 51:660–667, 1973

Safer D, Allen R, Barr E: Depression of growth in hyperactive children on stimulant drugs. N Engl J Med 287:217–220, 1972

Safer DJ, Allen RP, Barr E: Growth rebound after termination of stimulant drugs. J Pediatr 86:113–116, 1975

Safer DJ, Zito JM, Fine EM: Increased methylphenidate usage for attention deficit disorder in the 1990s. Pediatrics 98:1084–1088, 1996

Satterfield JH, Cantwell DP, Schell A, et al: Growth of hyperactive children treated with methylphenidate. Arch Gen Psychiatry 36:212–217, 1979

Schachar RJ, Tannock R: Childhood hyperactivity and psychostimulants: a review of extended treatment studies. J Child Adolesc Psychopharmacol 3:81–97, 1993

Schachar RJ, Tannock R, Cunningham C, et al: Behavioral, situational, and temporal effects of treatment of ADHD with methylphenidate. J Am Acad Child Adolesc Psychiatry 36:754–763, 1997

Schachter HM, Pham B, King J, et al: How efficacious and safe is short-acting methylphenidate for the treatment of attention-deficit disorder in children and adolescents? A meta-analysis. Can Med Assoc J 165:1475–1488, 2001

Simeon JG, Ferguson HB, Van Wyck FJ: Bupropion effects in attention deficit and conduct disorders. Can J Psychiatry 31:581–585, 1986

Solanto MV: Neuropharmacological basis of stimulant drug action in attention deficit disorder with hyperactivity: a review and synthesis. Psychol Bull 95:387–409, 1984

Spencer T, Wilens T, Biederman J, et al: A double-blind, crossover comparison of methylphenidate and placebo in adults with childhood-onset attention-deficit hyperactivity disorder. Arch Gen Psychiatry 52:434–443, 1995

Spencer TJ, Biederman J, Harding M, et al: Growth deficits in ADHD children revisited: evidence for disorder-associated growth delays? J Am Acad Child Adolesc Psychiatry 35:1460–1469, 1996

Spencer TJ, Adler LA, McGough JJ, et al: Efficacy and safety of dexmethylphenidate extended-release capsules in adults with attention-deficit/hyperactivity disorder. Biol Psychiatry 61:1380–1387, 2007a

Spencer TJ, Kratochvil CJ, Sangal RB, et al: Effects of atomoxetine on growth in children with attention-deficit hyperactivity disorder following up to five years of treatment. J Child Adolesc Psychopharmacology 17:689–700, 2007b

Spencer TJ, Greenbaum M, Ginsberg LD, et al: Safety and effectiveness of coadministration of guanfacine extended release and psychostimulants in children and adolescents with attention-deficit/hyperactivity disorder. J Child Adolesc Psychopharmacol 19:501–510, 2009

Sprague RL, Sleator EK: Methylphenidate in hyperkinetic children: differences in dose effects on learning and social behavior. Science 198:1274–1276, 1977

Steinhausen HC, Kreuzer EM: Learning in hyperactive children: are there stimulant-related and state-dependent effects? Psychopharmacology (Berl) 74:389–390, 1981

Stephens RS, Pelham WE, Skinner R: State-dependent and main effects of methylphenidate and pemoline on paired-associate learning and spelling in hyperactive children. J Consult Clin Psychol 52:104–113, 1984

Swanson J, Kinsbourne M: Stimulant-related state-dependent learning in hyperactive children. Science 192:1354–1357, 1976

Swanson J, Flockhart D, Udrea D, et al: Clonidine in the treatment of ADHD: questions about the safety and efficacy. J Child Adolesc Psychopharmacol 5:301–305, 1995a

Swanson J, Lerner M, Williams L: More frequent diagnosis of attention deficit-hyperactivity disorder. N Engl J Med 333:944, 1995b

Swanson JM, Wigal S, Greenhill LL, et al: Analog classroom assessment of Adderall in children with ADHD. J Am Acad Child Adolesc Psychiatry 37:519–526, 1998

Swanson JM, Kraemer HC, Hinshaw SP, et al: Clinical relevance of the primary findings of the MTA: success rates based on severity of ADHD and ODD symptoms at the end of treatment. J Am Acad Child Adolesc Psychiatry 40:168–179, 2001

Swanson J, Gupta S, Lam A, et al: Development of a new once-a-day formulation of methylphenidate for the treatment of attention-deficit/hyperactivity disorder: proof-of-concept and proof-of-product studies. Arch Gen Psychiatry 60:204–211, 2003

Swanson J, Wigal SB, Wigal T, et al: A comparison of once-daily extended-release methylphenidate formulations in children with attention-deficit/hyperactivity disorder in the laboratory school (the Comacs Study). Pediatrics 113:E206–E216, 2004

Swanson J, Greenhill L, Wigal T, et al: Effects of stimulant medication on growth rates across 3 years in the MTA Follow-up. J Am Acad Child Adolesc Psychiatry 46:1014–1026, 2007

Szatmari P: The epidemiology of attention-deficit hyperactivity disorders. Child and Adolescent Psychiatric Clinics 1:361–371, 1992

Szatmari P, Offord DR, Boyle MH: Ontario Child Health Study: Prevalence of attention deficit disorder with hyperactivity. J Child Psychol Psychiatry 30:219–230, 1989

Tannock R, Ickowicz A, Schachar R: Differential effects of methylphenidate on working memory in ADHD children with and without comorbid anxiety. J Am Acad Child Adolesc Psychiatry 34:886–896, 1995a

Tannock R, Schachar R, Logan G: Methylphenidate and cognitive flexibility: dissociated dose effects in hyperactive children. J Abnorm Child Psychol 23:235–266, 1995b

Taylor E, Schachar R, Thorley G, et al: Which boys respond to stimulant medication? A controlled trial of methylphenidate in boys with disruptive behaviour. Psychol Med 17:121–143, 1987

Taylor E, Sandberg S, Thorley G, et al: The epidemiology of childhood hyperactivity, in Child Psychiatry. Edited by Taylor E, Rutter M. London, Oxford University Press, 1991, pp 1–122

Thurber S, Walker CE: Medication and hyperactivity: a meta-analysis. J Gen Psychol 108:79–86, 1983

Tjon Pian Gi CV, Broeren JP, Starreveld JS, et al: Melatonin for treatment of sleeping disorders in children with attention deficit/hyperactivity disorder: a preliminary open label study. Eur J Pediatr 162:554–555, 2003

Velez CN, Johnson J, Cohen P: A longitudinal analysis of selected risk factors for childhood psychopathology. J Am Acad Child Adolesc Psychiatry 28:861–864, 1989

Verhulst F, Eussen M, Berden G: Pathways of problem behaviors from childhood to adolescence. J Am Acad Child Adolesc Psychiatry 32:388–392, 1992

Vikan A: Psychiatric epidemiology in a sample of 1510 ten-year-old children, I: prevalence. J Child Psychol Psychiatry 26:55–75, 1985

Visser SN, Lesesne CA: Mental health in the United States: prevalence of diagnosis and medication treatment for attention-deficit/hyperactivity disorder: United States, 2003. MMWR Morb Mortal Wkly Rep 54:842–847, 2006

Vitiello B: Research in child and adolescent psychopharmacology: recent accomplishments and new challenges. Psychopharmacology (Berl) 191:5–13, 2006

Vitiello B, Jensen PS: Developmental perspectives in pediatric psychopharmacology. Psychopharmacol Bull 31:75–81, 1995

Vitiello B, Jensen PS: Medication development and testing in children and adolescents: current problems, future directions. Arch Gen Psychiatry 54:871–876, 1997

Vitiello B, Elliot GR, Swanson JM, et al: Blood pressure and heart rate over 10 years in the multimodal treatment study of ADHD. Am J Psychiatry 169:167–177, 2012

Volkow ND, Ding YS, Fowler JS, et al: Is methylphenidate like cocaine? Studies on their pharmacokinetics and distribution in the human brain. Arch Gen Psychiatry 52:456–463, 1995

Volkow ND, Wang G, Fowler JS, et al: Therapeutic doses of oral methylphenidate significantly increase extracellular dopamine in the human brain. J Neurosci 21(2):RC121, 2001

Vyborova L, Nahunek K, Drtilkova I, et al: Intra-individual comparison of 21-day application of amphetamine and methylphenidate in hyperkinetic children. Act Nerv Super (Praha) 26:268–269, 1984

Weissman DH, Roberts KC, Visscher KM, et al: The neural bases of momentary lapses in attention. Nat Neurosci 9:971–978, 2006

Wesensten NJ, Belenky G, Kautz MA, et al: Maintaining alertness and performance during sleep deprivation: modafinil versus caffeine. Psychopharmacology (Berl) 159:238–247, 2002

Whalen CK, Henker B, Buhrmester D, et al: Does stimulant medication improve the peer status of hyperactive children? J Consult Clin Psychol 57:545–549, 1989

Wigal S, Swanson JM, Feifel D, et al: A double-blind, placebo-controlled trial of dexmethylphenidate hydrochloride and d,l-threo-methylphenidate hydrochloride in children with attention-deficit/hyperactivity disorder. J Am Acad Child Adolesc Psychiatry 43:1406–1414, 2004

Wilens TE, Biederman J: The stimulants. Psychiatr Clin North Am 15:191–222, 1992

Wilens TE, McBurnett K, Bukstein O, et al: Multisite controlled study of OROS methylphenidate in the treatment of adolescents with attention-deficit/hyperactivity disorder. Arch Pediatr Adolesc Med 160:82–90, 2006

Winsberg BG, Press M, Bialer I, et al: Dextroamphetamine and methylphenidate in the treatment of hyperactive-aggressive children. Pediatrics 53:236–241, 1974

Wolraich ML, Greenhill LL, Pelham W, et al: Randomized, controlled trial of OROS methylphenidate once a day in children with attention-deficit/hyperactivity disorder. Pediatrics 108:883–892, 2001

Woodruff TJ, Axelrad DA, Kyle AD, et al: Trends in environmentally related childhood illnesses. Pediatrics 113:1133–1140, 2004

Zametkin AJ, Rapoport JL: Neurobiology of attention deficit disorder with hyperactivity: where have we come in 50 years? J Am Acad Child Adolesc Psychiatry 26:676–686, 1987

Zuvekas S, Vitiello B: Stimulant medication use in children: a 12-year perspective. Am J Psychiatry 169:160–166, 2012

3

Disruptive Behavior Disorders and Aggression

Solomon G. Zaraa, D.O.

Natoshia Raishevich Cunningham, Ph.D.

Elizabeth Pappadopulos, Ph.D.

Peter S. Jensen, M.D.

Disruptive behavior disorders (DBDs)—oppositional defiant disorder (ODD), conduct disorder (CD), and disruptive behavior disorder not otherwise specified (DBD-NOS)—are among the most common and debilitating psychiatric ailments in children and adolescents (Bambauer and Connor 2005; Kazdin 1995). Various amounts of verbal and physical aggression often accompany each of these disorders. Notably, however, symptoms of aggression are often present in children with disorders across the array of DSM psychiatric disorders (American Psychiatric Association 2000), even when such children do not meet diagnostic criteria for a DBD. Given the public health importance of aggression and its salience to impairment, the conceptualization of DBDs and their response to treatment interventions require a comprehensive understanding of aggression, its impact, prevalence, and presentation across the DBD spectrum.

An emerging literature suggests that aggression can be categorized by two discrete subtypes: proactive aggression and reactive aggression (Dodge and Coie 1987). *Proactive aggression* is instrumental or deliberate, and occurs without provocation. *Reactive aggression* is an emotive form of aggression and attributes hostile intent to others. Proactive and reactive forms of aggression have also been described in the medical literature as *controlled-instrumental-predatory aggression* and *impulsive-hostile-affective aggression,* respectively (Vitiello and Stoff 1997).

These two forms of aggression and their relationship to the DBDs remain to be fully understood. This conceptual gap is largely a result of the failure to take aggressive subtypes into account in the assessment and treatment studies of DBDs. Instead, research trials tend to globally target symptoms of physical aggression, as opposed to proactive or reactive aggression, in the treatment of DBDs (Volavka and Citrome 1999). Furthermore, the callous-unemotional subtype of CD is under consideration for inclusion in the upcoming DSM-5 (Frick and Moffitt 2010; Moffitt et al. 2008). Callous-unemotional traits appear to be more highly associated with proactive aggression (Kimonis et al. 2006) and are correlated with poorer long-term outcomes (Fontaine et al. 2011; Pardini and Fite 2010; Pardini and Loeber 2008). Because the medical literature has largely failed to discriminate between proactive and reactive types of aggression, the potential clinical benefits of treatment of different forms of aggression have not yet been fully addressed (Pappadopulos et al. 2006). Some investigators have suggested that different subtypes of aggression may respond better to various forms of intervention (Gillberg and Hellgren 1986; Padhy et al. 2011; Steiner et al. 2011). As we discuss further in this chapter, youth with CD and impulsive aggression may greatly benefit from pharmacotherapy (Connor et al. 2004; Jensen et al. 2007; Steiner et al. 2003; Vitiello and Stoff 1997; Vitiello et al. 1990). However, it is unclear whether the psychopharmacological agents that have been proved efficacious in the treatment of CD actually ameliorate symptoms of proactive aggression (Jensen et al. 2007). Therefore, future randomized controlled trials (RCTs) may benefit from including a reliable measure of aggression that distinguishes between the aggressive subtypes (Brown et al. 1996), which may be used to help further refine treatment decisions. In this review, we address what is currently known about the treatment of DBDs and aggression and note where aggression has or has not been explicitly studied as a part of these conditions.

Epidemiology

Oppositional Defiant Disorder and Aggression

ODD is defined as a consistent pattern of defiance, disobedience, and hostility toward various authority figures and adults and persists for at least 6 months (Table 3–1) (American Psychiatric Association 2000). To meet diagnostic criteria for ODD, the youth must exhibit at least four of the following behaviors: losing his or her temper, arguing with adults, refusing to comply with authority figures, deliberately doing things to annoy other people, blaming others for his or her mistakes or behavior, being easily annoyed by others, being angry or resentful, and being spiteful or vindictive. For the individual to qualify for a diagnosis of ODD, the presenting behaviors must occur more frequently than is developmentally appropriate and must lead to a significant impairment in functioning. Approximately 2%–16% of children in the United States meet the criteria for ODD (American Psychiatric Association 2000).

Of note, ODD is only marginally predictive of proactive aggression (Lahey et al. 1998). This relationship, to the extent it is present, may be related to the diagnostic criteria of ODD that specify *spiteful* behaviors and *deliberate* attempts to annoy other people (American Psychiatric Association 2000). On the other hand, there may be numerous features of the disorder that may be indicative of verbal forms of reactive aggression, such as losing one's temper, being easily annoyed by others, arguing with adults, and being angry or resentful. Perhaps the relationship between aggressive subtypes and ODD diagnostic criteria suggests that there may be as-yet-undefined ODD subtypes, one of which may be a marker or precursor to more explicit, impulsive aggressive behaviors, whereas one or more other types might be related to more willful oppositional behaviors. This possibility should be explored in future research.

Table 3–1.   DSM-IV-TR diagnostic criteria for oppositional defiant disorder

A.   A pattern of negativistic, hostile, and defiant behavior lasting at least 6 months, during which four (or more) of the following are present:

(1)   often loses temper

(2)   often argues with adults

(3)   often actively defies or refuses to comply with adults' requests or rules

(4)   often deliberately annoys people

(5)   often blames others for his or her mistakes or misbehavior

(6)   is often touchy or easily annoyed by others

(7)   is often angry and resentful

(8)   is often spiteful or vindictive

Note: Consider a criterion met only if the behavior occurs more frequently than is typically observed in individuals of comparable age and developmental level.

B.   The disturbance in behavior causes clinically significant impairment in social, academic, or occupational functioning.

C.   The behaviors do not occur exclusively during the course of a psychotic or mood disorder.

D.   Criteria are not met for conduct disorder, and, if the individual is age 18 years or older, criteria are not met for antisocial personality disorder.

Source.   Reprinted from *Diagnostic and Statistical Manual of Mental Disorders,* 4th Edition, Text Revision. Washington, DC, American Psychiatric Association, 2000. Copyright © 2000 American Psychiatric Association. Used with permission.

Conduct Disorder

CD occurs in 6%–16% of males and 2%–9% of females (American Psychiatric Association 2000). CD is defined as a persistent pattern of maladaptive behavior in which the rights of others and/or societal norms are violated (Table 3–2) (American Psychiatric Association 2000). These behaviors fall into four main categories: aggressive behavior toward people and animals, destruction of property, deceitfulness or theft, and serious violations of societal norms or rules. As with ODD, it is possible that the features of this behavior disorder may correspond either to impulsive aggression or to proactive aggressive behaviors. Although some evidence suggests that proactive aggression, rather than reactive aggression, is a significant predictor of CD (Fite et al. 2009; Pardini and Fite 2010; Vitaro et al. 1998), this is an area in need of further study. In addition, compared with adolescent-onset CD, childhood-onset CD appears to be more associated with severe antisocial behaviors (Moffitt et al. 2008). Other features of CD, such as truancy and theft, may indicate quite a different clinical course, but these issues also remain in need of further study.

Differential Diagnosis

When a youth meets some but not all of the criteria for either ODD or CD and experiences significant impairment, a diagnosis of DBD-NOS may be appropriate (Table 3–3) (American Psychiatric Association 2000).

As noted earlier, aggression is relatively common across an array of psychiatric disorders, including major depression, bipolar disorder, attention-deficit/hyperactivity disorder (ADHD), posttraumatic stress disorder, and psychosis (Jensen et al. 2007). Aggression is also notable among youth with a primary diagnosis within the autism spectrum disorders. Thus, the high co-occurrence of aggression with other mental disorders appears to have important implications in the management and treatment of a broad range of mental disorders, not only the DBDs, in youth (Pappadopulos et al. 2003).

Course and Outcome

The occurrence of a DBD and/or aggressive behaviors in youth may lead to the subsequent development of other mental disorders. For example, a diagnosis of ODD may precede a diagnosis of CD. Loeber et al. (1993) found that youth who were diagnosed with ODD had a 43% chance of eventually developing CD. However, the emergence of CD does not necessarily mitigate or supersede a diagnosis of ODD; in fact, it is more common for ODD symptoms to persist even after full CD symptoms emerge.

One of the most serious outcomes of CD and other DBDs is the emergence of antisocial personality disorder. Studies indicate that 70%–90% of youth with CD will also develop antisocial personality disorder in adulthood (Loeber et al. 2002, 2003, 2009).

DSM-IV-TR (American Psychiatric Association 2000) categorizes antisocial personality disorder as a disregard for the rights of others, along with at

Table 3–2.   DSM-IV-TR diagnostic criteria for conduct disorder

A.   A repetitive and persistent pattern of behavior in which the basic rights of others or major age-appropriate societal norms or rules are violated, as manifested by the presence of three (or more) of the following criteria in the past 12 months, with at least one criterion present in the past 6 months:

Aggression to people and animals

(1)   often bullies, threatens, or intimidates others

(2)   often initiates physical fights

(3)   has used a weapon that can cause serious physical harm to others (e.g., a bat, brick, broken bottle, knife, gun)

(4)   has been physically cruel to people

(5)   has been physically cruel to animals

(6)   has stolen while confronting a victim (e.g., mugging, purse snatching, extortion, armed robbery)

(7)   has forced someone into sexual activity

Destruction of property

(8)   has deliberately engaged in fire setting with the intention of causing serious damage

(9)   has deliberately destroyed others' property (other than by fire setting)

Deceitfulness or theft

(10)   has broken into someone else's house, building, or car

(11)   often lies to obtain goods or favors or to avoid obligations (i.e., "cons" others)

(12)   has stolen items of nontrivial value without confronting a victim (e.g., shoplifting, but without breaking and entering; forgery)

Serious violations of rules

(13)   often stays out at night despite parental prohibitions, beginning before age 13 years

(14)   has run away from home overnight at least twice while living in parental or parental surrogate home (or once without returning for a lengthy period)

(15)   is often truant from school, beginning before age 13 years

B.   The disturbance in behavior causes clinically significant impairment in social, academic, or occupational functioning.

C.   If the individual is age 18 years or older, criteria are not met for antisocial personality disorder.

Table 3–2.   DSM-IV-TR diagnostic criteria for conduct disorder *(continued)*

Code based on age at onset:

312.81   **Conduct Disorder, Childhood-Onset Type:**   onset of at least one criterion characteristic of conduct disorder prior to age 10 years

312.82   **Conduct Disorder, Adolescent-Onset Type:**   absence of any criteria characteristic of conduct disorder prior to age 10 years

312.89   **Conduct Disorder, Unspecified Onset:**   age at onset is not known

Specify severity:

Mild: few if any conduct problems in excess of those required to make the diagnosis **and** conduct problems cause only minor harm to others

Moderate: number of conduct problems and effect on others intermediate between "mild" and "severe"

Severe: many conduct problems in excess of those required to make the diagnosis **or** conduct problems cause considerable harm to others

Source.   Reprinted from *Diagnostic and Statistical Manual of Mental Disorders,* 4th Edition, Text Revision. Washington, DC, American Psychiatric Association, 2000. Copyright © 2000 American Psychiatric Association. Used with permission.

Table 3–3.   DSM-IV-TR description of disruptive behavior disorder not otherwise specified

This category is for disorders characterized by conduct or oppositional defiant behaviors that do not meet the criteria for conduct disorder or oppositional defiant disorder. For example, include clinical presentations that do not meet full criteria either for oppositional defiant disorder or conduct disorder, but in which there is clinically significant impairment.

Source.   Reprinted from *Diagnostic and Statistical Manual of Mental Disorders,* 4th Edition, Text Revision. Washington, DC, American Psychiatric Association, 2000. Copyright © 2000 American Psychiatric Association. Used with permission.

least three of the following symptoms: disregard for the safety of oneself or others, failure to adhere to societal norms, impulsivity, irresponsibility, deceitfulness, lack of remorse, and physically aggressive behaviors. Antisocial personality disorder is associated with poor treatment outcomes, including an increased likelihood to commit violent acts or engage in illegal behaviors (Loeber et al. 2002). Thus, antisocial personality disorder, like CD, is linked by its diagnostic criteria to aggression. Proactive aggression, in and of itself, has also been shown to be related to later maladjustment (Dodge 1991) and increased levels of antisocial behaviors (Fite et al. 2009). Furthermore, proactive aggression is associated with callous-unemotional traits, which strongly predict serious and persistent criminal behaviors (Pardini and Fite 2010). Contrariwise, reactive aggression appears not to be associated with antisocial outcomes (Fite et al. 2009). Regardless of the primary psychiatric condition or nature of the aggressive behaviors, they are often accompanied by poor treatment outcome and the need for longer and more intensive treatment (Mannuzza et al. 1993, 1998; Werry 1997).

In general, the prognosis for DBDs is especially poor if the youth fails to respond to behavioral interventions, which are often considered the first line of treatment for behavior disorders and/or symptoms of aggression. Because of the limitations of current psychotherapeutic interventions, however, a growing body of literature has focused on the outcomes of psychopharmacological treatment of aggressive symptoms in youth with DBDs (Connor et al. 1999, 2002; DosReis et al. 2003; Pappadopulos et al. 2003; Schur et al. 2003; Steiner et al. 2003), which is the focus of this chapter.

Rationale and Justification for Psychopharmacological Treatment

As reviewed in subsequent sections of this chapter, psychotropic agents may be beneficial for the treatment of DBDs and/or aggression in youth. However, given the highly overlapping nature of DBDs and the aggressive subtypes with other conditions such as ADHD or bipolar disorder, decisions about which psychopharmacological treatments are appropriate depend on which "underlying" conditions are present. Not surprisingly then, the literature is sometimes unclear about whether psychotropic interventions are targeting a specific DBD or aggressive symptoms that may nor may not be co-occurring with other disorders. Although this distinction is often unclear, current research on the treatment efficacy of varying psychotropic agents does offer evidence and a preliminary framework to determine optimal use of psychopharmacological agents in the treatment of aggression and DBDs in youth.

Issues in Study Design and Interpretation

Treatment efficacy is most rigorously established through RCTs, which are studies in which participants are randomly assigned to differing treatment conditions, including administration of psychopharmacological agents, behavioral interventions, and/or placebo. These conditions are used to compare treatment outcomes among groups.

As RCTs of psychotropic agents continue to emerge, the systematic evaluation of treatment outcomes across all of the studies becomes necessary. One useful and objective technique to compare efficacy across RCTs is through the evaluation of reported *effect sizes* (Pappadopulos et al. 2006). Comparing effect sizes allows for a broadband comparison across studies involving RCTs. Thus, we use effect sizes as a comparative measure in the following review of treatment studies. However, because effect sizes are not necessarily sensitive to other factors, such as treatment duration, side effects, and number of studies or participants, we also review the efficacy of the various agents in terms of the *strength of evidence,* grading the overall strength of evidence of each agent in three hierarchical levels (Jensen et al. 1999; Jobson and Potter 1995; Vitiello and Stoff 1997): *Level A* denotes the highest level of empirical support, as demonstrated by two or more RCTs showing the agent's efficacy; *Level B* constitutes moderate support for a given agent, evidenced by at least one RCT with or without data from open trials and case studies; and *Level C* is assigned to those agents for which evidence is based only on expert opinion, case studies, open-label trials, or data from adult samples. A fourth level, *Level D,* is reserved for instances in which trials have been done but findings have been negative.

In the following sections, we principally review key RCTs, as well as safety information, on the major classes of psychopharmacological agents that have been studied in relation to management of aggression and/or DBDs in youth. These classes include atypical antipsychotics, typical antipsychotics, stimulants, mood stabilizers, α_2 agonists, β-blockers, and norepinephrine reuptake inhibitors. Please note that we do not attempt to review all RCTs for each class of agents; rather, we seek to provide an overview of several key RCTs for each agent. When RCTs are not available, we provide other sources of evidence, such as open-label or uncontrolled trials, to assess the efficacy of a particular class of agents.

Atypical Antipsychotics: Review of Treatment Studies

Risperidone

Risperidone is currently the most extensively studied medication in the treatment of aggression in youth, with RCTs testing short- and long-term benefits of this agent in behaviorally disordered and/or aggressive youth. These studies include larger-scale, multisite trials and small-scale RCTs.

Short-Term Efficacy

Two industry-sponsored, multisite RCTs were conducted in parallel to test the efficacy of risperidone in the treatment of aggressive symptoms and/or DBDs in youth with low-normal or subaverage intelligence. The first RCT evaluated 118 children (ages 5–12) with subaverage intelligence and a primary diagnosis of DBD, including ODD, CD, or DBD-NOS (Aman et al. 2002). Compared with subjects receiving placebo, risperidone-treated youth experienced significant reduction in aggressive symptoms as measured by the Conduct Problem subscale of the Nisonger Child Behavior Rating Form (NCBRF), with an effect size of 0.7. The second industry-sponsored study achieved comparable results in an identically designed RCT (Snyder et al. 2002).

Several smaller trials have yielded similar results. For example, Findling et al. (2000) demonstrated significant reductions in aggressive behaviors as measured by the Rating of Aggression Against People and/or Property (RAAPP) scale in a sample of 20 youths with CD (ages 5–15) receiving outpatient treatment. Similar reductions were noted in an RCT that specifically targeted symptoms of severe aggression during a 6-week trial of 38 inpatient adolescents with subaverage intelligence and DBDs (Buitelaar et al. 2001). Their aggressive symptoms were measured by the Clinical Global Impression (CGI) Severity of Illness subscale and the Aberrant Behavior Checklist (ABC). Moreover, during the 2-week washout trial following the 6 weeks of treatment, the risperidone group experienced a statistically significant worsening of aggressive behaviors as measured by the CGI Severity of Illness subscale, the ABC, and the Overt Aggression Scale—Modified (OAS-M).

The efficacy of risperidone in the treatment of aggressive symptoms has also been documented in an 8-week, double-blind RCT of 101 youths with autism (McCracken et al. 2002). Risperidone treatment was associated with significant reductions in aggression as indicated by scores on the ABC and the CGI within 4 weeks of receiving treatment. Moreover, a significant treatment-by-time interaction effect indicated that the risperidone group continued to improve through weeks 4–8, whereas the placebo group deteriorated.

Unfortunately, many of these studies are limited in that they involve atypical samples (e.g., inpatients, subjects with low or subaverage intelligence, subjects with pervasive developmental disorders). Furthermore, the aforementioned risperidone trials were designed to evaluate short-term treatment outcome. As such, these findings may not be generalizable to the treatment of chronic aggression in youth. Similarly, it is less likely that serious adverse effects would occur during the relatively brief course of these studies. Therefore, other studies must document if adverse effects emerge more frequently with long-term use. In spite of these limitations, available data suggest that risperidone appears to be effective in the short-term treatment of aggressive symptoms and/or behavior disorders in youth. For specific dosage information pertaining to the effective use of risperidone in the treatment of aggression in youth, see Table 3–4.

Long-Term and Maintenance Efficacy

In addition to the evidence for short-term efficacy of risperidone for symptoms of aggression and/or DBDs, emerging evidence suggests that risperidone may also be beneficial in the long-term maintenance of treatment gains. In one study of long-term efficacy (Reyes et al. 2006a), 335 youths ages 5–17 who had responded to open-label risperidone treatment over 12 weeks were then blindly and randomly assigned to receive 6 additional months of either a continuation of risperidone or placebo. The NCBRF was used to assess both proactive and reactive aggressive behaviors, On average, longer treatment maintenance periods were documented in the risperidone group. Significant aggressive symptom recurrence occurred after 119 days in 25% of patients in the risperidone group and in 47.1% of patients in the placebo group. Notably, the results indicate that more than half the placebo group did not experience a recurrence of symptoms. Therefore, psychopharmacological discontinuation may be a plausible treatment option for some youth with symptoms of aggression and/or DBD. Reyes et al. (2006a) also reported significant treatment gains in hyperactive, compliant, and adaptive social behaviors in the risperidone group as compared

Table 3–4. Selected agents prescribed for treatment of aggressive youth with disruptive behavior disorders

Class	Generic name	Trade name	Typical dosage
Antipsychotics, atypical	Aripiprazole	Abilify	2.5–15 mg/day
	Clozapine	Clozaril	150–600 mg/day
	Olanzapine	Zyprexa	2.5–20 mg/day
	Quetiapine	Seroquel	100–600 mg/day
	Risperidone	Risperdal	1–4 mg/day
	Ziprasidone	Geodon	40–160 mg/day
Antipsychotics, typical	Haloperidol	Haldol	0.5–10 mg/day
	Thioridazine	Mellaril	25–400 mg/day
Stimulants	Dexmethylphenidate	Focalin, Focalin XR	5–30 mg/day
	Dextroamphetamine	Dexedrine	10–40 mg/day
	Lisdexamfetamine	Vyvanse	20–70 mg/day
	Methylphenidate	Ritalin, Ritalin LA, Ritalin-SR, Metadate, Metadate CD, Metadate ER, Methylin	5–60 mg/day
		Concerta	18–72 mg/day
	Methylphenidate	Daytrana, transdermal	10–30 mg/9 hours
	Mixed amphetamine salts	Adderall, Adderall XR	5–40 mg/day
Mood stabilizers	Carbamazepine	Tegretol	10–20 mg/kg/day[a]
	Lithium, lithium carbonate	Eskalith, Lithobid	10–30 mg/kg/day[b]
	Valproic acid	Depakene, Depakote	15–60 mg/kg/day[c]

Table 3–4.   Selected agents prescribed for treatment of aggressive youth with disruptive behavior disorders *(continued)*

Class	Generic name	Trade name	Typical dosage
Alpha$_2$ agonists	Clonidine	Catapres, Kapvay	0.025–0.4 mg/day
	Guanfacine	Tenex, Intuniv	0.5–4 mg/day
Beta-blockers	Nadolol	Corgard	20–200 mg/day
	Propranolol	Inderal	2–8 mg/kg/day

Note.   See Jensen et al. 2004 and Martin et al. 2003 for additional information.
[a]Carbamazepine doses optimally adjusted based on blood levels, 4–14 µg/L.
[b]Lithium doses optimally adjusted based on blood levels, 0.6–1.1 mEq/L.
[c]Valproic acid doses optimally adjusted based on blood levels 50–125 µg/L.

with the placebo group. After the completion of this yearlong study, an additional 1-year open-label expansion study was conducted involving 48 responders, and maintenance of the original treatment gains was again demonstrated (Reyes et al. 2006b). Overall, these studies suggest that risperidone may be efficacious in the treatment of DBDs and/or aggression in children for a cumulative period of 2 years.

Findings from the studies by Reyes et al. (2006a, 2006b) are also supported by other yearlong, open-label trials assessing the sustained safety and efficacy of risperidone in youth of subaverage intelligence with symptoms of aggression and other disruptive behaviors (Aman et al. 2004; Croonenberghs et al. 2005; Turgay et al. 2002). In general, across these yearlong, open-label, follow-on studies of initial RCTs, youth maintained treatment gains reported in the initial waves of the study (see preceding section on short-term effectiveness of risperidone). Of particular interest within the aggressive subtype literature, there was a highly significant decrease in scores on the secondary outcome measure (the Vineland Adaptive Behavior Scales) used to assess physical aggression and emotional outbursts (Turgay et al. 2002). Therefore, preliminary evidence appears to indicate the utility of risperidone in the treatment of impulsive aggression.

Furthermore, some evidence has documented the efficacy of long-term use of risperidone in aggressive youth who have a primary diagnosis of autism or other pervasive developmental disorders. In the Research Units on Pediatric Psychopharmacology follow-up study (Research Units on Pediatric Psychopharmacology Autism Network 2005), two-thirds of patients maintained behavioral improvements for 6 months following the initial risperidone treatment, after being reassigned to receive either risperidone or placebo. Notably, however, 37.5% of youth who had taken risperidone in the original study did not relapse even while taking placebo in the follow-up study. Similarly, Troost et al. (2005) studied 36 children with autism spectrum disorders (ages 5–17) who had symptoms of severe aggression or self-injurious behavior. These youth were initially placed on an 8-week, open-label trial of risperidone. Those who responded continued treatment for another 16 weeks, and then a double-blind discontinuation ($n=24$) was carried out, consisting of either 3 weeks of tapering and 5 weeks of placebo or continued use of risperidone. Only 25% of patients who continued taking risperidone relapsed, compared with 66.67% of youth who were switched to placebo. Thus, both studies suggest that risperidone was more efficacious than placebo in preventing relapse, but findings from both studies also imply that at least a subset of initially treated children may not relapse when their risperidone is switched to placebo, suggesting that consideration of medication discontinuation may be appropriate for children who have done well for a substantial period of time.

Overall, there is increasing evidence to suggest that risperidone is efficacious in the long-term treatment of aggressive symptoms and/or behavior disorders in youth. However, the literature is limited in that it primarily focuses on samples of youth with low-normal or subaverage intelligence and/or autism.

Olanzapine

Several studies of olanzapine indicate preliminary success as a treatment in the management of aggressive disorders in youth (see Table 3–4 for dosage information). In a study by Stephens et al. (2004), 10 children with Tourette syndrome and aggression were treated in single-blind fashion (after a 2-week placebo run-in) with olanzapine over 8 weeks. The authors demonstrated significant reductions in both aggressive symptoms and tic severity, as assessed with standard rating scales. In one open-label trial of olanzapine in children, adolescents, and adults with pervasive developmental disorders, significant behavioral improvement was documented within the first several weeks of treatment (Potenza et al. 1999). Similarly, a case report by Horrigan et al. (1997) concluded that olanzapine was associated with decreased aggression toward people and property and a decreased number of explosive outbursts in youth. Even though these reports suggest that olanzapine may have a role in treating aggression and/or DBDs, firm conclusions about the potential efficacy of olanzapine cannot be reached without further studies.

Quetiapine

A 7-week RCT involving 19 adolescents with CD provides data that quetiapine may be beneficial in the treatment of CD (Connor et al. 2008). An 8-week open-label trial involving 16 youths with CD suggests that quetiapine may be of benefit in the treatment of aggression in that population (Findling et al. 2006). In the 26-week open-label extension of that trial, the benefit of quetiapine was found to be sustained and well tolerated with adjunctive stimulants (Findling et al. 2007). Finally, an open-label trial of quetiapine and methylphenidate found reduction in aggression and ADHD symptoms in youth with severe aggression who did not respond to methylphenidate monotherapy (Kronenberger et al. 2007). At this time, further research on quetiapine in the treatment of aggression and DBDs is needed. (See Table 3–4 for dosage information.)

Aripiprazole

An 8-week RCT involving 98 youths with autistic disorder found that treatment with aripiprazole was efficacious in reducing irritability (Owen et al. 2009). A 52-week open-label study of aripiprazole in youth with autistic disorder supports the medication's efficacy in long-term reduction of irritable symptoms (Marcus et al. 2011). In addition, an open-label study of youth with CD suggests that aripiprazole is generally well tolerated and is associated with improvements in aggressive behaviors. Study data also found that lower starting dosages of aripiprazole improved tolerability and reduced side effects in youth (Findling et al. 2009). Further evaluation of aripiprazole in the treatment of DBDs is warranted. (See Table 3–4 for dosage information.)

Clozapine

To date, no RCTs have evaluated the efficacy of clozapine in the treatment of aggressive symptoms in children or adults. However, there are several case studies that suggest clozapine is an effective treatment for aggression in adult samples (Rabinowitz et al. 1996; Volavka and Citrome 1999). Significant reductions in physical and verbal aggression were observed in 75 adults with schizophrenia during 6 months of treatment. Few studies have evaluated clozapine's effectiveness in the treatment of aggression in youth (Chalasani et al. 2001; Kranzler et al. 2005). In a chart review of six children and adolescents with schizophrenic disorders, violent episodes were significantly reduced and global functions improved significantly (Chalasani et al. 2001). Similarly, an open-label study by Kranzler et al. (2005) indicated that clozapine yielded significant pre-post benefits in patients with treatment-refractory schizophrenia and aggression. Finally, findings from a retrospective cohort study of patients with autism spectrum disorders and severe DBDs suggest that clozapine may decrease aggressiveness in treatment-resistant patients (Beherec et al. 2011).

Nonetheless, additional research is needed to assess the efficacy of clozapine in the treatment of aggression and/or behavior disorders in youth. (See Table 3–4 for dosage information.)

Other Atypical Antipsychotics

Currently, available data have not demonstrated efficacy of ziprasidone in the management of aggressive symptoms in youth with DBDs. One RCT of low-dose ziprasidone in youth with DBDs found no significant difference between treatment and placebo groups (Fleischhaker et al. 2011). Therefore, additional research is needed to further assess the comparative efficacy of other atypical antipsychotics. This research may be especially beneficial in treatment planning for youth with behavior disorders and/or aggression in light of the reported efficacy of the other atypical antipsychotics (principally risperidone) that have been extensively studied. Moreover, it would be of great clinical relevance to assess the different side-effect profiles of the various atypical antipsychotics to meet the need for a wider array of safe and effective therapeutic agents in the management of aggressive symptoms and/or behavior disorders in youth. (See Table 3–4 for dosage information.)

Benefits of Atypical Antipsychotics

Overall, atypical antipsychotics have a notably large effect on aggression (mean effect size = 0.9) that generally increases with the length of the study (Table 3–5). However, it should be noted that apart from risperidone and aripiprazole, little evidence is available on the efficacy of atypical antipsychotics in the treatment of aggressive symptoms and/or behavior disorders in youth. Risperidone may be the most appropriate treatment option, compared with the other atypical antipsychotics, because of the number of RCTs supporting its efficacy (Table 3–6).

Furthermore, risperidone is noted for its efficacy both as a monotherapy and in combination with other agents and, compared with typical antipsychotics, may also be associated with fewer extrapyramidal side effects (EPS) over the long term. As a result of the potential for decreased adverse side effects in child and adolescent samples, risperidone has largely replaced conventional antipsychotics in the treatment of aggression in youth (Connor et al. 2001; McConville and Sorter 2004).

Table 3–5. Effect sizes of various psychotropic agents for the treatment of aggression and/or disruptive behavior disorders in youth

Agent	Effect size	Total N across studies
Atypical antipsychotics	0.9	973
Risperidone	0.9	875
Aripiprazole	0.87	98
Typical antipsychotics	0.7	136
Haloperidol	0.8	53
Thioridazine	0.35	30
Stimulants	0.78	1,057
Methylphenidate	0.9	844
Mood stabilizers	0.4	217
Lithium	0.5	195
Alpha$_2$ agonists	0.5	259
Clonidine	1.1	8
Guanfacine	0.5	251
Beta-blockers	ND	ND
Mean effect size	0.7	

Note. See Pappadopulos et al. 2006, Owen et al. 2009, Connor et al. 2010 for additional information. ND = no data.

Risks of Atypical Antipsychotics

Although the adverse effects of atypical antipsychotics may be milder than those of typical antipsychotics, studies have indicated that atypical antipsychotics are nonetheless associated with mild-to-moderate side effects, including EPS, somnolence, headache, increases in prolactin levels, and increases in weight (Aman et al. 2004; Snyder et al. 2002). Of particular importance to pediatric care providers, youth treated with these agents appear to experience significantly greater weight gain than adults using atypical antipsychotics, even at low dosages (Sikich et al. 2004). Less commonly reported problems in youth may include type 2 diabetes and cardiac rhythm abnormalities, but more studies may be necessary to address concerns about these possible side effects (Schur et al. 2003). A retrospective cohort of over 9,000 children and adolescents suggests a significant increase in the incidence of diabetes mellitus in

Table 3–6. Efficacy levels of various psychotropic agents for the treatment of aggression and/or disruptive behavior disorders in youth

Class	Agent	Short-term efficacy	Long-term efficacy
Atypical antipsychotics	Risperidone	A	A
	Aripiprazole	A	ND
	Olanzapine	C	ND
	Clozapine	C	ND
	Quetiapine	C	ND
	Ziprasidone	ND	ND
Typical antipsychotics	Haloperidol	A	B
	Thioridazine	A	B
Stimulants	Methylphenidate	A	B
	Dextroamphetamine	B	ND
	Pemoline	B	ND
Norepinephrine reuptake inhibitor	Atomoxetine	B	ND
Mood stabilizers	Lithium	A	C
	Divalproex	A	C
	Carbamazepine	C	ND
Alpha$_2$ agonists	Clonidine	A	ND
	Guanfacine	A	ND
Beta-blockers	Nadolol	C	ND

Note. A = highest level of empirical support, two or more randomized controlled trials (RCTs); B = moderate support by at least one RCT plus or minus data from open trials and case studies; C = support based only on expert opinion, case studies, or open-label trials; D = data from completed trials report negative findings; ND = no data.

those treated with atypical antipsychotics (Andrade et al. 2011). In children and adolescents, long-term risks that are typically associated with atypical antipsychotic use also include withdrawal, tardive dyskinesia, parkinsonism, and neuroleptic malignant syndrome. Table 3–7 provides additional information on the potential side effects of atypical antipsychotics.

Because atypical antipsychotics are associated with an array of serious side effects, the U.S. Food and Drug Administration (FDA) has required that these

Table 3–7.   Common and serious side effects for various classes of psychopharmacological agents

Class	Common side effects	Serious or uncommon side effects
Atypical antipsychotics	Insomnia, agitation, extrapyramidal symptoms, headache, anxiety, rhinitis, constipation, nausea/vomiting, dyspepsia, dizziness, tachycardia, somnolence, increased dream activity, dry mouth, diarrhea, weight gain, visual disturbance, sexual dysfunction, hyperprolactinemia, menstrual irregularities	Hypotension, severe syncope (rare), extrapyramidal symptoms, severe tardive dyskinesia, neuroleptic malignant syndrome, hyperglycemia, severe diabetes mellitus, seizures (rare), priapism (rare), stroke, transient ischemic attack
Typical antipsychotics	Extrapyramidal symptoms, tardive dyskinesia, akathisia, insomnia, anxiety, drowsiness, lethargy, weight changes, anticholinergic effects, gynecomastia, breast tenderness, galactorrhea, menstrual irregularities, injection site reaction (depot), elevated prolactin levels	Neuroleptic malignant syndrome, tardive dyskinesia, pneumonia, arrhythmia, hypotension, hypertension, seizures, jaundice, hyperpyrexia, heat stroke, dystonia
Stimulants	Nervousness, insomnia, abdominal pain, nausea, anorexia, motor tics, headache, palpitations, dizziness, blurred vision, tachycardia, weight loss, fever, depression, transient drowsiness, dyskinesia, angina, rash, urticaria, blood pressure changes	Growth suppression (long term), seizures, dependency, abuse, arrhythmia, leukopenia (rare), thrombocytopenic purpura (rare), toxic psychosis (rare), Tourette syndrome (rare), exfoliative dermatitis (rare), erythema multiforme (rare), neuroleptic malignant syndrome (rare), cerebral arteritis (rare), hepatotoxicity (rare)

Table 3–7. Common and serious side effects for various classes of psychopharmacological agents *(continued)*

Class	Common side effects	Serious or uncommon side effects
Mood stabilizers	Enuresis, fatigue, ataxia, increased thirst, nausea, vomiting, urinary frequency, gastrointestinal upset, sleepiness, weight gain (Bassarath 2003; Malone et al. 2000)	Disruption in hepatic, hematological, and metabolic functioning (Cummings and Miller 2004)
Alpha$_2$-agonists	Drowsiness and dizziness (Cantwell et al. 1997), dry mouth, irritability, dysphoria, rebound hypertension (Martin et al. 2003), abdominal pain, headache (Connor et al. 2010)	Syncope (rare) (Cantwell et al. 1997), hypotension (rare) (Martin et al. 2003)
Beta-blockers	Sedation, mild hypotension, lowered heart rate, bronchoconstriction, dizziness, sleep disruption (Riddle et al. 1999)	Hypoglycemia (in patients with diabetes), growth-hormone regulation issues (Riddle et al. 1999)

Note. Side effects for specific medications may vary within classes; specific details of differences among specific agents can be found elsewhere (Connor et al. 2001; Pappadopulos et al. 2003; Weiner 1996).

Source. Center for the Advancement of Children's Mental Health, Office of Mental Health: "10 Tips: Navigating Child and Adolescent Inpatient and Residential Services in New York State." Unpublished document.

medications carry warning labels to specifically indicate their potential risk for increased weight gain and disruption of metabolic functioning (Stigler et al. 2004; U.S. Food and Drug Administration 2005). Given the concerns about side effects and the increasing rates at which atypical antipsychotics are being prescribed to youth with symptoms of aggression (Olfson et al. 2006), additional studies are necessary to examine the safety of these agents in the treatment of aggression in youth.

Typical Antipsychotics: Review of Treatment Studies

Haloperidol

Prior to the emergence of atypical antipsychotics, conventional antipsychotics were considered first-line agents in the treatment of aggression and/or behavior disorders in youth (for a review, see Campbell et al. 1999). Notably, haloperidol was considered an effective means to treat aggression. For example, during the course of a double-blind study of treatment-resistant inpatient youth (ages 5.2–12.9 years) with CD, a significant reduction in aggressive symptoms was seen in those taking haloperidol (Campbell et al. 1984). On the other hand, a double-blind, placebo-controlled study of haloperidol in the treatment of aggression in adolescents of subaverage intelligence found that the treatment only led to moderate behavioral improvements (Aman et al. 1989). Interestingly, haloperidol was considered most effective in treating youth with aggressive symptoms of irritability, thereby suggesting that haloperidol may be useful in the treatment of reactive aggression in youth (Campbell et al. 1999). (See Table 3–4 for dosage information.)

Thioridazine

Several early studies of thioridazine suggest its efficacy in managing aggressive symptoms in youth. For example, an RCT of thioridazine demonstrated modest clinical improvements in symptoms of aggression in youth (Aman et al. 1991) and led to a reduction in hyperactivity and conduct problems. Although thioridazine has shown superiority over placebo for treatment of youth meeting criteria for ADHD, it also may be less effective in maintaining treatment gains (Gittelman-Klein et al. 1976). Specifically, thioridazine appeared to be less effective at week 12 than at week 4 of the treatment. (See Table 3–4 for dosage information.)

Benefits of Typical Antipsychotics

Early studies suggested that low dosages of typical antipsychotics were effective for managing aggressive behaviors in youth, with a moderate effect size (mean = 0.7) (see Table 3–5) (Pappadopulos et al. 2006). Typical antipsychotics may also be beneficial when an aggressive youth experiences comorbid psychotic disorder (see Table 3–6).

Risks of Typical Antipsychotics

Available evidence indicates that typical antipsychotics can produce debilitating side effects in youth (see Table 3–7), including an increased occurrence of EPS and tardive dyskinesia (Connor et al. 2001; McConville and Sorter 2004). The risks associated with typical antipsychotics may outweigh the benefits of prescribing these agents in the treatment of aggression in youth. Therefore, typical antipsychotics should not be used to treat aggressive symptoms and/or DBDs in youth prior to a trial in which an atypical agent is used (Pappadopulos et al. 2003). In specific instances, however, if the patient is being treated with an atypical agent, emergent problems with weight gain or diabetes may warrant case-by-case use of typical antipsychotics.

Stimulants: Review of Treatment Studies

Methylphenidate

Short-Term Efficacy

To date, a growing number of short-term RCTs have provided evidence for the efficacy of methylphenidate and other stimulants in the treatment of aggression and DBDs in youth. For example, one meta-analysis of 28 studies occurring over the past 30 years examined the efficacy of stimulants on covert and overt aggressive behavior in ADHD, with largely promising findings with regard to short-term efficacy (Connor et al. 2002). Moreover, the use of methylphenidate and other stimulants to treat aggression appears to have a substantial treatment effect that is independent from effects on core ADHD symptoms in youth with ADHD and aggressive behavior. For example, one RCT of methylphenidate in 18 children with ADHD found significant improvement in aggressive behaviors and symptoms of hyperactivity and inattention (Bukstein and Kolko 1998). Moreover, notable improvements in peer relations were demonstrated. Similarly, an RCT testing the efficacy of methylphenidate in 84 children with CD with or without ADHD found significant reductions in core behaviors associated with CD, independent of the effects of the children's ADHD symptoms (Klein et al. 1997). Finally, an RCT of methylphenidate in 31 children with ADHD and comorbid tic disorder found improvement of oppositional behavior and peer aggression (Gadow et al. 2008).

Long-Term and Maintenance Efficacy

Several reports from the National Institute of Mental Health (NIMH) Multimodal Treatment of ADHD (MTA) study have explored longer-term treatment for youth experiencing comorbid impulsive aggression and ADHD. For example, the MTA's 14-month follow-up indicated that stimulants (principally methylphenidate) not only alleviated core symptoms of ADHD but also reduced the secondary symptoms of ODD and aggression in youth (MTA Cooperative Group 1999), as rated on the Swanson, Nolan, and Pelham Version IV (SNAP-IV) scale (Swanson et al. 2001). However, symptoms of aggression and oppositionality that are present along with internalizing disorders, such as depression or anxiety, may improve most with psychopharmacological treatment that is combined with a behavioral intervention (Jensen et al. 2001). Overall, the evidence suggests that methylphenidate may be efficacious in treating aggressive symptoms associated with DBDs and ADHD.

Other Stimulants

Although methylphenidate is the most commonly prescribed stimulant for the treatment of ADHD and co-occurring aggressive symptoms, some evidence suggests that other stimulants may also be efficacious in the treatment of youth with comorbid symptoms of aggression and ADHD (see also Chapter 2, "Attention-Deficit/Hyperactivity Disorder," in this manual). These agents include a combination of methylphenidate and mixed amphetamine salts, and a combination of methylphenidate, dextroamphetamine, and pemoline (Pappadopulos et al. 2004). Given the small number of studies available for evaluation, however, it is unclear whether the efficacy of these other stimulants on the treatment of aggression is comparable to that of methylphenidate. (See Table 3–4 for dosage information for these other stimulants.)

Benefits of Stimulants

Stimulants are recommended as a first-line treatment in youth with comorbid ADHD and aggression (Pappadopulos et al. 2006). The rationale for stimulant use in the management of aggressive symptoms of ADHD or behavior disorder is based on the number of controlled trials demonstrating its efficacy and its large overall effect size (0.78–0.9; see Tables 3–5 and 3–6) (Connor et al. 2002; Pappadopulos et al. 2006). Therefore, the use of stimulants may be an appropriate treatment option for the management of aggression in youth in instances of comorbidity with the DBDs and other psychiatric disorders that are also typically treated with stimulants (MTA Cooperative Group 1999). In contrast to earlier concerns regarding stimulant usage, MTA data also suggest that stimulant use is effective in treating ADHD, even among youth who present with co-occurring symptoms of mania and aggression (Galanter et al. 2004). Youth with comorbid ADHD and aggression may be more likely than nonaggressive youth to experience insufficient response to stimulant monotherapy and may require more rigorous dosing for symptom remission (Blader et al. 2010). Stimulant treatment also appears to yield improvements in global functioning and social interaction (Bukstein and Kolko 1998; MTA Cooperative Group 1999; Swanson et al. 2001).

Risks of Stimulants

Despite their efficacy, stimulants are associated with several adverse effects, including insomnia, reduced appetite, stomachache, headache, and dizziness. Stimulants have also been linked to long-term adverse effects, including height and weight suppression (Lisska and Rivkees 2003). MTA analyses support the potential for a growth-suppression effect in youth who were systematically treated with stimulants. However, findings are also consistent with the interpretation that growth is merely delayed, as opposed to reduced, in youth taking stimulants, compared with youth who are not taking stimulant medications (MTA Cooperative Group 2004). Further long-term follow-up studies must address the lingering questions.

Of note, the FDA has recommended that stimulants be labeled with a black box warning that indicates their potential for adverse cardiac effects in children (U.S. Food and Drug Administration 2006). One retrospective case-control study suggests a link between stimulant use and rare events of sudden unexplained death in children and adolescents (Gould et al. 2009). Although the possibility of causing adverse cardiac effects remains unproven, caution should be taken in prescribing stimulants to youth with preexisting or family history of heart conditions. (See Table 3–7 for additional information pertaining to the potential adverse effects associated with stimulant usage.)

Mood Stabilizers: Review of Treatment Studies

Lithium

Most existing literature on the efficacy of mood stabilizers in the treatment of aggression in youth has focused on the use of lithium in patients with CD. Overall, these results suggest that lithium is associated with reduction in aggressive behavior in youth with CD (Campbell et al. 1995; Malone et al. 2000). For example, in one RCT, inpatient children with a primary diagnosis of CD received either lithium or placebo (Campbell et al. 1995). Lithium was associated with reduction in aggressive behaviors across several standardized measures, including the Children's Psychiatric Rating Scale (CPRS). In an RCT comparing lithium and placebo among 40 youths with CD, improvements were found in aggressive behaviors, as measured by the Overt Aggression Scale (OAS), for those treated with lithium (Malone et al. 2000).

Overall, lithium has been shown to reduce bullying, fighting, and temper outbursts in severely aggressive, inpatient youth with CD (Campbell et al. 1984, 1995; Carlson et al. 1992; Malone et al. 2000). This evidence implies that lithium may have an important role in the treatment of reactive or affective aggression in youth. However, the necessity of frequent monitoring and blood draws associated with this treatment, as well as lithium's potential for side effects, may render it a second-line choice after pharmacological agents such as the atypical antipsychotics (Pappadopulos et al. 2003). (See Table 3–4 for dosage information.)

Divalproex

Some evidence indicates that divalproex is effective in reducing aggressive symptoms and/or behavior disorders in youth. For example, in one RCT, improvement in impulse control was demonstrated in incarcerated male youth given high doses of divalproex; moreover, global improvements among the subjects, as measured by the CGI Scale (Steiner 2003), were also noted. Similarly, another trial found that divalproex was associated with a reduction in aggressive symptoms in youth with CD (Donovan et al. 2000, 2003). Evidence also suggests that divalproex may be especially beneficial to youth who present with explosive and severe aggression (Donovan et al. 1997), as well as for treating impulsive aggression symptoms in youth with pervasive developmental disorders (Hollander et al. 2001). A 12-week, open-label trial of divalproex sodium in 25 youths with bipolar disorder indicated a significant reduction in aggressive symptoms as measured by the OAS (Saxena et al. 2006). Another RCT found that when treated with stimulant and divalproex adjunctive treatment, 30 youths with ADHD and chronic aggression refractory to stimulant monotherapy demonstrated higher rates of remission of aggressive behavior (Blader et al. 2009). Finally, an RCT involving 58 males with severe CD in the juvenile justice system found significantly higher response to divalproex in males with reactive aggression than in those with proactive aggression (Padhy et al. 2011). Therefore, evidence suggests that divalproex may be efficacious in treating youth with an array of psychiatric disorders, including CD, ADHD, and bipolar disorder, whose behavior includes severe impulsive aggression. (See Table 3–4 for dosage information.)

Carbamazepine

The use of carbamazepine and other mood stabilizers/anticonvulsants in the treatment of aggressive disorders has increased twofold over the past decade and a half (Hunkeler et al. 2005). Preliminary research indicates that carbamazepine produces statistically significant decreases in aggressiveness and explosiveness in youth, with a moderate effect size (Evans et al. 1987; Kafantaris et al. 1992; Pappadopulos et al. 2006). On the other hand, countervailing evidence suggests that carbamazepine does not differ from placebo in reducing aggression in youth (Cueva et al. 1996). Thus, the results are inconclusive with regard to the efficacy of carbamazepine. (See Table 3–4 for dosage information.)

Benefits of Mood Stabilizers

In general, mood stabilizers appear to be beneficial in the treatment of aggression in youth with behavior disorders. Overall, the mean effect size for mood stabilizers appears to be moderate (0.4; see Table 3–5) (Pappadopulos et al. 2006). A mood stabilizer may be a suitable alternative when a youth does not respond to the more rigorously tested atypical antipsychotics or stimulants.

Lithium, in particular, can be considered an evidence-based treatment in aggressive behaviors in youth with DBDs (see Table 3–6). Moreover, lithium should be considered as the first-line treatment option for severe aggressive symptoms in youth who have received a primary diagnosis of a mood disorder, such as bipolar disorder. Lithium may also be a suitable treatment option when the youth has a sole diagnosis of CD in addition to showing severe aggressive symptoms, given that RCTs have demonstrated the efficacy of lithium in treating CD among children and adolescents.

Overall, the current evidence largely supports mood stabilizers' efficacy in the treatment of reactive aggression in youth with CD. However, because many of the symptoms of CD correspond to proactive aggression, additional research is needed to determine whether either subtype of aggression responds differentially to mood stabilizers.

Risks of Mood Stabilizers

To date, studies pertaining to mood stabilizers in the treatment of aggression in youth have been limited in that they have measured short-term treatment outcomes. Therefore, certain adverse effects may not become evident during the limited duration of these studies, but may appear in trials spanning longer periods. Furthermore, these studies have been limited in scope, given that they have largely relied on inpatient data. Therefore, additional research is needed to measure the risks, benefits, and efficacy of mood stabilizers in aggressive youth in an array of settings (e.g., outpatient and emergency care).

Mood stabilizers are associated with a variety of adverse side effects (see Table 3–7). Common side effects of lithium include enuresis, fatigue, ataxia, increased thirst, nausea, vomiting, urinary frequency, and weight gain (Bassarath 2003; Malone et al. 2000). Moreover, frequent blood draws for dosage monitoring are needed; thus, lithium may be less suitable for the treatment of aggressive symptoms in children (Malone et al. 2000). Side effects associated with divalproex include gastrointestinal upset and sleepiness (Steiner et al. 2003). Carbamazepine may carry the greatest risk for adverse side effects among mood stabilizers and has been linked to disruption in hepatic, hematological, and metabolic functioning (Cummings and Miller 2004). In 2008, the FDA found that patients treated with anticonvulsants had nearly twice the risk of suicidal ideation or behavior compared with those given placebo, and therefore mandated warning labeling for anticonvulsant medications (U.S. Food and Drug Administration 2008).

Other Agents

Alpha$_2$-Adrenergic Agonists

Clonidine

Some evidence supports the use of α_2-adrenergic agonists in the treatment of aggressive symptoms and/or DBDs among children and adolescents. Specifically, clonidine has demonstrated efficacy in the treatment of aggression in youth, according to a meta-analysis of 11 double-blind, controlled, randomized studies (Connor et al. 1999). More recently, Hazell and Stuart (2003) reported gains in a 6-week randomized, double-blind, placebo-controlled trial of a combined clonidine-plus-stimulant treatment. Specifically, conduct problems were improved in youth with ADHD and comorbid ODD or CD. Further research on clonidine in the treatment of aggression and DBDs is needed. (For dosage information, see Table 3–4.)

Guanfacine

Guanfacine has demonstrated efficacy in the treatment of aggressive symptoms in an 8-week RCT involving 34 youths, ages 7–15 years, each having ADHD and a tic disorder (Scahill et al. 2001). A 9-week RCT of extended-release guanfacine in 217 youths with ADHD and oppositional symptoms resulted in significant reduction in both oppositional and ADHD symptoms (Connor et al. 2010). Thus, it appears that guanfacine may be beneficial in the treatment of aggressive symptoms in youth with comorbid psychiatric disorders; however, further research is needed to provide conclusive support for the use of this agent in the treatment of DBDs in youth. (See Table 3–4 for dosage information.)

Benefits of Alpha₂-Adrenergic Agonists

Overall, α_2-adrenergic agonists have been shown to produce medium effect sizes, ranging from 0.5 to 1.1 (see Table 3–5) (Pappadopulos et al. 2006). Interestingly, α_2 agonists may reduce the side effects associated with stimulant treatments. Therefore, this agent may be most useful when combined with stimulants in the treatment of aggressive symptoms (see Table 3–6 for detailed efficacy assessment of this class). Additional research is needed to compare the efficacy of α_2 agonists with that of other psychotropic agents in the treatment of aggressive symptoms in youth with behavior disorders.

Risks of Alpha₂-Adrenergic Agonists

α_2-Adrenergic agonists are associated with several adverse side effects, including drowsiness and dizziness (Cantwell et al. 1997). These agents may also be associated with serious adverse risks. Specifically, Cantwell et al. (1997) reported harmful and potentially life-threatening side effects in several children who were treated with clonidine. One child in the study died as a result of an exercise-related syncope, which may have been related to the clonidine treatment. Caution should be executed in administering α_2 agonists to youth with symptoms of aggression and/or DBDs. (See Table 3–7 for additional details on the potential adverse effects associated with α_2 agonists.)

Beta-Blockers

Current literature on the efficacy of β-blockers in the treatment of aggression in youth is sparse. In a 1999 review of β-blockers, Connor et al. (1997) reported treatment gains for over 80% of children and adults who took β-blockers for management of symptoms of aggression. Specifically, an open-label study found that nadolol, in particular, may be useful in the treatment of aggression and comorbid ADHD in youth with developmental delays. (See Table 3–4 for dosage information.)

Risks of Beta-Blockers

To date, no RCTs of the use of β-blockers in the treatment of youth have been conducted. Therefore, firm conclusions about the efficacy of these agents cannot be drawn (see Table 3–6). Some of the adverse effects associated with β-blockers include sedation, mild hypotension, lowered heart rate, bronchoconstriction, hypoglycemia (in patients with diabetes), dizziness, sleep disruption, and potential growth-hormone regulation disturbances (see Table 3–7) (Riddle et al. 1999). Further research on the benefits and risks associated with using β-blockers to treat youth with aggressive symptoms is needed.

Norepinephrine Reuptake Inhibitors

Atomoxetine

In an RCT evaluating atomoxetine treatment of comorbid ADHD and ODD, Newcorn et al. (2005) found that atomoxetine improves ADHD and ODD symptoms and suggested that higher dosages may be needed to treat youth who meet criteria for both conditions. However, a meta-analysis of aggression in RCTs of atomoxetine found that the risk of aggressive or hostile events in youth taking atomoxetine was not statistically significant from that of youth given placebo (Polzer et al. 2007). A randomized, placebo-controlled, double-blind study in 180 youths with ADHD and comorbid ODD found significant reductions in symptoms of ADHD and ODD after 9 weeks of treatment (Dittmann et al. 2011). Further research on the long-term benefits and risks associated with using atomoxetine to treat youth with disruptive behavior disorders is needed.

Risks of Norepinephrine Reuptake Inhibitors

Children and adolescents who take atomoxetine may experience dry mouth, fatigue, irritability, nausea, appetite change, constipation, dizziness, sweating, dysuria, urinary retention or hesitancy, priapism, increased obsessive behaviors, weight changes, palpitations, suicidal ideation, hepatic injury, increased heart rate, and increased blood pressure. Six cases of drug-induced liver injury were reported from 2005 to 2008 (U.S. Food and Drug Administration 2009). The FDA has mandated a black box warning for atomoxetine due to increased risk of suicidal ideation in children and adolescents (U.S. Food and Drug Administration 2010).

Safety Issues

Monitoring

Antipsychotics

Height and weight should be thoroughly monitored throughout the course of treatment using antipsychotic agents. If weight gain is identified in a child or adolescent who is taking these agents, the physician should implement a diet and exercise plan. Vital signs, with particular attention to cardiac function, should also be routinely assessed in a youth who is taking atypical antipsychotics (Schur et al. 2003). If cardiac symptoms emerge, the physician should consider consulting with a cardiology specialist.

In youth taking typical or atypical antipsychotics, the physician should carefully monitor for EPS such as akathisia, akinesia, tremor, dystonia, and emergent tardive dyskinesia (Connor et al. 2001; McConville and Sorter 2004). Furthermore, the youth should be routinely screened for abnormalities in liver function and lipid production, particularly in the presence of weight gain. Monitoring glucose metabolism is important, given that certain agents may be linked to juvenile diabetes (Clark and Burge 2003). Furthermore, prolactin levels should be monitored in the case of endocrine symptoms (Wudarsky et al. 1999). Patients should be monitored for rare but life-threatening side effects, including neuroleptic malignant syndrome, seizures, and heat stroke.

Stimulants

Children and adolescents who are taking stimulants should be routinely monitored for adverse symptoms, including insomnia, reduced appetite, stomachache, headache, and dizziness (Lisska and Rivkees 2003; MTA Cooperative Group 1999). Of note, stimulant use has been linked to long-term adverse effects, including height and weight suppression; therefore, it is important that vital signs, height and weight, and abnormalities in metabolic function be thoroughly monitored throughout the course of treatment. Although concerns have been raised about the possibility of cardiac side effects, such effects remain unproven, and electrocardiography or other cardiac monitoring procedures are not indicated in otherwise healthy youth treated for aggression or DBDs. However, if the stimulant is being taken concurrently with another psychopharmacological agent, such as clonidine, cardiac monitoring is recommended (Fenichel and Lipicky 1994).

Mood Stabilizers

Certain mood-stabilizing agents, such as lithium, require frequent blood draws for dosage monitoring and therefore may be less suitable in the treatment of aggressive symptoms and/or behavior disorders in youth (Bassarath 2003; Malone et al. 2000). In addition, common side effects associated with mood stabilizers include enuresis, fatigue, ataxia, increased thirst, nausea, vomiting, and urinary frequency. Therefore, careful monitoring of these symptoms is required. Moreover, because weight gain is associated with use of mood stabilizers, height and weight should be monitored during the treatment course. Importantly, because carbamazepine has been linked to serious adverse effects, including hepatotoxic, hematological, and metabolic reactions, comprehensive assessment of these systems is important (Cummings and Miller 2004).

Alpha$_2$-Adrenergic Agonists

Careful consideration is needed before prescribing α_2 agonists to youth with symptoms of aggression. Concerns regarding the safety of α_2 agonists have been raised because of reports of harmful and potentially life-threatening side effects in several children treated with clonidine (Cantwell et al. 1997). Moreover, because clonidine can produce drowsiness and dizziness, patients should be routinely monitored for these symptoms (Hazell and Stuart 2003).

Beta-Blockers

Careful attention should be given to the potential side effects most commonly associated with use of β-blockers in youth, including sedation, mild hypotension, lowered heart rate, bronchoconstriction, hypoglycemia (in patients with diabetes), dizziness, and sleep disruption (Hazell and Stuart 2003). As with antipsychotics, stimulants, and mood stabilizers, vital signs, height, and weight should be thoroughly monitored throughout the treatment process.

Norepinephrine Reuptake Inhibitors

All pediatric patients treated with atomoxetine should be closely monitored for suicidal thoughts, sudden changes in behavior, hepatic function, vital signs, height, and weight throughout the treatment process (U.S. Food and Drug Administration 2009).

Preventing Adverse Effects

Conservative dosing procedures may prevent the possible occurrence of adverse effects in youth taking psychopharmacological agents. The general rule of thumb is to "start low, go slow, and taper slowly" (Pappadopulos et al. 2003). Moreover, potential side effects should be monitored on a systematic basis with rating scales or structured assessment methods (Pappadopulos et al. 2003).

To prevent adverse effects, the physician should avoid prescribing multiple agents whenever possible. In addition, the physician should evaluate and adjust the treatment regimen in youth who do not experience a decrease in aggressive symptoms. Finally, the physician should consider tapering the agent if the youth demonstrates a good response. If the treatment response is maintained during the tapering of a medication, the physician may consider discontinuing the agent.

Interventions to Address Adverse Effects of Psychotropic Agents

Side effects of pharmacological interventions range in severity from life-threatening, irreversible, and acutely distressing effects, to those effects that are merely uncomfortable. In Table 3–7, we separate the potential side effects of various psychotropic agents into two categories: common and uncommon but serious.

As a general rule of thumb, if the side effect is considered serious, the physician should generally discontinue use of the agent. Once the serious adverse event is resolved, the physician may consider starting a different psychopharmacological intervention. When appropriate to do so, the physician should consult with specialists (e.g., those in emergency internal medicine, hematology, pediatrics) in the care management of youth experiencing serious adverse side effects.

Practical Management Strategies

Treatment Guidelines

Clearly, any conclusions that can be drawn from this review on the pharmacotherapy of aggression are limited by the current scope of the literature. For example, RCTs evaluating the efficacy of atypical medications are a rarity in the current literature. Therefore, until the results of additional RCTs become available, a combination of evidence-based treatment recommendations and expert consensus guidelines may serve to guide the use of psychopharmacological agents in the treatment of youth with aggression. Algorithms "provide the framework for facilitating thinking about clinical problems" (Margolis 1983, p. 631). Available evidence suggests that patients whose doctors generally follow practice guidelines get better outcomes (Emslie et al. 2004; Pliszka et al. 2003; Rush et al. 1995, 1999).

The American Academy of Child and Adolescent Psychiatry has developed several practice parameters geared toward specific mental health issues in children that are based on expert consensus and review of the scientific literature. Several relevant parameters address the assessment and treatment of symptoms of aggression in youth with CD (Steiner 1997), autism (Volkmar et al. 1999), and mental retardation (Szymanski and King 1999). Overall, these parameters stress the importance of using standardized screening instruments and empirically supported multimodal interventions.

Currently, practice parameters are under development with regard to the use of atypical antipsychotics in the treatment of ODD, CD, aggression, and an array of other psychiatric symptoms and disorders in youth (Findling et al., in press). The focus on the use of atypical agents in the treatment of aggression and/or DBDs in youth is particularly important because aggression is the most common target symptom for which atypical antipsychotics are prescribed (Cooper et al. 2004; DelBello and Grcevich 2004; Pappadopulos et al. 2003; Simeon et al. 2002; Stigler et al. 2001; Turgay 2005).

Overall, these practice parameters for atypical antipsychotics cite the importance of considering both the age of the study population and the specific diagnosis evaluated in determining whether research findings are applicable to the treatment of child and adolescent psychiatric disorders in clinical cases (Findling et al., in press). Recommendations for screening, assessment, drug titration, dosage, and other management issues are also addressed (Findling et al., in press). Of particular importance in the consideration of aggression typologies, these parameters also note that although atypical antipsychotics have been most rigorously tested as a treatment for impulsive aggression in youth with DBDs, the effectiveness of atypical agents in treating other aspects of DBDs has not been as clearly demonstrated. Thus, further research is needed to assess the efficacy of antipsychotics and other psychotropic agents in the treatment of a multitude of aggressive subtypes.

In addition, specific clinical guidelines have been developed for the treatment of aggression and DBDs in youth (Pappadopulos et al. 2003). The Treatment Recommendations for the Use of Antipsychotic Medications for

Aggressive Youth (TRAAY) (Jensen et al. 2004) were created using a combination of evidence- and consensus-based methodologies. Moreover, recommendations were developed from three primary sources of information: current scientific evidence, the expressed needs for guidelines as reported by physicians in focus groups, and consensus of clinical and research experts. Although these guidelines focus primarily on the use of atypical antipsychotics, the use of other classes and agents is addressed. Fourteen treatment recommendations on the use of atypical antipsychotics for aggression in youth with comorbid psychiatric conditions were developed. Each recommendation corresponds to one of the phases of care: evaluation, treatment, stabilization, and maintenance.

The TRAAY guidelines can be briefly summarized as follows: Physicians should conduct an initial diagnostic evaluation (preferably using a standardized assessment tool) before using a pharmacological or psychosocial treatment to manage aggressive symptoms. Typically, a physician should begin with an evidence-based psychosocial intervention as a first-line method of treatment in an aggressive youth. If the youth does not make gains in psychotherapy after an adequate time period, the clinician may then consider psychopharmacological treatment, tailoring the agent choice to the individual's primary disorder. If the youth fails to make treatment gains with the agent best suited for his or her primary disorder, the physician should then consider tapering or switching the agent. Regardless of the psychopharmacological approach, the physician should strive to use a conservative dosing strategy. During the course of treatment, the physician should routinely and systematically assess the youth for potential adverse effects. Even for some cases in which adverse effects develop, it is important to ensure an adequate trial of the agent before modifying the treatment plan. Furthermore, the physician should consider tapering and discontinuing medications in youth who show a reduction in aggressive symptoms for a period of 6 months or more. (For additional information about the TRAAY guidelines, see Pappadopulos et al. 2003.)

Role of Nonmedication Interventions

Whether or not a psychopharmacological intervention is ultimately used, psychoeducation is a critical component of the successful treatment of aggressive disorders in youth. Psychoeducation enables the youth and family to understand and identify aggressive behaviors. Moreover, it helps the youth and family members learn about plausible treatment options, including psychopharmacological treatments and behavioral interventions.

As noted in the TRAAY guidelines (see "Treatment Guidelines" above), empirically supported behavioral interventions should typically constitute the first-line treatment approach for aggressive youth (Pappadopulos et al. 2003). Evidence-based psychosocial interventions for aggression in youth include cognitive-behavioral therapy for aggressive disorders and parent management training. These evidence-based treatments work to increase positive time that youth and family members spend together, help set rules and consequences, and provide training on problem-solving and social skills. However, moderate-to-severe aggressive symptoms in youth typically require a combination of psychoeducation, cognitive and behavioral management strategies, and pharmacological agents.

Involvement of Others

The clinician needs to solicit help from everybody involved and sometimes outsiders to achieve the best possible outcome. From the outset, particularly in difficult cases, the clinician should indicate to parents and youth that treating DBDs and aggression with medication can be helpful but is rarely sufficient. As with treatment of diabetes or severe allergies, changes in family lifestyle are needed. The family and clinician must work as partners to address situations that escalate the child's aggression or DBD symptoms.

If the family is close to even a medium-sized city, the clinician can encourage or require parents to attend parent support groups. Organizations that offer such groups include the following: National Alliance on Mental Illness (NAMI) (www.nami.org), Children and Adults With Attention-Deficit/ Hyperactivity Disorder (CHADD) (www.chadd.org), Depression and Bipolar Support Alliance (DBSA) (www.dbsalliance.org), National Federation of Families for Children's Mental Health (www.ffcmh.org), and Mental Health America (formerly National Mental Health Association) (www.nmha.org, www.mentalhealthamerica.net), among others.

A clinician who cannot provide evidence-based psychotherapeutic support would be wise to get a partner who can. Such support is a must. Various psychosocial interventions have been developed for treating aggression and related conduct problems, including parent management training (Brestan and Eyberg 1998; Burke et al. 2002; Kazdin et al. 1989, 1992), Parent-Child Interaction Therapy (Schuhmann et al. 1998), some school- and community-based programs (Farmer et al. 2004), and some individual cognitive-behavioral treatments, including anger management training and problem-solving skills training (Brestan and Eyberg 1998; Lochman and Curry 1986; Lochman and Lampron 1988).

Conclusions

Additional RCTs are needed to assess the short-term and long-term efficacy, safety, and tolerability of the psychotropic agents used to manage symptoms of aggression and DBDs in youth. More RCTs are also needed to establish the comparative efficacy of the varying psychotropic agents in the treatment of aggression and/or behavior disorders in youth.

Authors describing future RCTs should routinely publish effect size values to enhance the clinical interpretation of research findings. Thus far, it appears that the largest effects for the treatment of aggression in youth have been demonstrated with methylphenidate for youth with ADHD and comorbid disruptive behavior problems (mean effect size = 0.90) and with risperidone for youth with CD and subaverage intelligence (mean effect size = 0.90) (Pappadopulos et al. 2006); however, additional RCTs are needed to test these agents in the management of aggressive youth with nonprimary diagnoses of ADHD and aggressive youth with normal intelligence, respectively.

Additional research is necessary to systematically assess and treat symptoms of proactive and reactive aggression in youth. Because these two forms of aggression may have different etiological pathways, they may respond differently to different forms of treatment. Thus far, there is some, albeit limited, evidence to suggest that certain psychopharmacological agents may be best suited to manage impulsive aggression in youth; however, additional research is needed. Moreover, the development of a standardized measure of aggression subtypes would assist in the goal of understanding and successfully treating the subtypes of aggression.

Although the pharmacological study of aggression and the DBDs is challenged by the severity and chronicity of these conditions, there is some hope that several of the current treatments are among the most effective, in terms of effect sizes, in all of pediatric psychopharmacology. New ways of understanding and assessing aggression, and perhaps the DBDs as well, should be readily available more generally. Overall, although we appear to be making progress in the treatment of severe aggression in youth, this burgeoning area of study and interest bears careful watch in the coming decades.

Clinical Pearls

- Carefully consider using and following currently available evidence- and consensus-based guidelines to achieve the best possible outcomes.
- Always try to use fewer rather than more medications. Do not add a medication if changing the dose of the current medication is likely to achieve comparable benefit. Do not assume that smaller dosages of two or more medications are preferable to higher, appropriate dosages of a single medication.
- Do not assume that a given medication does not work until you have tested it throughout the dose range. As a general rule, in the absence of side effects and lack of response, continue to cautiously raise the dose until you see treatment effects or side effects.
- Always start low, go slow, and taper slowly.
- Address compliance and adherence issues.
- Help children and adolescents to take active roles and responsibility for controlling and redirecting their behaviors.
- Encourage parents to put optimal parenting and milieu strategies into place when managing aggression and DBDs.

References

Aman MG, Teehan CJ, White AJ, et al: Haloperidol treatment with chronically medicated residents: dose effects on clinical behavior and reinforcement contingencies. Am J Ment Retard 93:452–460, 1989

Aman MG, Marks RE, Turbott SH, et al: Clinical effects of methylphenidate and thioridazine in intellectually subaverage children. J Am Acad Child Adolesc Psychiatry 30:246–256, 1991

Aman MG, De Smedt G, Derivan A, et al: Double-blind, placebo-controlled study of risperidone for the treatment of disruptive behaviors in children with subaverage intelligence. Am J Psychiatry 159:1337–1346, 2002

Aman MG, Binder C, Turgay A: Risperidone effects in the presence/absence of psychostimulant medicine in children with ADHD, other disruptive behavior disorders, and subaverage IQ. J Child Adolesc Psychopharmacol 14:243–254, 2004

American Psychiatric Association: Diagnostic and Statistical Manual of Mental Disorders, 4th Edition, Text Revision. Washington, DC, American Psychiatric Association, 2000

Andrade SE, Lo JC, Roblin D, et al: Antipsychotic medication use among children and risk of diabetes mellitus. Pediatrics 128:1135–1141, 2011

Bambauer KZ, Connor DF: Characteristics of aggression in clinically referred children. CNS Spectr 10:709–718, 2005

Bassarath L: Medication strategies in childhood aggression: a review. Can J Psychiatry 48:367–373, 2003

Beherec L, Lambrey S, Quilici G, et al: Retrospective review of clozapine in the treatment of patients with autism spectrum disorder and severe disruptive behaviors. J Clin Psychopharmacol 31:341–344, 2011

Blader JC, Schooler NR, Jensen PS, et al: Adjunctive divalproex versus placebo for children with ADHD and aggression refractory to stimulant monotherapy. Am J Psychiatry 166:1392–1401, 2009

Blader JC, Pliszka SR, Jensen PS, et al: Stimulant-responsive and stimulant-refractory aggressive behaviors among children with ADHD. Pediatrics 126:E796–E806, 2010

Brestan EV, Eyberg SM: Effective psychosocial treatments of conduct-disordered children and adolescents: 29 years, 82 studies, and 5,272 kids. J Clin Child Psychol 27:180–189, 1998

Brown K, Atkins MS, Osborne ML, et al: A revised teacher rating scale for reactive and proactive aggression. J Abnorm Child Psychol 24:473–480, 1996

Buitelaar JK, van der Gaag RJ, Cohen-Kettenis P, et al: A randomized controlled trial of risperidone in the treatment of aggression in hospitalized adolescents with subaverage cognitive abilities. J Clin Psychiatry 62:239–248, 2001

Bukstein OG, Kolko DJ: Effects of methylphenidate on aggressive urban children with attention deficit hyperactivity disorder. J Clin Child Psychol 27:340–351, 1998

Burke JD, Loeber R, Birmaher B: Oppositional defiant disorder and conduct disorder: a review of the past 10 years, part II. J Am Acad Child Adolesc Psychiatry 41:1275–1293, 2002

Campbell M, Small AM, Green WH, et al: Behavioral efficacy of haloperidol and lithium carbonate: a comparison in hospitalized aggressive children with conduct disorder. Arch Gen Psychiatry 41:650–656, 1984

Campbell M, Adams PB, Small AM, et al: Lithium in hospitalized aggressive children with conduct disorder: a double-blind and placebo-controlled study. J Am Acad Child Adolesc Psychiatry 34:445–453, 1995

Campbell M, Rapoport JL, Simpson GM: Antipsychotics in children and adolescents. J Am Acad Child Adolesc Psychiatry 38:537–545, 1999

Cantwell DP, Swanson J, Connor DF: Case study: adverse response to clonidine. J Am Acad Child Adolesc Psychiatry 36:539–544, 1997

Carlson GA, Rapport MD, Pataki CS, et al: Lithium in hospitalized children at 4 and 8 weeks: mood, behavior and cognitive effects. J Child Psychol Psychiatry 33:411–425, 1992

Chalasani L, Kant R, Chengappa KN: Clozapine impact on clinical outcomes and aggression in severely ill adolescents with childhood-onset schizophrenia. Can J Psychiatry 46:965–968, 2001

Clark C, Burge MR: Diabetes mellitus associated with atypical anti-psychotic medications. Diabetes Technol Ther 5:669–683, 2003

Connor DF, Ozbayrak KR, Benjamin S, et al: A pilot study of nadolol for overt aggression in developmentally delayed individuals. J Am Acad Child Adolesc Psychiatry 36:826–834, 1997

Connor DF, Fletcher KE, Swanson JM: A meta-analysis of clonidine for symptoms of attention-deficit hyperactivity disorder. J Am Acad Child Adolesc Psychiatry 38:1551–1559, 1999

Connor DF, Fletcher KE, Wood JS: Neuroleptic-related dyskinesias in children and adolescents. J Clin Psychiatry 62:967–974, 2001

Connor DF, Glatt SJ, Lopez ID, et al: Psychopharmacology and aggression, I: a meta-analysis of stimulant effects on overt/covert aggression-related behaviors in ADHD. J Am Acad Child Adolesc Psychiatry 41:253–261, 2002

Connor DF, Steingard RJ, Cunningham JA, et al: Proactive and reactive aggression in referred children and adolescents. Am J Orthopsychiatry 74:129–136, 2004

Connor DF, McLaughlin TJ, Jeffers-Terry M: Randomized controlled pilot study of quetiapine in the treatment of adolescent conduct disorder. J Child Adolesc Psychopharmacol 18:140–156, 2008

Connor DF, Findling RL, Kollins SH, et al: Effects of guanfacine extended release on oppositional symptoms in children aged 6–12 years with attention-deficit hyperactivity disorder and oppositional symptoms: a randomized, double-blind, placebo-controlled trial. CNS Drugs 24:755–768, 2010

Cooper WO, Hickson GB, Fuchs C, et al: New users of antipsychotic medications among children enrolled in TennCare. Arch Pediatr Adolesc Med 158:753–759, 2004

Croonenberghs J, Fegert JM, Findling RL et al: Risperidone in children with disruptive behavior disorders and subaverage intelligence: a 1-year, open-label study of 504 patients. J Am Acad Child Adolesc Psychiatry 44:969–970, 2005

Cueva JE, Overall JE, Small AM, et al: Carbamazepine in aggressive children with conduct disorder: a double-blind and placebo-controlled study. J Am Acad Child Adolesc Psychiatry 35:480–490, 1996

Cummings MR, Miller BD: Pharmacologic management of behavioral instability in medically ill pediatric patients. Curr Opin Pediatr 16:516–522, 2004

DelBello M, Grcevich S: Phenomenology and epidemiology of childhood psychiatric disorders that may necessitate treatment with atypical antipsychotics. J Clin Psychiatry 65:12–19, 2004

Dittmann RW, Schacht A, Helsberg K: Atomoxetine versus placebo in children and adolescents with attention-deficit/hyperactivity disorder and comorbid oppositional defiant disorder: a double-blind, randomized, multicenter trial in Germany. J Child Adolesc Psychopharmacol 21:97–110, 2011

Dodge K: The structure and function of reactive and proactive aggression, in The Development and Treatment of Childhood Aggression. Edited by Pepler DJ, Rubin KH. Hillsdale, NJ, Erlbaum, 1991, pp 201–208

Dodge K, Coie JD: Social-information processing factors in reactive and proactive aggression in children's peer groups. J Pers Soc Psychol 52:1146–1158, 1987

Donovan SJ, Susser ES, Nunes EV, et al: Divalproex treatment of disruptive adolescents: a report of 10 cases. J Clin Psychiatry 58:12–15, 1997

Donovan SJ, Stewart JW, Nunes EV, et al: Divalproex treatment for youth with explosive temper and mood lability: a double-blind, placebo-controlled crossover design. Am J Psychiatry 157:818–820, 2000

Donovan SJ, Nunes EV, Stewart JW, et al: Outer-directed irritability: a distinct mood syndrome in explosive youth with a disruptive behavior disorder? J Clin Psychiatry 64:698–701, 2003

DosReis S, Barnett S, Love RC: A guide for managing acute aggressive behavior of youths in residential and inpatient treatment facilities. Psychiatr Serv 54:1357–1363, 2003

Emslie GJ, Hughes CW, Crismon ML, et al: A feasibility study of the childhood depression medication algorithm: the Texas Children's Medication Algorithm Project (CMAP). J Am Acad Child Adolesc Psychiatry 43:519–527, 2004

Evans RW, Clay TH, Gualtieri CT: Carbamazepine in pediatric psychiatry. J Am Acad Child Adolesc Psychiatry 26:2–8, 1987

Farmer EM, Dorsey S, Mustillo SA: Intensive home and community interventions. Child Adolesc Psychiatr Clin N Am 13:857–884, 2004

Fenichel RR, Lipicky RJ: Combination products as first-line pharmacotherapy. Arch Intern Med 154:1429–1430, 1994

Findling RL, McNamara NK, Branicky LA, et al: A double-blind pilot study of risperidone in the treatment of conduct disorder. J Am Acad Child Adolesc Psychiatry 39:509–516, 2000

Findling RL, Reed MD, O'Riordan MA, et al: Effectiveness, safety, and pharmacokinetics of quetiapine in aggressive children with conduct disorder. J Am Acad Child Adolesc Psychiatry 45:792–800, 2006

Findling RL, Reed MD, O'Riordan MA, et al: A 26-week open-label study of quetiapine in children with conduct disorder. J Child Adolesc Psychopharmacol 17:1–9, 2007

Findling RL, Kauffman R, Sallee FR, et al: An open-label study of aripiprazole: pharmacokinetics, tolerability, and effectiveness in children and adolescents with conduct disorder. J Child Adolesc Psychopharmacol 19:431–439, 2009

Findling RL, Drury SS, Jensen PS, et al: Practice parameter for the use of atypical antipsychotic medications in children and adolescents. J Am Acad Child Adolesc Psychiatry (in press)

Fite PJ, Raine A, Stouthamer-Loeber M, et al: Reactive and proactive aggression in adolescent males: examining differential outcomes 10 years later in early adulthood. Crim Justice Behav 37:141–157, 2009

Fleischhaker C, Hennighausen K, Schneider-Momm K, et al: Ziprasidone for severe conduct and other disruptive behavior disorders in children and adolescents—a placebo-controlled, randomized, double-blind clinical trial. Poster presented at the joint annual meeting of the American Academy of Child and Adolescent Psychiatry and the Canadian Academy of Child and Adolescent Psychiatry, Toronto, Canada, October 2011

Fontaine NM, McCrory EJ, Boivin M, et al: Predictors and outcomes of joint trajectories of callous-unemotional traits and conduct problems in childhood. J Abnorm Psychol 120:730–742, 2011

Frick PJ, Moffitt TE: A proposal to the DSM-V Childhood Disorders and the ADHD and Disruptive Behavior Disorders Work Groups to include a specifier to the diagnosis of conduct disorder based on the presence of callous-unemotional traits. 2010. Available at: www.dsm5.org/Proposed%20Revision%20Attachments/Proposal%20for%20Callous%20and%20Unemotional%20Specifier%20of%20Conduct%20Disorder.pdf. Accessed May 12, 2012.

Gadow KD, Nolan EE, Sverd J, et al: Methylphenidate in children with oppositional defiant disorder and both comorbid chronic multiple tic disorder and ADHD. J Child Neurol 23:981–990, 2008

Galanter CA, Carlson GA, Jensen PS, et al: Response to methylphenidate in children with attention deficit hyperactivity disorder and manic symptoms in the multimodal treatment study of children with attention deficit hyperactivity disorder titration trial. J Child Adolesc Psychopharmacol 13:123–136, 2004

Gillberg C, Hellgren L: Mental disturbances in adolescents: a knowledge review. Nord Med 101:49–53, 1986

Gittelman-Klein R, Klein DF, Katz S, et al: Comparative effects of methylphenidate and thioridazine in hyperkinetic children, I: clinical results. Arch Gen Psychiatry 33:1217–1231, 1976

Gould MS, Walsh BT, Munfakh JL, et al: Sudden death and use of stimulant medications in youths. Am J Psychiatry 166:992–1001, 2009

Hazell PL, Stuart JE: A randomized controlled trial of clonidine added to psychostimulant medication for hyperactive and aggressive children. J Am Acad Child Adolesc Psychiatry 42:886–894, 2003

Hollander E, Dolgoff-Kaspar R, Cartwright C, et al: An open trial of divalproex sodium in autism spectrum disorders. J Clin Psychiatry 62:530–534, 2001

Horrigan JP, Barnhill LJ, Courvoisie HE: Olanzapine in PDD. J Am Acad Child Adolesc Psychiatry 36:1666–1667, 1997

Hunkeler EM, Fireman B, Lee J, et al: Trends in use of antidepressants, lithium, and anticonvulsants in Kaiser Permanente–insured youths, 1994–2003. J Child Adolesc Psychopharmacol 15:26–37, 2005

Jensen PS, Kettle L, Roper MT, et al. Are stimulants overprescribed? Treatment of ADHD in four U.S. communities. J Am Acad Child Adolesc Psychiatry 38:797–804, 1999

Jensen PS, Hinshaw SP, Kraemer HC, et al: ADHD comorbidity findings from the MTA study: comparing comorbid subgroups. J Am Acad Child Adolesc Psychiatry 40:147–158, 2001

Jensen PS, MacIntyre JC, Pappadopulos EA (eds): Treatment Recommendations for the Use of Antipsychotic Medications for Aggressive Youth (TRAAT): Pocket Reference Guide for Clinicians in Child and Adolescent Psychiatry. New York, New York State Office of Mental Health and Center for the Advancement of Children's Mental Health at Columbia University, Department of Child and Adolescent Psychiatry, 2004

Jensen PS, Youngstrom EA, Steiner H, et al: Consensus report on impulsive aggression as a symptom across diagnostic categories in child psychiatry: implications for medication studies. J Am Acad Child Adolesc Psychiatry 46:309–322, 2007

Jobson KO, Potter WZ: International psychopharmacology algorithm project report. Psychopharmacol Bull 31:457–459, 491–500, 1995

Kafantaris V, Campbell M, Padron-Gayol MV, et al: Carbamazepine in hospitalized aggressive conduct disorder children: an open pilot study. Psychopharmacol Bull 28:193–199, 1992

Kazdin AE: Child, parent and family dysfunction as predictors of outcome in cognitive-behavioral treatment of antisocial children. Behav Res Ther 33:271–281, 1995

Kazdin AE, Bass D, Siegel T, et al: Cognitive-behavioral therapy and relationship therapy in the treatment of children referred for antisocial behavior. J Consult Clin Psychol 57:522–535, 1989

Kazdin AE, Siegel TC, Bass D: Cognitive problem-solving skills training and parent management training in the treatment of antisocial behavior in children. J Consult Clin Psychol 60:733–747, 1992

Kimonis ER, Frick PJ, Boris NW, et al: Callous-unemotional features, behavioral inhibition, and parenting: independent predictors of aggression in a high-risk preschool sample. J Child Fam Stud 15:745–756, 2006

Klein RG, Abikoff H, Klass E, et al: Clinical efficacy of methylphenidate in conduct disorder with and without attention deficit hyperactivity disorder. Arch Gen Psychiatry 54:1073–1080, 1997

Kranzler H, Roofeh D, Gerbino-Rosen G, et al: Clozapine: its impact on aggressive behavior among children and adolescents with schizophrenia: clinical trial. J Am Acad Child Adolesc Psychiatry 44:55–63, 2005

Kronenberger WG, Giauque AL, Lafata DE, et al: Quetiapine addition in methylphenidate treatment-resistant adolescents with comorbid ADHD, conduct/oppositional-defiant disorder, and aggression: a prospective, open-label study. J Child Adolesc Psychopharmacol 17:334–347, 2007

Lahey BB, Loeber R, Quay HC, et al: Validity of DSM-IV subtypes of conduct disorder based on age of onset. J Am Acad Child Adolesc Psychiatry 37:435–442, 1998

Lisska MC, Rivkees SA: Daily methylphenidate use slows the growth of children: a community based study. J Pediatr Endocrinol Metab 16:711–718, 2003

Lochman JE, Curry JF: Effects of social problem-solving training and self-instruction training with aggressive boys. J Clin Child Psychol 15:159–164, 1986

Lochman JE, Lampron LB: Cognitive-behavioral interventions for aggressive boys: seven months follow-up effects. J Child Adolesc Psychotherapy 5:15–23, 1988

Loeber R, Keenen K, Lahey BB, et al: Evidence for developmentally based diagnoses of oppositional defiant disorder and conduct disorder. J Abnorm Child Psychol 21:377–410, 1993

Loeber R, Burke JD, Lahey BB: What are adolescent antecedents to antisocial personality disorder? Crim Behav Ment Health 12:24–36, 2002

Loeber R, Green SM, Lahey BB: Risk factors for antisocial personality, in Primary Prevention of Adult Antisocial Personality. Edited by Coid J, Farrington DP. Cambridge, UK, Cambridge University Press, 2003

Loeber R, Burke J, Pardini DA: Perspectives on oppositional defiant disorder, conduct disorder, and psychopathic features. J Child Psychol Psychiatry 50:133–142, 2009

Malone RP, Delaney MA, Luebbert JF, et al: A double-blind placebo-controlled study of lithium in hospitalized aggressive children and adolescents with conduct disorder. Arch Gen Psychiatry 57:649–654, 2000

Mannuzza S, Klein RG, Bessler A, et al: Adult outcome of hyperactive boys: educational achievement, occupational rank, and psychiatric status. Arch Gen Psychiatry 50:565–576, 1993

Mannuzza S, Klein RG, Bessler A, et al: Adult psychiatric status of hyperactive boys grown up. Am J Psychiatry 155:493–498, 1998

Marcus RN, Owen R, Manos G, et al: Aripiprazole in the treatment of irritability in pediatric patients (aged 6–17 years) with autistic disorder: results from a 52-week, open-label study. J Child Adolesc Psychopharmacol 21:229–236, 2011

Margolis CZ: Uses of clinical algorithms. JAMA 249:627–632, 1983

Martin A, Scahill L, Charney DS, et al (eds): Pediatric Psychopharmacology: Principles and Practice. Oxford, UK, Oxford University Press, 2003

McConville BJ, Sorter MT: Treatment challenges and safety considerations for antipsychotic use in children and adolescents with psychoses. J Clin Psychiatry 65:20–29, 2004

McCracken JT, McGough J, Shah B: Risperidone in children with autism and serious behavioral problems. N Engl J Med 347:314–321, 2002

Moffitt TE, Arseneault L, Jaffee SR, et al: Research review: DSM-V conduct disorder: research needs for an evidence base. J Child Psychol Psychiatry 49:3–33, 2008

MTA Cooperative Group: A 14-month randomized clinical trial of treatment strategies for attention-deficit/hyperactivity disorder. The MTA Cooperative Group. Multimodal Treatment Study of Children With ADHD. Arch Gen Psychiatry 56:1073–1086, 1999

MTA Cooperative Group: National Institute of Mental Health Multimodal Treatment Study of ADHD follow-up: 24-month outcomes of treatment strategies for attention-deficit/hyperactivity disorder. Pediatrics 113:754–761, 2004

Newcorn JH, Spencer TJ, Biederman J, et al: Atomoxetine treatment in children and adolescents with attention-deficit/hyperactivity disorder and comorbid oppositional defiant disorder. J Am Acad Adolesc Psychiatry 44:240–248, 2005

Olfson M, Blanco C, Liu L, et al: National trends in the outpatient treatment of children and adolescents with antipsychotic drugs. Arch Gen Psychiatry 63:679–685, 2006

Owen R, Sikich L, Marcus RN, et al: Aripiprazole in the treatment of irritability in children and adolescents with autistic disorder. Pediatrics 124:1533–1540, 2009

Padhy R, Saxena K, Remsing L, et al: Symptomatic response to divalproex in subtypes of conduct disorder. Child Psychiatry Hum Dev 42:584–593, 2011

Pappadopulos E, Macintyre JC, Crismon ML, et al: Treatment Recommendations for the Use of Antipsychotics for Aggressive Youth (TRAAY), Part II. J Am Acad Child Adolesc Psychiatry 42:145–161, 2003

Pappadopulos E, Tate Guelzow B, Wong C, et al: A review of the growing evidence base for pediatric psychopharmacology. Child Adolesc Psychiatr Clin N Am 13:817–855, 2004

Pappadopulos EA, Woolston S, Chait A, et al: Pharmacotherapy of aggression in children and adolescents: efficacy and effect size. J Can Acad Child Adolesc Psychiatry 15:27–39, 2006

Pardini DA, Fite PJ: Symptoms of conduct disorder, oppositional defiant disorder, and callous-unemotional traits as unique predictors of psychosocial maladjustment in boys: advancing an evidence base for DSM-V. J Am Acad Child Adolesc Psychiatry 49:1134–1144, 2010

Pardini DA, Loeber R: Interpersonal callousness trajectories across adolescence: early social influences and adult outcomes. Crim Justice Behav 35:173–196, 2008

Pliszka SR, Lopez M, Crismon ML, et al: A feasibility study of the Children's Medication Algorithm Project (CMAP) algorithm for the treatment of ADHD. J Am Acad Child Adolesc Psychiatry 42:279–287, 2003

Polzer J, Bangs ME, Zhang S, et al: Meta-analysis of aggression or hostility events in randomized, controlled clinical trials of atomoxetine for ADHD. Biol Psychiatry 61:713–719, 2007

Potenza MN, Holmes JP, Kanes SJ, et al: Olanzapine treatment of children, adolescents, and adults with pervasive developmental disorders: an open-label pilot study. J Clin Psychopharmacol 19:37–44, 1999

Rabinowitz J, Avnon M, Rosenberg V: Effect of clozapine on physical and verbal aggression. Schizophr Res 22:249–255, 1996

Research Units on Pediatric Psychopharmacology Autism Network: Risperidone treatment of autistic disorder: longer-term benefits and blinded discontinuation after 6 months. Am J Psychiatry 162:1361–1369, 2005

Reyes M, Buitelaar J, Toren P, et al: A randomized, double-blind, placebo-controlled study of risperidone maintenance treatment in children and adolescents with disruptive behavior disorders. Am J Psychiatry 163:402–410, 2006a

Reyes M, Croonenberghs J, Augustyns I, et al: Long-term use of risperidone in children with disruptive behavior disorders and subaverage intelligence: efficacy, safety, and tolerability. J Child Adolesc Psychopharmacol 16:260–272, 2006b

Riddle MA, Berstein GA, Cook EH, et al: Anxiolytics, adrenergic agents, and naltrexone. J Am Acad Child Adolesc Psychiatry 38:546–556, 1999

Rush AJ, Kupfer DJ: Strategies and Tactics in the Treatment of Depression, Vol 1, 2nd Edition. Washington, DC, American Psychiatric Press, 1995

Rush AJ, Rago WV, Crismon ML, et al: Medication treatment for the severely and persistently mentally ill: the Texas Medication Algorithm Project. J Clin Psychiatry 60:284–291, 1999

Saxena K, Howe M, Simeonova D, et al: Divalproex sodium reduces overall aggression in youth at high risk for bipolar disorder. J Child Adolesc Psychopharmacol 16:252–259, 2006

Scahill L, Chappell PB, Kim YS, et al: A placebo-controlled study of guanfacine in the treatment of children with tic disorders and attention deficit hyperactivity disorder. Am J Psychiatry 158:1067–1074, 2001

Schuhmann EM, Foote RC, Eyberg SM, et al: Efficacy of Parent-Child Interaction Therapy: interim report of a randomized trial with short-term maintenance. J Clin Child Psychol 27:34–45, 1998

Schur SB, Sikich L, Findling RL, et al: Treatment Recommendations for the Use of Antipsychotics for Aggressive Youth (TRAAY), part I: a review. J Am Acad Child Adolesc Psychiatry 42:132–144, 2003

Sikich L, Hamer RM, Bashford RA, et al: A pilot study of risperidone, olanzapine, and haloperidol in psychotic youth: a double-blind, randomized, 8-week trial. Neuropsychopharmacology 29:133–145, 2004

Simeon J, Milin R, Walker S: A retrospective chart review of risperidone use in treatment-resistant children and adolescents with psychiatric disorders. Prog Neuropsychopharmacol Biol Psychiatry 26:267–275, 2002

Snyder R, Turgay A, Aman M, et al: Effects of risperidone on conduct and disruptive behavior disorders in children with subaverage IQs. J Am Acad Child Adolesc Psychiatry 41:1026–1036, 2002

Steiner H: Practice parameters for the assessment and treatment of children and adolescents with conduct disorder. American Academy of Child and Adolescent Psychiatry. J Am Acad Child Adolesc Psychiatry 36(suppl):122S–139S, 1997

Steiner H: Divalproex sodium for the treatment of conduct disorder: a randomized clinical trial. J Clin Psychiatry 64:1183–1191, 2003

Steiner H, Saxena K, Chang K: Psychopharmacologic strategies for the treatment of aggression in juveniles. CNS Spectr 8:298–308, 2003

Steiner H, Silverman M, Karnik NS, et al: Psychopathology, trauma and delinquency: subtypes of aggression and their relevance for understanding youth offenders. Child Adolesc Psychiatry Ment Health 5:21, 2011

Stephens RJ, Bassel C, Sandor P: Olanzapine in the treatment of aggression and tics in children with Tourette's syndrome: a pilot study. J Child Adolesc Psychopharmacol 14:255–266, 2004

Stigler KA, Potenza MN, McDougle CJ: Tolerability profile of atypical antipsychotics in children and adolescents. Paediatr Drugs 3:927–942, 2001

Stigler KA, Potenza MN, Posey DJ, et al: Weight gain associated with atypical antipsychotic use in children and adolescents: prevalence, clinical relevance, and management. Paediatr Drugs 6:33–44, 2004

Swanson JM, Kraemer HC, Hinshaw SP, et al: Clinical relevance of the primary findings of the MTA: success rates based on severity of ADHD and ODD symptoms at the end of treatment. J Am Acad Child Adolesc Psychiatry 40:168–179, 2001

Szymanski L, King BH: Practice parameters for the assessment and treatment of children, adolescents, and adults with mental retardation and comorbid mental disorders. American Academy of Child and Adolescent Psychiatry Working Group on Quality Issues. J Am Acad Child Adolesc Psychiatry 38(suppl):5S–31S, 1999

Troost PW, Lahuis BE, Steenhuis MP, et al: Long-term effects of risperidone in children with autism spectrum disorders: a placebo discontinuation study. J Am Acad Child Adolesc Psychiatry 44:1137–1144, 2005

Turgay A: Treatment of comorbidity in conduct disorder with attention-deficit hyperactivity disorder (ADHD). Essent Psychopharmacol 6:277–290, 2005

Turgay A, Binder C, Snyder R, et al: Long-term safety and efficacy of risperidone for the treatment of disruptive behavior disorders in children with subaverage IQs. Pediatrics 110:E34, 2002

U.S. Food and Drug Administration: Antidepressant use in children, adolescents, and adults. Rockville, MD, U.S. Food and Drug Administration. 2005. Available at: www.fda.gov/cder/drug/antidepressants/default.htm. Accessed May 12, 2012.

U.S. Food and Drug Administration: Drug Safety and Risk Management Advisory Committee (DSaRM), Vol 1. Rockville, MD, U.S. Department of Health and Human Services, Food and Drug Administration, Center for Drug Evaluation and Research. 2006. Available at: www.fda.gov/ohrms/dockets/ac/06/transcripts/2006-4202t1.pdf. Accessed May 10, 2012.

U.S. Food and Drug Administration: Statistical review and evaluation: antiepileptic drugs and suicidality. Rockville, MD, U.S. Food and Drug Administration. 2008. Available at: www.fda.gov/ohrms/dockets/ac/08/briefing/2008-4372b1-01-fda.pdf. Accessed May 10, 2012.

U.S. Food and Drug Administration: Drug safety newsletter, Vol 2. Rockville, MD, U.S Food and Drug Administration, Center for Drug Evaluation and Research (CDER). 2009. Available at: www.fda.gov/downloads/Drugs/DrugSafety/DrugSafetyNewsletter/ucm107318.pdf. Accessed May 10, 2012.

U.S. Food and Drug Administration: FDA alert [09/05]: suicidal thinking in children and adolescents. Rockville, MD, U.S. Food and Drug Administration. January 27, 2010. Available at: www.fda.gov/Drugs/DrugSafety/PostmarketDrugSafetyInformationforPatientsandProviders/ucm124391.htm. Accessed May 12, 2012.

Vitaro F, Gendreau PL, Tremblay RE, et al: Reactive and proactive aggression differentially predict later conduct problems. J Child Psychol Psychiatry 39:377–385, 1998

Vitiello B, Stoff DM: Subtypes of aggression and their relevance to child psychiatry. J Am Acad Child Adolesc Psychiatry 36:307–315, 1997

Vitiello B, Behar D, Hunt J, et al: Subtyping aggression in children and adolescents. J Neuropsychiatry Clin Neurosci 2:189–192, 1990

Volavka J, Citrome L: Atypical antipsychotics in the treatment of the persistently aggressive psychotic patient: methodological concerns. Schizophr Res 35:23–33, 1999

Volkmar F, Cook EH Jr, Pomeroy J, et al: Practice parameters for the assessment and treatment of children, adolescents, and adults with autism and other pervasive developmental disorders. American Academy of Child and Adolescent Psychiatry Working Group on Quality Issues. J Am Acad Child Adolesc Psychiatry 38 (suppl): 32S–54S, 1999

Weiner B (ed): Physician's Desk Reference Generics, 2nd Edition. Montvale, NJ, Medical Economics, 1996

Werry JS: Severe conduct disorder: some key issues. Can J Psychiatry 42:577–583, 1997

Wudarsky M, Nicolson R, Hamburger SD, et al: Elevated prolactin in pediatric patients on typical and atypical antipsychotics. J Child Adolesc Psychopharmacol 9:239–245, 1999

4

Anxiety Disorders

Moira A. Rynn, M.D.

Olga Jablonka, B.A.

Lourival Baptista Neto, M.D.

Pablo H. Goldberg, M.D.

Anxiety disorders begin in childhood and often continue into adulthood, resulting in lifelong impairment in multiple areas, such as school achievement, work, relationships, and health. Anxiety disorders are insidious in nature and can lead to a person's experiencing of chronic symptoms, often without relief, due to a lack of identification and treatment of the anxiety problem. The illness can have a waxing and waning course. The lack of acknowledgment and, consequently, treatment is partly due to the belief on the part of patients and clinicians that symptoms of anxiety are an expected part of a normal life. A bias seems to exist among health care providers that suffering from an anxiety disorder is not as serious as suffering from other psychiatric disorders, such as major depression.

The sense that anxiety disorders are less serious than other disorders is reflected in the DSM definitions. Anxiety disorders were all classified as *psychoneurotic disorders* (reactions) in DSM-I (American Psychiatric Association 1952) and as neuroses in DSM-II (American Psychiatric Association 1968). It was not until DSM-III (American Psychiatric Association 1980) that anxiety disorders started to take shape with delineated criteria for children, including the diagnosis of separation anxiety disorder. In DSM-IV and DSM-IV-TR (American Psychiatric Association 1994, 2000), most childhood anxiety disorders are subsumed under the adult definitions for generalized anxiety disorder (GAD), obsessive-compulsive disorder (OCD), posttraumatic stress disorder (PTSD), social anxiety disorder, and panic disorder (Rickels and Rynn 2001). For example, children who in the past may have been diagnosed with overanxious disorder in childhood would currently receive the diagnosis of GAD on the basis of contemporary psychiatric nosology.

Epidemiology

Anxiety disorders, such as overanxious disorder, GAD, and social anxiety disorder, are among the most common diagnoses reported in childhood and adolescent epidemiological studies (Feehan et al. 1994; Lewinsohn et al. 1993; McGee et al. 1990). Beesdo et al. (2009) found that the lifetime prevalence rate of a child or adolescent meeting criteria for any anxiety disorder is about 15%–20%. In community epidemiological studies, the prevalence rates for overanxious disorder have ranged from 2.9% to 4.6%, and rates for separation anxiety disorder have ranged from 2.4% to 4.1% (Anderson et al. 1987; Bowen et al. 1990; Costello 1989). In a general pediatric clinical sample, 8%–10% of children met criteria for any anxiety disorder (Costello et al. 1988; Egger and Angold 2006).

In addition, social avoidance that interferes with functioning and is manifested in worries, isolation, hypersensitivity, sadness, and self-consciousness has been reported in 10%–20% of school-age children (Orvaschel and Weissman 1986; Werry 1986). Prevalence rates for internalizing disorders are greater in clinical samples, with 14% of patients being diagnosed with an anxiety disorder (Keller et al. 1992).

For specific anxiety disorders, the reported prevalence rates are variable (for review, see Costello et al. 2005): GAD/overanxious disorder is the most common, and separation anxiety disorder is the second most common. OCD and panic disorder each have a prevalence approaching 1% in population studies. However, these reported rates vary depending on whether the level of functional impairment is included in the definition. A child with some impaired functioning may not exhibit every symptom to satisfy the full diagnostic criteria and, unfortunately, may not be recommended to receive treatment.

Prevalence rates do not differ significantly between young boys and girls, but differences become noticeable in adolescence, when girls become two to three times more likely than boys to have an anxiety disorder (Costello et al. 2003; Rockhill et al. 2010).

Course and Outcome

Children with anxiety disorders often have low self-esteem and experience social isolation, which fosters inadequate social skills (Strauss 1988). These children also report higher rates of physical symptoms, such as headaches, stomachaches, and irritable bowel syndrome (Livingston et al. 1988). These symptoms can then increase visits to the pediatrician, leading to an increase in medical costs. Furthermore, the presence of anxiety disorders early in childhood may provide the pathway for developing subsequent mood and substance abuse disorders (Weissman et al. 1999). Pine and Grun (1998) reported that children with a history of long-term anxiety disorders exhibit increased rates of other psychiatric disorders, psychiatric hospitalization, and suicide attempts as adults.

Anxiety disorders and symptoms are not simply transitory but persist over time (Beidel et al. 1996; Cantwell and Baker 1989; Keller et al. 1992). Dadds et al. (1997) performed a school-based prevention study in which untreated anxious children were identified by self-report and/or teachers' ratings as having features of an anxiety disorder but not meeting the full diagnosis. Results revealed that 54% of those children developed a full anxiety disorder over the remaining 6 months of the study. Children with GAD/overanxious disorder have also been found to be at a higher risk for concurrent additional anxiety disorder (Last et al. 1987a). A prospective 3- to 4-year follow-up study by Last et al. (1996) showed that children with anxiety disorders, although free from their initial anxiety diagnosis at follow-up, were more likely than control subjects to develop new psychiatric disorders, usually a different anxiety disorder, over the time course.

An association also appears to exist between childhood disorders and the presence of adult anxiety disorders. A large number of adults diagnosed with anxiety report childhood histories of separation anxiety or overanxious disorders (Aronson and Logue 1987; Last et al. 1987b, 1987c). One of the few prospective studies that have assessed anxious children's adjustment to early adulthood found that anxious children, especially those with comorbid depression, were less likely than control subjects with no history of psychiatric illness to be living independently, working, or attending school (Last et al. 1997). In an outpatient setting, approximately 30% of children with an anxiety disorder have comorbid depression (for review, see Brady and Kendall 1992).

The Great Smoky Mountains Study (GSMS), a longitudinal study examining the development of emotional and behavioral disorders and the need for mental health treatment in North Carolina, has also provided valuable data regarding outcome predictions (Costello et al. 1996). Bittner et al. (2007) reported that within the GSMS sample, childhood separation anxiety was associated with subsequent separation anxiety in adolescence; childhood overanxious disorder was associated with the development of overanxious disorder, panic attacks, depression, and conduct disorder in adolescence; GAD was associated with conduct disorder; and social phobia in childhood was related to later social phobia, overanxious disorder, and attention-deficit/hyperactivity disorder (ADHD) in adolescence. Furthermore, the presence of comorbid anxiety and depression increased the chance of high-risk of substance use and suicidality (Federman et al. 1997; Foley et al. 2006).

In addition, some evidence suggests that up to 41% of children or adolescents with major depression had an anxiety disorder that preceded the depression (Brady and Kendall 1992; Kovacs et al. 1989). The presence of an anxiety disorder was found to predict a worse prognosis for the depression and, at times, had an effect on the length of or recovery from the depressive episode. Furthermore, after treatment of and recovery from depression, the anxiety disorder usually persisted (Kovacs et al. 1989). Early treatment intervention for anxiety disorders may prevent and alter the course of developing depression and other psychiatric disorders, leading to an improved opportunity for a successful adulthood.

Rationale and Justification for Psychopharmacological Treatment

In recent history, there have been major developments in the treatment of pediatric anxiety disorders with medications. Strong evidence suggests that antidepressants, particularly selective serotonin reuptake inhibitors (SSRIs), are safe and efficacious for treating these disorders. In addition, an extensive literature supports the use of cognitive-behavioral therapy (CBT) for the treatment of pediatric anxiety disorders. The American Academy of Child and Adolescent Psychiatry (2007) practice parameters for treating anxiety recommend that psychosocial treatments such as CBT, if available, be considered first for the treatment of anxious children. Unfortunately, one of the challenges often faced by clinicians recommending CBT is the limited availability of this treatment in many communities, in which case medication treatment is initiated instead.

Another consideration concerning the use of medications is the risk-benefit profile. The available safety data from completed randomized controlled trials (RCTs) demonstrate that the adverse-effect profiles of SSRIs in children resemble those in adults and that, overall, these medications are safe and well tolerated. However, the U.S. Food and Drug Administration (FDA) has required a black box warning on all antidepressants because of concern for a potentially increased risk of suicidal ideation and/or behaviors for children taking these medications. In contrast to the pediatric depression RCTs, the majority of pediatric anxiety studies did not show evidence of increased suicidal thinking or behaviors for children taking medications compared with placebo. An alternative option is combined treatment of CBT with medication. An emerging literature, reviewed later in "Combination Treatment," suggests that combined treatment may provide some advantages.

Medications for Pediatric Anxiety Disorders: Review of Treatment Studies

Selective Serotonin Reuptake Inhibitors

To date, the most widely researched pharmacological treatments for pediatric anxiety disorders are SSRIs (Table 4–1). The class of SSRIs includes fluox-

Table 4–1. Medications for pediatric anxiety disorders

Drug	TDD	Dosing schedule	Main indications	Side effects/prescribing considerations
ANTIDEPRESSANTS				
Selective serotonin reuptake inhibitors				
Citalopram	20–40 mg	qd (A.M.)	Social phobia	Gastrointestinal side effects, weight gain and loss, sweating, dry mouth, headaches, irritability, insomnia, fatigue, hypersomnia, restlessness, increased hyperactivity, tremor, increased risk for self-injury and self-injurious behaviors, mania, withdrawal effects, sexual side effects
Fluoxetine	10–60 mg	qd (A.M.)	OCD, GAD, SAD, SOC	
Fluvoxamine	50–300 mg	qd (A.M.)	OCD, GAD, SAD, SOC	
Paroxetine	10–40 mg	qd (A.M.)	SAD, SOC	
Sertraline	25–200 mg	qd (A.M.)	Panic disorder	
Serotonin-norepinephrine reuptake inhibitors				
Venlafaxine XR	37.5–225 mg	qd	GAD, SAD, SOC	Gastrointestinal side effects, headache, weight loss, fatigue, insomnia, irritability, hypersomnia Monitor blood pressure
Tricyclic antidepressants				
Tertiary amines				
Clomipramine	2.0–5.0 mg/kg	qd or bid	OCD, school refusal	Anticholinergic effects such as dizziness, drowsiness, and dry mouth
Imipramine	2.0–5.0 mg/kg	qd or bid	GAD, panic disorder	Requires electrocardiographic monitoring
Secondary amines				
Desipramine	2.0–5.0 mg/kg	qd or bid	OCD	Potential for cardiac toxicity

Table 4–1. Medications for pediatric anxiety disorders *(continued)*

Drug	TDD	Dosing schedule	Main indications	Side effects/prescribing considerations
BENZODIAZEPINES				
Long-acting				
Clonazepam[a]	0.25–2 mg	qd, bid, tid	GAD, panic disorder	Sedation, drowsiness, decreased alertness, disinhibition Requires taper
Short- to intermediate-acting				
Alprazolam[a]	0.25–4 mg	prn, qd, bid, tid	GAD, panic disorder	Sedation, drowsiness, decreased alertness, disinhibition Requires taper
Lorazepam[a]	0.25–6 mg	prn, qd, bid, tid	GAD, panic disorder	Sedation, drowsiness, decreased alertness, disinhibition Requires taper
NONBENZODIAZEPINES				
Buspirone	0.2–0.6 mg/kg	bid or tid	OCD, GAD, SOC	Light-headedness, dizziness, nausea, sedation

Note. GAD = generalized anxiety disorder; OCD = obsessive-compulsive disorder; SAD = separation anxiety disorder; SOC = social anxiety disorder; TDD = total daily dose.
[a]Adjunct treatment.

etine (Prozac), sertraline (Zoloft), fluvoxamine (Luvox), paroxetine (Paxil), and citalopram (Celexa), among others. Although SSRIs are characterized as antidepressants, they are unique in that they specifically inhibit the reuptake of the neurotransmitter serotonin, therefore resulting in increased amounts of serotonin in the synapses of the brain. Decreased serotonin levels are attributed to various disorders, including depression (Roy et al. 1989) and anxiety disorders (Nutt and Lawson 1992; Pigott 1996; Tancer 1993). Extensive empirical literature supports the efficacy of SSRIs in treating adult anxiety disorders (Katzelnick et al. 1995; Liebowitz et al. 2002; Pohl et al. 1998; Pollack et al. 2001).

Efficacy of Acute Treatment

The use of SSRIs and other, newer antidepressants in the U.S. population under age 18 years increased significantly from 0.8% in 1997 to 1.6% in 2002 ($P<0.001$; Vitiello et al. 2006). As a result of the evidence presented in the current literature and the relatively minimal side effects, SSRIs are presently considered the first-line pharmacotherapy choice for childhood anxiety disorders. Although numerous promising open-label studies have been conducted (Birmaher et al. 1994; Compton et al. 2001), the RCTs discussed in the following subsections are those that demonstrate the most compelling evidence for the acute treatment with SSRIs.

Fluoxetine.   To date, numerous well-designed fluoxetine studies for the treatment of pediatric anxiety disorders have been reported. Black and Uhde (1994) conducted a double-blind, placebo-controlled trial to examine the efficacy of fluoxetine in treating children (ages 5–16) with the primary diagnosis of elective mutism. Sixteen children were given a placebo run-in for 2 weeks. The nonresponders were then randomly assigned to receive either placebo ($n=9$) or fluoxetine (n=6; mean maximum dosage=21.4 mg/day, range=12–27 mg/day) for another 12 weeks.

By the end of the trial, although the subjects in the fluoxetine group showed great improvement over time on all parent, patient, and clinician ratings, an analysis of variance (ANOVA) indicated few significant results. The fluoxetine group, compared with the placebo group, showed significantly greater improvement in one symptom—namely, mutism—as reflected by change in ratings on two of the nine parent scales, the mutism (Clinical Global Impression [CGI]) scale ($P<0.0003$) and global CGI scale ($P<0.04$), and on one teacher rating, the Conners Anxiety Scale ($P<0.02$). The proportion of subjects rated as treatment responders based on the parent's rating of mutism change ($P<0.03$) and global change ($P<0.03$) was also significantly greater in the fluoxetine group. Side effects were minimal and did not differ significantly between treatment groups (Black and Uhde 1994).

Several reasons may account for the lack of significant results in Black and Uhde's (1994) study. The sample size was relatively small, and the length of the trial may not have been long enough to show the effects of fluoxetine, given that treatment response did not increase markedly until weeks 8–12. In addition, the investigators note that timing may have affected treatment response. Clinical response in an earlier case report (Black and Uhde 1992), in which treatment began before the start of the school year, was more striking than in the 1994 study, which was carried out in the last half of the school year, when children with elective mutism may have already known what to expect from their teachers and peers and were less motivated to improve.

In a later, double-blind, placebo-controlled trial, Geller et al. (2001) studied response to fluoxetine in children and adolescents diagnosed with OCD. Subjects were randomly assigned to receive fluoxetine ($n=71$; mean total daily dose [TDD] = 24.6 mg) or placebo ($n=32$) for 13 weeks; the fluoxetine was initiated at 10 mg/day for the first 2 weeks, and the dosage was then increased to 20 mg/day. If subjects were unresponsive to treatment, as indicated by no change or worsening on the CGI Severity of Illness subscale (CGI-S), the medication could be titrated to 40 mg/day at week 4 and again to 60 mg/day at week 7.

In an intent-to-treat analysis, Geller et al. (2001) found that subjects randomly assigned to receive fluoxetine showed a greater reduction of OCD severity on the primacy efficacy measure, the Children's Yale-Brown Obsessive Compulsive Scale (CY-BOCS) total score ($P=0.026$), with the reduction tending toward significance at week 5 ($P=0.086$) and reaching significance thereafter ($P<0.05$). Almost half (49%) of the subjects in the fluoxetine group were considered responders (with response defined as a 40% or greater reduction of symptoms on the CY-BOCS), compared with 25% in the placebo group (Mantel-Haenszel exact $P=0.030$). In addition, significantly more subjects in the fluoxetine group than in the placebo group were rated as *much improved* or *very much improved* on the CGI Improvement (CGI-I) scale

(55% vs. 18.8% placebo, P<0.001). Patient and parent improvement ratings also reflected this trend (P<0.001). Fluoxetine was well tolerated in this trial, with no adverse effects occurring significantly more often in the fluoxetine group than in the placebo group.

Although the results of this study by Geller et al. (2001) do support the efficacy of fluoxetine in treating children and adolescents with OCD, there are some notable limitations in these findings. The investigators point out that the week in which treatment differences became significant occurred slightly later in this trial than in similar trials using different SSRIs. Also, the study design did not allow for a comparison of efficacy between fixed doses of fluoxetine, so it is difficult to determine whether the higher dosage caused treatment effects or whether subjects would have improved at a later point in the study while taking a lower dose. Results are supported by a similar crossover trial (Riddle et al. 1992).

Birmaher et al. (2003) completed a fluoxetine treatment study involving children and adolescents diagnosed with separation anxiety disorder, social phobia, and/or GAD. Seventy-four individuals (ages 7–17) were randomly assigned to receive placebo or fluoxetine (maximum dosage = 20 mg/day) for 12 weeks. The investigators found that at treatment end the fluoxetine group showed significantly more improvement on the CGI-I, the primary outcome variable (61% vs. 35% placebo, $\chi^2 = 4.93$). Fluoxetine-treated subjects diagnosed with social phobia seemed to have the best outcome, with significantly higher scores on the CGI-I ($\chi^2 = 12.13$) and the Children's Global Assessment Scale (CGAS) ($\chi^2 = 6.01$) than those given placebo. Side effects in this study were minimal for the most part but included occasional headaches, drowsiness, abdominal pain, nausea, and agitation. The investigators noted that by the end of the trial, approximately half of the subjects remained symptomatic, and suggested that some subjects may have required a higher dosage or may have fared better with concurrent psychotherapy.

Sertraline.   RCTs using sertraline as treatment have focused on pediatric populations diagnosed with OCD and GAD. In a double-blind, placebo-controlled trial, March et al. (1998) tested the efficacy of sertraline for 107 children (ages 6–12) and 80 adolescents (ages 13–17) with OCD. Subjects were randomly assigned to receive placebo ($n = 95$) or sertraline ($n = 92$) for 12 weeks, with the dosage starting at 25 mg/day for children and 50 mg/day for adolescents and then titrated upward (in a forced design) by 50 mg/week to a maximum of 200 mg/day (mean TDD = 167 mg). Efficacy analyses revealed that by the end of week 2, subjects treated with sertraline showed significantly greater improvement than subjects taking placebo on the primary outcome measures, the CY-BOCS ($P=0.005$) and the National Institute of Mental Health Global Obsessive Compulsive Scale (NIMH-GOCS, $P=0.002$). In addition, 53% of the sertraline-treated subjects were considered responders compared with 37% of the placebo group ($P=0.03$) as indicated by the CY-BOCS. Results were similar on the NIMH-GOCS (42% vs. 26%, $P=0.02$). Side effects in this trial were generally mild to moderate, with sertraline-treated subjects reporting significantly more incidences of insomnia, nausea, agitation, and tremor ($P<0.05$).

The results of this study by March et al. (1998) indicate that sertraline is efficacious in treating children and adolescents with OCD in the short term. As in other studies, some subjects continued to exhibit symptoms at the end of the trial, which may indicate the need for concurrent psychotherapy.

Rynn et al. (2001) subsequently conducted a double-blind, placebo-controlled trial assessing the efficacy of a lower daily dose of sertraline (50 mg/day) in children and adolescents diagnosed with GAD ($N=22$, ages 5–17). An analysis of covariance (ANCOVA) on the primary outcome variables revealed that significant treatment differences were apparent by week 4 and continued until the end of the study. At the end of week 9, compared with subjects taking placebo, the subjects receiving sertraline were rated as endorsing fewer symptoms on all Hamilton Anxiety Rating Scale scores (Total, $F=15.3$, $P<0.001$; Psychic Factor, $F=22.6$, $P<0.001$; Somatic Factor, $F=8.9$, $P<0.01$), measuring less severity on the CGI-S ($F=30.5$, $P<0.001$), and showing greater improvement on the CGI-I ($F=14.9$, $P<0.001$). At treatment endpoint, 90% of sertraline-treated subjects were considered improved based on CGI-I scores (1 or 2), as opposed to 10% of subjects taking placebo ($P<0.001$, Fisher exact test). However, only 18% of the subjects in the improved sertraline group were rated as markedly improved, which represents a small remission rate. Side effects did not differ significantly between the sertraline and placebo groups. This trial suggests that 50 mg/day of sertraline may be an effective, safe dosage for short-term use in young patients diagnosed with GAD, resulting in a reduction in both psychic and somatic symptoms of anxiety with mild side effects.

Fluvoxamine.   In a multisite, randomized, placebo-controlled study, Riddle et al. (2001) examined the effects of fluvoxamine in pediatric OCD. Following a 1- to 2-week single-blind screening period, eligible subjects ($N=120$, ages 8–17) were randomly assigned to receive placebo or fluvoxamine (maximum dosage of 200 mg/day) for 10 weeks. Investigators found that fluvoxamine was significantly more effective than placebo in ameliorating OCD symptoms on all measures. A two-way ANOVA on the CY-BOCS total score revealed significant treatment effects at weeks 1, 2, 3, 4, 6, and 10. At the end of the study, 42% of subjects taking fluvoxamine were defined as treatment responders, having had a 25% reduction of symptoms on the CY-BOCS since baseline, compared with 25% of subjects taking placebo ($P=0.065$, Cochran-Mantel-Haenszel test). Responder analysis on the CGI-Clinician also revealed that significantly more fluvoxamine-treated subjects had a meaningful response to treatment (*much improved* or *very much improved*) at the end of 10 weeks (29.8% vs. 17.5% placebo, $P=0.078$, Cochran-Mantel-Haenszel test). Adverse effects that were significantly more prevalent in the fluvoxamine group included asthenia (fatigue, loss of energy, or weakness) and insomnia.

Riddle et al. (2001) demonstrated that fluvoxamine is both fast acting and effective as a short-term pediatric OCD treatment. A limitation of the study is that most subjects did not have comorbid diagnoses, and therefore the sample differs somewhat from the typical OCD population, in which psychiatric comorbidity is high.

In another large-scale study, the Research Units on Pediatric Psychopharmacology (RUPP) Anxiety Study Group ("Fluvoxamine for the Treatment of Anxiety Disorders in Children and Adolescents" 2001) assessed the efficacy of fluvoxamine treatment in children and adolescents ($N=128$, ages 6–17) who met the criteria for social phobia, separation anxiety disorder, or GAD. The children were randomly assigned to receive fluvoxamine ($n=63$) or placebo ($n=65$) for 8 weeks. Fluvoxamine was titrated upward 50 mg/week to a maximum of 300 mg/day for adolescents and 250 mg/day for children ages 12 years and younger. From an intent-to-treat analysis, the investigators found that fluvoxamine-treated subjects had a greater reduction of anxiety symptoms and higher rates of clinical response than did subjects in the placebo group. Treatment differences on one primary outcome variable, the Pediatric Anxiety Rating Scale (PARS), reached significance by week 3 and increased through week 6. By the end of the study, the fluvoxamine group showed significantly lower PARS scores, indicating mild symptoms of anxiety ($P<0.001$). The CGI-I score, which defines meaningful clinical response to treatment as scores of 3 (*improved*), 2 (*much improved*), or 1 (*free of symptoms*), revealed that at study endpoint, significantly more fluvoxamine-treated participants than subjects given placebo received scores of <4 (76% vs. 29% placebo, $P<0.001$). Fluvoxamine-treated subjects reported significantly more abdominal discomfort ($P=0.02$) and showed a trend for increased motor activity ($P=0.06$).

Following the acute trial, the RUPP group investigated possible moderators and mediators of pharmacological treatment in children and adolescents with anxiety disorders (Walkup et al. 2003). Even though no significant moderators were found, analyses revealed that subjects presenting with social phobia ($P<0.05$) and a greater severity of baseline illness ($P<0.001$) were less likely to improve, regardless of treatment group.

Paroxetine.   In a placebo-controlled, multicenter trial, Wagner et al. (2004) evaluated the effects of paroxetine in children and adolescents diagnosed with social anxiety disorder ($N=319$, ages 8–17). Subjects were randomly assigned to receive either paroxetine ($n=163$, mean dosage=24.8 mg/day) or placebo ($n=156$) for a 16-week trial. Results at week 16 demonstrated that 77.6% of paroxetine-treated subjects were defined as treatment responders, having a score of *improved* or *much improved* on the CGI-I, compared with 38.3% of subjects taking placebo ($P<0.001$). This trend appeared even within the first 4 weeks of treatment. Adverse effects were rated from mild to moderate in severity, with insomnia ($P=0.02$), decreased appetite ($P=0.11$), and vomiting ($P=0.07$) considered treatment-emergent effects. Because paroxetine treatment exhibited a greater response rate than placebo and treatment differences reached significance on all five secondary outcome variables, Wagner et al. (2004) supported the use of paroxetine in treating pediatric social anxiety disorder. Another interesting finding is that the children and adolescents in this study (77.6%) demonstrated a greater response to treatment than did socially anxious adults treated with paroxetine (55%; Stein et al. 1998). The investigators acknowledged that commonly occurring comorbid disorders, such as major depression, were identified as exclusions and that, therefore, their findings cannot be generalized to a broader population. Similar findings were presented in another large-scale, multisite trial (Geller et al. 2004).

Meta-analytic data.   No meta-analyses of trials using SSRIs on a short-term basis to treat pure pediatric anxiety disorders have been reported to date. However, a meta-analysis of pediatric OCD trials conducted by Geller et al. (2003) reveals a highly significant pooled effect for each SSRI and clomipramine against placebo ($P<0.001$). There were no significant pooled mean differences between one SSRI and another, indicating that no one SSRI was more efficacious than another in treating pediatric OCD. There was, however, a significant pooled mean difference favoring clomipramine over the SSRIs ($P=0.002$, χ^2 test), indicating that clomipramine was more effective in reducing OCD symptoms across studies.

Although this analysis showed clomipramine to be superior to the SSRIs, Geller et al. (2003) did not recommend using clomipramine as a first-line pharmacological agent because of its side-effect profile and association with cardiac toxicity. The investigators suggest that in less severe cases, SSRIs should be the first-choice medication, specifying that the choice of individual SSRI should be based more on adverse-effect profiles and pharmacokinetic properties such as half-life than on efficacy.

Risks of Selective Serotonin Reuptake Inhibitors

Currently, the FDA has approved only the following SSRIs for the treatment of pediatric OCD: fluoxetine, sertraline, and fluvoxamine. The consensus is that in most cases, the benefits of SSRIs outweigh their risks. However, the use of psychopharmaceuticals, including SSRIs, for child and adolescent disorders is not without risk. SSRI-related side effects include nausea, diarrhea, gastrointestinal distress, headaches, lack of energy, sweating, dry mouth, restlessness, initial insomnia, sleepiness, increased hyperactivity, and tremor. These problems are usually short-lived, are dose related, and tend to resolve with time.

The possibility of discontinuation symptoms exists, however, with some SSRIs, such as paroxetine, which has increasingly been associated with a withdrawal syndrome upon discontinuation (Leonard et al. 1997). Withdrawal symptoms do not generally occur with fluoxetine because of its long half-life, and they are of less concern with sertraline because of the presence of its one weak metabolite. Some trials (Geller et al. 2001; Riddle et al. 2001) also reported cases of subjects who showed abnormal vital signs, an unsurprising finding given that medication has been associated with changes in weight and decreases in blood pressure. As with any medication, there is always a risk of allergic reaction.

In addition to these issues, the FDA issued an advisory to physicians that the use of antidepressants may lead to suicidal thinking or attempts in youth. This warning highlights the need for close observation for signs of worsening symptoms and the emergence of suicidality in children treated with these medications.

Efficacy of Long-Term Treatment and Maintenance

Benefits.   Following their acute trial described above in the section on flu-voxamine, the RUPP group conducted a 6-month, open-label extension study (Walkup et al. 2002) to examine the effects of continuing fluvoxamine treatment or treatment with a second SSRI in remaining subjects. The study design was such that active treatment responders from the acute trial continued with fluvoxamine treatment (Group I, $n=35$), active nonresponders switched to fluoxetine treatment (Group II, $n=14$), and placebo nonresponders began fluvoxamine treatment (Group III, $n=48$), with dosage schedules that varied according to treatment group.

This study was not controlled, and therefore data analyses are suggestive and pertain more to clinical functioning. Using the CGI-I as a primary outcome measure, the investigators found that 94% of subjects who continued taking open-label fluvoxamine (mean final dosage=131 mg/day) were considered responders, with scores of ≤ 3 after 24 weeks, and maintained response. After 24 weeks, 71% of subjects who were administered fluoxetine (mean final dosage=24 mg/day) met the criteria for response. Finally, 56% of placebo nonresponders initiated on open-label fluvoxamine (135 mg/day) were considered responders at week 24. Side effects were mild and generally transient. Data from this extension study suggest that relapse rates for anxious children maintained on SSRI treatment are low and that extended SSRI treatment is generally safe.

In addition to the RUPP extension study, data from long-term OCD trials can provide some indication of the efficacy and safety of maintenance treatment with SSRIs. Following a 12-week double-blind study (March et al. 1998), Cook et al. (2001) conducted a 52-week sertraline extension trial for subjects who completed the acute phase. Dosages for subjects ($N=137$, ages 6–18) were titrated to and maintained at the level at which the subjects exhibited satisfactory clinical response (not to exceed 200 mg/day). Data analysis was performed according to age (children: $n=72$, mean dosage = 108 mg/day; adolescents: $n=65$, mean dosage = 132 mg/day). Response rates, with response defined as a greater than 25% decrease in the baseline CY-BOCS score and a CGI-I score of 1 or 2 at trial endpoint, were 67% for the combined age groups, 72% for children, and 61% for adolescents. Significant improvements over treatment were evident on all outcome measures ($P<0.05$). By the end of the study, 85% of active treatment responders who completed the full 52 weeks maintained responder status as compared with 43% of nonresponders. Side effects were common, with an incidence of 77% among all subjects, and included headache, insomnia, nausea, diarrhea, somnolence, abdominal pain, hyperkinesias, nervousness, dyspepsia, and vomiting.

These results provide support for long-term sertraline treatment in youths with OCD. The most striking feature of the analyses is that of those subjects who did not respond to sertraline in the acute phase, 43% were considered responders by the end of the extension trial. Although side effects generally improved as treatment continued, the percentage of subjects withdrawing because of adverse events (12%) seems somewhat high in comparison with other trials.

A smaller trial assessing the long-term effects of citalopram concurrent with CBT on adolescents with OCD (Thomsen et al. 2001) revealed similar results. After a 10-week, open-label trial ($N=23$) of citalopram (maximum dosage = 40 mg/day, Thomsen 1997), subjects given citalopram ($N=30$, ages 13–18) continued in an open trial (mean dosage = 46.5 mg/day, range = 20–80 mg/day) for a 6-month to 2-year period. Although 28 subjects continued taking citalopram for 1 year, only 14 completed the 2-year study. Analyzing data from baseline to the 2-year endpoint, investigators found that the decrease in scores on the CY-BOCS or Yale-Brown Obsessive Compulsive Scale (Y-BOCS) was statistically significant for each time period (baseline to 10 weeks, 10 weeks to 6 months, 6 months to 1 year, and baseline to 2 years, $P=0.000$) except for the time from the 1-year endpoint to the 2-year endpoint. This finding indicates that subjects maintaining citalopram treatment for 4.5 months following the acute trial continued to exhibit a reduction of symptoms on the CY-BOCS or Y-BOCS, with an even greater reduction in the next 6 months, and that symptom reduction did not continue in the second year of treatment. Side effects, similar to those reported in other SSRI trials, were generally mild and decreased with continued treatment. Only sexual dysfunction and sedation were reported as persistent, causing two subjects to drop out of the trial.

In addition to these trial reports, review articles provide guidance on long-term SSRI use in children and adolescents. In his review of acute-anxiety trials and adult and animal studies, Pine (2002) argued that children who have shown satisfactory response to SSRI treatment should be given a medication-free trial instead of maintaining long-term treatment, and should be promptly returned to medication if they show a relapse. Evidence from longitudinal data suggests that mood and anxiety disorders evident in childhood carry a significant risk for mood and anxiety disorders later in life; if left untreated, these disorders may have considerable harmful effects on development, with possible long-term implications. Pine stated that this finding must be weighed against potential risks in using long-term SSRI medication. Evidence from animal studies also provides an interesting dilemma. Although serotonin plays a role in neural plasticity, and long-term SSRI use may adversely affect cellular processes that involve serotonin, stress in early life can also greatly impact brain development. Thus, Pine (2002) put forth the recommendation that another treatment be selected following successful SSRI treatment to minimize risks and still maximize benefit.

Risks.   Side effects reported in studies of long-term SSRI use were similar to those reported in acute trials. These effects, which included gastrointestinal disturbance, headache, and insomnia, were often mild in nature and decreased with continued treatment. Overall, adverse effects did not typically lead to study withdrawal, and most trials had relatively low dropout rates. However, some long-term studies included reports of hyperkinesia (Cook et al. 2001) that was severe enough to warrant study withdrawal, in addition to persistent complaints of sexual dysfunction and sedation (Thomsen et al. 2001). There have also been reports (Weintrob et al. 2002) documenting a decrease in growth rate among children treated with various SSRIs at dosages of 20–100 mg/day for a period ranging from 6 months to 5 years.

Serotonin-Norepinephrine Reuptake Inhibitors

Pharmacological treatments tend to focus on several neurotransmitter systems believed to form the biological foundation of anxiety disorders, such as serotonin and γ-aminobutyric acid (GABA). Another class of medications that shows promise in the treatment of pediatric anxiety disorders is the selective serotonin-norepinephrine reuptake inhibitors (SNRIs), which target both the serotonergic and noradrenergic systems. The SNRI venlafaxine XR (extended release) has been shown to be effective in adult GAD at TDDs between 75 and 225 mg in several large, double-blind, placebo-controlled trials (Davidson et al. 1999; Gelenberg et al. 2000; Rickels et al. 2000). As has been the case with SSRI use, children with anxiety disorders appear to respond to venlafaxine XR in the same manner as adults (Rynn et al. 2004). Duloxetine, another SNRI, is also considered effective for adult major depression and possibly for adult GAD (Rynn et al. 2007), although investigation continues.

Efficacy of Acute Treatment

Benefits.   Rynn et al. (2007) reported the results of a pooled analysis of two combined multisite, 8-week studies examining the efficacy and safety of venlafaxine XR ($n=154$) compared with placebo ($n=159$) in the treatment of GAD in children ages 6–17 ($P<0.001$). Exclusions included concurrent psychiatric disorders, such as major depressive disorder, social anxiety disorder, and separation anxiety disorder. Dosing for venlafaxine XR began with 37.5 mg/day, and the TDD was increased on the basis of body weight (children ≥50 kg, maximum dose = 225 mg; children 40–49 kg, dose range = 75–150 mg; children 25–39 kg, dose range = 37.5–112.5 mg). Analysis revealed that one of the two studies showed statistically significant improvement favoring venlafaxine XR on both primary ($P<0.001$) and secondary ($P<0.01$) outcome measures. The other study showed significant improvement for venlafaxine XR in some secondary outcome measures, but not in the primary measure ($P=0.06$). Pooled analysis indicated a greater mean decrease on the primary outcome for venlafaxine XR versus placebo (–17.4 vs. –12.7; $P<0.001$). Rates of response (defined as a CGI-I score <3) were also significantly greater for venlafaxine XR than for placebo (69% vs. 48%; $P=0.004$).

Tourian et al. (2004) found similar results when comparing venlafaxine XR ($n=137$) and placebo ($n=148$) in children and adolescents (ages 8–17) with social anxiety disorder ($P<0.001$) over 16 weeks. Subjects with scores ≥50 on the Social Anxiety Scale (SAS), a CGI-S score ≥4, and no concurrent psychiatric disorder were eligible. Results showed that baseline-to-endpoint improvement in total SAS scores was significantly higher for the venlafaxine

XR group compared with the placebo group (22.5 vs.14.9 points, adjusted change; $P < 0.001$).

Risks. In the Rynn et al. (2007) study, the incidence of asthenia, pain, anorexia, and somnolence in subjects treated with venlafaxine XR ($\geq 5\%$) was twice that of the placebo group. Only the development of anorexia differed significantly between the venlafaxine XR (13%) and placebo groups (3%); also, two medication-treated subjects displayed suicidal ideation and behavior, leading to their removal from the study. In addition, those children treated with venlafaxine XR had statistically significant mean increases from baseline cholesterol serum levels, as well as statistically significant mean changes from baseline in vital signs, with a difference in pulse rate of approximately 4 beats/minute and a difference in blood pressure (supine diastolic and systolic) of approximately 2 mm Hg for those children treated with venlafaxine XR. The venlafaxine XR–treated group had a height increase from baseline of 0.3 cm ($P < 0.05$), compared with 1.0 cm ($P < 0.001$) in children receiving placebo (difference between groups: $P = 0.041$).

In Tourian et al.'s (2004) study, the most common adverse effects among venlafaxine XR–treated patients were flu, anorexia, asthenia, weight loss, nausea, and pharyngitis. Three adolescents in the medication group also displayed suicidal ideation, as opposed to none in the placebo arm. The venlafaxine XR–treated patients experienced significant mean weight loss compared with placebo ($P < 0.001$); in several cases, the weight loss was considered clinically significant ($n = 8$).

Efficacy of Long-Term Treatment and Maintenance

Two adult venlafaxine XR studies (Allgulander et al. 2001; Gelenberg et al. 2000) were conducted to assess response to 6 months of treatment with venlafaxine XR compared with placebo. Results indicated no tolerance to the efficacy of venlafaxine XR over the 6-month treatment period. Although neither study was designed to assess relapse rates after treatment discontinuation as a function of long-term treatment, both suggest that patients with GAD can benefit from at least 6 months of continuous treatment. Presently, there are no pediatric anxiety studies that evaluate the long-term use of this class of compound, and the risks are unknown.

Benzodiazepines

Benzodiazepines have been used as effective anxiolytics and sedatives in adults since they first appeared in clinical practice in the early 1960s, before their mechanism of action was understood. It was not until almost two decades later that researchers discovered specific benzodiazepine receptors on the neurons of the brain and began to understand how benzodiazepines produce their varying effects. Following this discovery, researchers posited that benzodiazepines function by activating GABA, an inhibitory neurotransmitter, which slows the response of neural activity in the brain and produces an overall sedating effect.

Although the exact chemical process by which benzodiazepines produce anxiolytic effects has yet to be determined, the effect of benzodiazepines is strongly linked to the relationship between benzodiazepines and the GABAergic system. Bernstein and Shaw (1993) hypothesized that because abnormalities in norepinephrine and GABA levels in the brain are thought to underlie anxiety disorders, correcting these levels with agents such as benzodiazepines should lead to a reduction of anxiety symptoms. Future research in the field should indicate the precise mechanism.

Benzodiazepines vary widely in terms of what are considered to be their effective daily dose and half-life, which represents how fast the drug is metabolized by the body. Although, according to the cited literature, some benzodiazepines, such as clonazepam, can be effective in adults at a TDD of 0.5–3.0 mg, others, such as lorazepam, are effective at a dosage of 1–6 mg/day (Witek et al. 2005). Clonazepam also has a much longer half-life (18–50 hours) than lorazepam (10–20 hours), indicating that clonazepam remains in the body for a longer period of time. This means that clonazepam is long acting and, in addition to perhaps being useful in relieving long-term anxiety, it may lengthen the incidence for side effects.

Justification for using benzodiazepines in clinical practice for treatment of anxious children is provided by adult studies on GAD and panic disorder. In a large, multisite, placebo-controlled study, Ballenger et al. (1988) examined the effects of alprazolam on 481 adults diagnosed with panic disorder in an 8-week trial. According to the endpoint analysis, subjects in the alprazolam group were judged to have significantly higher physician and patient global improvement scores ($P<0.0001$) and fewer phobic ($P<0.0001$) and anxiety

($P<0.0001$) symptoms on the Overall Phobia Rating Scale and clinician-rated Hamilton Anxiety Rating Scale, respectively, and they reported significantly fewer panic attacks.

Benzodiazepines have also been effective in treating adults with GAD. Rickels et al. (1983) found that anxious adults ($N=151$) randomly assigned to receive alprazolam or diazepam greatly improved over a 4-week trial when compared with those given placebo. Although more patients dropped out of the placebo group, subjects in the medication groups had significantly more improvement on patient and physician ratings as early as 1 week into the study (mean dosages: alprazolam=1.2 mg/day, diazepam=20 mg/day). Significance was also apparent on many of the rating scales at endpoint analysis, indicating that effects were maintained throughout the trial.

Efficacy of Acute Treatment

Benefits.   Unlike in the substantial literature available on treatment with SSRIs, there are relatively few published, structured investigations assessing the efficacy of benzodiazepines in pediatric anxiety disorders. In one of the earliest RCTs measuring the efficacy of benzodiazepines in children with anxiety disorders, Bernstein et al. (1990) examined the effect of alprazolam and imipramine on young school refusers. Encouraged by the positive results of an open-label trial, in which 67% of patients randomly assigned to receive alprazolam showed marked or moderate improvement and 55% returned to school, the researchers created a double-blind crossover study. Participants were randomly assigned to receive alprazolam, imipramine, or placebo for 8 weeks, and then the medication was tapered for 1–2 weeks and discontinued. The investigators discovered that the treatments did show statistically significant differences at week 8 on the Anxiety Rating for Children (ARC) measure; participants randomly assigned to receive alprazolam (maximum dosage=3 mg/day) showed the most improvement. However, these results failed to reach significance once the baseline scores were factored in as covariates in an ANCOVA.

Simeon et al. (1992) conducted an RCT following the results of their open study (Simeon and Ferguson 1987). As in the Bernstein et al. (1990) trial, the follow-up, placebo-controlled, double-blind study failed to corroborate Simeon's earlier open-label findings. The subjects were 30 children meeting DSM-III criteria for anxiety and avoidance. The children were given placebo for 1 week and randomly assigned to receive alprazolam or placebo for 4 weeks (mean maximum dosage = 1.57 mg/day, range = 0.5–3.5 mg/day); then the medication was tapered for 2 additional weeks and replaced with a placebo. Although their evaluations, administered after the double-blind trial (day 28), seemed to indicate improvement among children who were administered alprazolam, Simeon et al. (1992) found that differences in clinical global ratings were not statistically significant.

Following the Simeon et al. (1992) trial, Graae et al. (1994) conducted a double-blind, crossover pilot study involving children with similar anxiety diagnoses (N = 15). All but one child had a diagnosis of separation anxiety disorder according to the DSM-III criteria, and all but two presented with comorbid anxiety disorders. In this study, unlike the Simeon et al. study, subjects were immediately randomly assigned to receive either clonazepam (at a maximum dosage of 2 mg/day) or placebo for a 4-week double-blind trial. Although at the end of the study half of the children no longer met the criteria for an anxiety disorder, treatment-effect comparisons did not reach significant levels. There were no significant treatment differences related to the frequency and severity of anxiety symptoms identified by the other measures, the Diagnostic Interview Schedule for Children and the Children's Manifest Anxiety Scale. Graae et al. (1994) did not support using clonazepam at the dosing schedule of 2 mg/day in children and adolescents with anxiety disorders.

Risks.　Side effects for most benzodiazepines were reported as infrequent and mild, although they varied in severity across studies. The most common side effects were dry mouth and drowsiness. Simeon et al. (1992) also reported that sedation and disinhibition, manifested by aggressivity, irritability, and incoordination, were common. In addition, 71% of subjects in the Bernstein et al. (1990) trial presented with abdominal pain, dizziness, and headaches.

Graae et al. (1994), in their study, reported the most severe side effects. The authors pointed out that disinhibition, irritability, and oppositionalism were notable in their sample; in three cases, these side effects were severe enough to cause the subjects to drop out of the study at Phase I. Benzodiazepines can lead to dependency with chronic use, which is usually defined as longer than 8 weeks of treatment (Nishino et al. 1995). Although none of the reviewed studies indicate withdrawal symptoms during the tapering period, it would be wise to monitor children closely during this period and not administer benzodiazepines on a long-term basis. Although the review findings indicate that benzodiazepine treatment offers some benefits for anxious children and adolescents, there have not been enough well-designed clinical trials with large sample sizes to clearly evaluate this class of compounds.

Efficacy of Long-Term Treatment and Maintenance

Because of concern that dependence will develop as a result of long-term treatment with benzodiazepines, many of the published RCTs have been acute studies, and no long-term studies that evaluate treatment for anxious children and adolescents have been done. However, there have been numerous long-term studies using benzodiazepines in adults diagnosed with anxiety disorders, especially panic disorder, because the chronic nature of panic disorder tends to require longer treatment duration.

For example, in a large, placebo-controlled study, Schweizer et al. (1993) investigated the treatment effect of the long-term use of alprazolam (mean dosage = 5.7 mg/day) or imipramine (mean dosage = 175 mg/day) in adults diagnosed with panic disorder, with or without agoraphobia (N = 106, ages 18–65). Following an acute trial, subjects who improved were randomly assigned to receive alprazolam (n = 27), imipramine (n = 13), or placebo (n = 11) for an additional 6 months of maintenance treatment. Monthly assessments included measures of panic attack frequency and severity, generalized anxiety, and phobias. Results indicated that following maintenance treatment, panic attack frequency declined for all patients except one in the placebo group. At week 32, only 9% of the alprazolam group, 0% of the imipramine group, and 22% of the placebo group still reported experiencing minor symptom attacks. Subjects receiving maintenance treatment with alprazolam who showed tolerance to adverse events such as sedation, a common side effect for benzodiazepines, declined from 49% incidence during the acute trial to 7% incidence.

Although this study had a high attrition rate from the acute trial to the maintenance phase, with significantly more subjects remaining in the alprazolam group, the results are striking. Compared with imipramine- and placebo-treated subjects, alprazolam-treated patients showed significantly more difficulty in discontinuing medication. In addition, the investigators noted that after 1-year follow-up, patients who had originally been treated with imipramine or placebo did just as well on clinical measures as those who had been treated with alprazolam but without exhibiting any of the physical dependence or withdrawal symptoms. This finding indicates that the sustained treatment effects of long-term therapy with benzodiazepines might not be worth the risk, especially in the pediatric population.

Tricyclic Antidepressants

Tricyclic antidepressants (TCAs), named for their three-ring structure, are known for their mood-elevating effects. For this reason, they have been used as a front-line pharmacological treatment for adults with depression and anxiety since the mid-1960s (Potter et al. 1995). Precursors to the safer SSRIs, TCAs act by binding to presynaptic transporter proteins in the brain and inhibiting the reuptake of norepinephrine and serotonin in the presynaptic terminal. Although all TCAs are equally effective in inhibiting both norepinephrine and serotonin, some are more preferential to one or the other, causing them to be referred to as "noradrenergic" or "serotonergic," respectively (Meyer and Quenzer 2005).

TCAs may be helpful for long-term treatment of anxiety, because inhibition of norepinephrine and serotonin extends the duration of the transmitter action at the synapse and changes both the presynaptic and postsynaptic receptors. This adaptation over time may increase the potential for clinical improvement, but it also extends the potential for side effects. In terms of half-life, most TCAs remain in the body for approximately 24 hours, allowing for once-a-day dosing (Potter et al. 1995). In adults, TCAs are used for the treatment of major depression, anxiety disorders (GAD, panic disorder, and OCD), and pain syndromes.

Efficacy of Acute Treatment

Benefits.   Although some RCTs (Bernstein et al. 2000; Gittelman-Klein and Klein 1971) indicated significant treatment differences between TCAs and placebo, a number of studies were unable to replicate and support these findings (Berney et al. 1981; Bernstein et al. 1990; Klein et al. 1992). Additionally, investigators have reported serious side effects in children taking TCAs, suggesting that the risk involved may outweigh the potential benefits.

Gittelman-Klein and Klein (1971) performed the first RCT evaluating the effect of TCAs on children with school phobia. In their double-blind, placebo-controlled study, the investigators randomly assigned school-phobic children ($N=35$) to receive either imipramine (mean dosage = 152 mg/day, range = 100–200 mg/day) or placebo for 6 weeks. Assessments included measures of global improvement on a 7-point scale, school attendance, and psychiatric ratings of symptoms. At the end of the 6-week trial, the investigators found that imipramine was significantly more effective than placebo in increasing school attendance and indicated greater improvement on all other measures. Of children taking medication, 81% returned to school, as opposed to 47% who were given placebo ($P<0.05$), and reports indicated a significantly greater frequency of improvement in the imipramine group.

Berney et al. (1981) followed Gittelman-Klein and Klein's (1971) study with a 12-week trial assessing the efficacy of clomipramine in child and adolescent school refusers ($N=46$). Subjects were randomly selected to receive placebo or clomipramine, prescribed according to age (40 mg/day for ages 9–10, 50 mg/day for ages 11–12, 75 mg/day for ages 13–14). Although the investigators discovered a significant shift toward improvement on global scores within both the placebo and the medication groups, they found that this significance disappeared when the groups were compared in an ANCOVA. By the end of the study, more than one-third of the sample still had serious difficulty returning to school.

In a double-blind, placebo-controlled study comparing the use of alprazolam and imipramine in treating school-refusing children and adolescents ($N=24$), Bernstein et al. (1990) found similar effects. An ANOVA showed that subjects randomly assigned to receive imipramine (mean TDD = 164.29 mg) for the full 8 weeks showed significantly less improvement on the ARC scale than those in the alprazolam group, but demonstrated significantly more improvement than those given placebo ($P=0.03$). However, these results were no longer significant after ANCOVAs were performed.

Following this trial, Klein et al. (1992) conducted another RCT comparing imipramine and placebo in children with separation anxiety disorder ($N=20$). If subjects did not respond to a 4-week behavioral treatment, they were randomly assigned to receive placebo or imipramine (mean dosage = 153 mg/day; range = 75–275 mg/day) for a 6-week trial. By the end of the study, results were not significant on any of the ratings, which included parent and child self-reports, teacher and psychiatrist ratings, and global improvement scores. Although half the subjects in this study improved, these results do not appear to support use of TCAs as a monotherapy for pediatric anxiety disorders. The targeted sample had pure separation anxiety without comorbid depression, not school phobia, yet the medication did not prove to be any more effective than placebo. Also, children in the medication group reported some severe side effects and were still receiving psychotherapy as an adjunctive treatment.

Studies assessing the efficacy of the serotonergic TCA clomipramine in children with OCD also give some insight into the overall efficacy of TCAs for anxiety disorders. In a 10-week, double-blind, crossover trial ($N=48$), Leonard et al. (1989) compared two TCAs: clomipramine, which has been shown to be effective in children with OCD, and desipramine, which is less potent in inhibiting serotonin reuptake (Ross and Renyi 1975). Following a 2-week, single-blind, placebo phase to assess efficacy, subjects were randomly assigned to receive either clomipramine or desipramine for the first 5 weeks (Phase A), and then their medication was switched to the alternate treatment for another 5 weeks (Phase B). Dosages were on a fixed schedule, with a target TDD of 3 mg/kg, and were based on weight (mean dosages: clomipramine= 150 mg/day, desipramine= 153 mg/day; range= 50–250 mg/day). ANCOVA showed that clomipramine, but not desipramine, produced a significant decrease in all obsessive-compulsive ratings (NIMH-GOCS, $P=0.0002$) and depression ratings (Hamilton Rating Scale for Depression, $P=0.006$; NIMH depression scales, $P=0.0001$), as well as an increase in a measure of global functioning ($P=0.001$).

Drug order was also shown to have a significant effect. Of the subjects who switched from clomipramine in Phase A to desipramine in Phase B, 64% showed a sign of relapse, defined as at least a 1-point decline on the NIMH-GOCS by the fifth week of Phase B. This relapse would indicate that desipramine did not produce the same positive clinical effects as clomipramine and could not sustain those effects following clomipramine treatment. DeVeaugh-Geiss et al. (1992) found similar results in their 8-week, multisite study assessing clomipramine use in children and adolescents with OCD ($N=60$). Subjects were randomly assigned to receive clomipramine (maximum dosage by body weight: 25–30 kg, 75 mg/day; 31–45 kg, 100 mg/day; 46–60 kg, 150 mg/day; >60 kg, 200 mg/day) or to continue with placebo. Subjects in the clomipramine group had a 37% mean reduction of symptoms on the Y-BOCS compared with 8% for those receiving placebo, and a 34% mean reduction on the NIMH-GOCS compared with 6% for the placebo group. Both findings were significant using ANCOVA ($P<0.05$).

Risks.   Side effects for TCAs ranged in severity across studies. Gittelman-Klein and Klein (1971) reported that most side effects disappeared without requiring a dosage change. The most common side effects were drowsiness, dizziness, dry mouth, and constipation. Similarly, Berney et al. (1981) found that although side effects were reported, they were usually not severe. No subject in the Bernstein et al. (1990) study had side effects that rated higher than mild, the most common being headache, dizziness, dry mouth, abdominal pain, and nausea.

Klein et al. (1992) reported the most severe side effects, the most frequent being irritability or angry outbursts and dry mouth. Children in the imipramine group experienced considerably more side effects than did children in the placebo group ($\chi^2=5.05$, $P<0.03$), with all complaints lasting at least 3 days and two-thirds reported in the moderate-to-severe range. This finding is troubling, given that the mean daily dose in this trial was similar to that administered by Gittelman-Klein and Klein (1971), although their sample was significantly smaller. Side effects in studies using clomipramine and desipramine to treat children with OCD were similar. Leonard et al. (1989) reported dry mouth, tiredness, and dizziness as the most common adverse effects. However, subjects taking clomipramine experienced more tremor and other side effects, such as chest pain, hot flashes, heartburn, rash, and acne.

In addition to these side effects, sudden unexplained death in children taking TCA medications has been reported in some case studies (Biederman 1991; Riddle et al. 1993; Varley and McClellan 1997). In many of the reported cases, the children were being treated with desipramine at varying but therapeutic or even subtherapeutic levels for attention-deficit disorder or ADHD. Monitoring seems to have been inconsistent among the cases, but the cause of death was usually linked to adverse cardiac events. Because of the possibility of cardiac toxicity in young children, clinicians are advised to monitor very closely the effects of TCA levels on their subjects and to follow serial electrocardiograms (ECGs) over the course of treatment to ensure that plasma levels are not above the therapeutic threshold.

Overall, there does not yet appear to be enough evidence to support the frequent use of TCAs as a monotherapy for children and adolescents with anxiety disorders, with the exception of OCD.

Efficacy of Long-Term Treatment and Maintenance

Although there have not been many long-term studies assessing the efficacy of TCAs in children with pure anxiety disorders, evidence from long-term OCD trials provides some indication of effects. Following their short-term, placebo-controlled trial (see preceding section "Efficacy of Acute Treatment"), DeVeaugh-Geiss et al. (1992) continued with an open-label extension study for 1 year. They found that efficacy was maintained in subjects who elected to participate and completed the whole year ($N=25$). By the end of the year, the mean Y-BOCS score was 9.5, compared with 23 at the beginning of the extension. The investigators reported that clomipramine was still well tolerated.

Leonard et al. (1991) also performed an 8-month trial similar in design to their previous short-term crossover trial (also described in the preceding section). Children and adolescents from the previous trial receiving maintenance clomipramine treatment ($N=26$) for OCD entered into the study and continued to receive clomipramine (mean dosage = 143 mg/day) for 3 months. At month 4, subjects were randomly assigned to receive desipramine substitution (mean dosage = 123 mg/day) or to continue with clomipramine for 2 months. For the final 3-month phase, all subjects continued to receive clomipramine treatment. For those subjects completing the entire trial ($N=20$), results revealed that during the months of the substitution, those randomized to receive desipramine showed greater impairment across ratings than those continuing with clomipramine. These results were only significant, however, on the NIMH-GOCS scale once the investigators controlled for the error rate. This study would seem to indicate that efficacy was maintained in subjects receiving long-term TCA treatment, given that few subjects in the clomipramine group relapsed. However, even those subjects receiving clomipramine for the full 8 months still experienced OCD symptoms, which varied in severity over time. Thus, long-term clomipramine treatment for children and adolescents with OCD seems to be effective in decreasing symptoms, but it does not completely eliminate troubling symptoms.

Buspirone

Buspirone, a nonbenzodiazepine anxiolytic, has been shown to be effective in reducing anxiety symptoms without the side effects of benzodiazepines. Unlike the sedative-hypnotics, buspirone does not enhance the GABAergic system but instead acts as an agonist at the serotonin $5\text{-}HT_{1A}$ presynaptic receptors and as a partial agonist at the $5\text{-}HT_{1A}$ postsynaptic receptors. This process is meant to reduce both the flow of serotonin away from the presynaptic neuron and serotonergic activity in the central nervous system (CNS) overall. Buspirone is also not accompanied by the sedation, confusion, or withdrawal that can appear with sedative-hypnotic use (Robinson et al. 1990) and does not enhance the effects of CNS depressants, such as alcohol, making it relatively safe.

Efficacy of Acute Treatment

Currently, there are no well-designed, controlled trials assessing the efficacy of buspirone in treating pediatric anxiety disorders. Much of the available information stems from case reports, case series, and open-label trials. Although individual case reports (Alessi and Bos 1991; Balon 1994; Kranzler 1988) seem to indicate some usefulness of buspirone in relieving anxiety symptoms, they do not provide evidence of its efficacy.

In a small open-label study, Pfeffer et al. (1997) investigated the treatment effects of buspirone for child psychiatric inpatients exhibiting symptoms of anxiety and moderate aggression ($N = 25$, ages 5–12). Subjects who received high scores on the Revised Children's Manifest Anxiety Scale (RCMAS) and the Measure of Aggression, Violence, and Rage in Children (MAVRIC) were eligible to receive buspirone treatment. The TDD was titrated up 5–10 mg every 3 days (maximum dose = 50 mg) for 3 weeks (Phase II), after which the medication was kept at the optimum dosage for a 6-week maintenance period (Phase III). Results indicated that by the end of the 9-week trial, subjects had a significant reduction of symptoms on the social anxiety factor of the RCMAS ($P < 0.04$) but not on the total RCMAS. There was also a significant reduction in overall aggression, as measured by the MAVRIC ($P < 0.02$), and in the number of seclusions and daily physical restraints used ($P < 0.01$). Some children ($N = 6$) had to discontinue use of buspirone because of severe side effects, including agitation, increased aggressivity, euphoric symptoms, increased impulsivity, and out-of-control behavior.

Although the results of this study are limited by its open-label design, they do show some efficacy in treating pediatric social phobia with buspirone. The 19 subjects who completed the trial tolerated buspirone (mean dosage = 28 mg/day) well, reporting few side effects other than headache. However, as the investigators noted, it is troubling that almost 25% of the sample had to discontinue treatment due to interfering adverse events.

A later case series (Thomsen and Mikkelson 1999) also seems to indicate support for the addition of buspirone to SSRI treatment in adolescents diagnosed with OCD ($N=6$, ages 15–19). If patients did not show improvement following past SSRI treatment with or without CBT, they were treated with buspirone (mean dosage=20 mg/day). Although the cases varied in severity, the investigators reported that buspirone in combination with continuing SSRI treatment showed a positive reduction effect on obsessive-compulsive symptoms, especially anxiety and distress. In addition, dramatic clinical improvement, as measured by the Y-BOCS, was observed in three of the six cases. Buspirone was well tolerated, inasmuch as no patients reported severe side effects or had to discontinue combined treatment.

Safety Issues

Monitoring

Prior to starting medication treatment in a child or adolescent, the clinician needs to review the family's medical and psychiatric history, as well as laboratory results and previous medical evaluations. When prescribing a medication, the clinician should document the child's baseline weight, height, and vital signs and then monitor them over time. It is important for the clinician to consult with the child's primary care physician to obtain additional medical information, such as concomitant medication history and last physical examination, and to establish a collaborative treatment relationship. Informed consent/assent should be obtained from the parent and child following a full explanation of the risks and benefits of the selected medication treatment. The clinician should review with the child and parent a list of the most impairing anxiety symptoms, which they can track over time with the expectation that the medication will lead to improvement in these symptoms over time.

No laboratory tests are required for the use of SSRIs. SSRIs are well tolerated by children and adolescents, and the pediatric side-effect profile is similar to what is seen in adult clinical studies. The main side effects of concern are the following: gastrointestinal discomfort, drowsiness, headaches, insomnia, nervousness, hyperkinesia, and hostility (Waslick 2006). There are reports of withdrawal symptoms accompanying the discontinuation of SSRIs. The child may experience the following symptoms: gastric distress, headache, dizziness, irritability, and agitation (Labellarte et al. 1998). Given this possibility, it is recommended that these medications not be abruptly discontinued.

As discussed earlier in the section on the risks of treatment with SNRIs, acute-treatment studies have shown that children receiving venlafaxine XR had statistically significant changes in blood pressure, heart rate, weight, height, and total cholesterol. From these results, it is unclear what impact long-term exposure to this medication would have on these clinical parameters. When prescribing this compound for acute or long-term treatment, clinicians should monitor vital signs, weight, and height, and conduct a periodic laboratory assessment of cholesterol.

TCA use in children has the potential for cardiac risk. When this medication is prescribed, the child should have baseline vital signs, including sitting and standing blood pressure with pulse and ECG. Once the clinician has titrated the medication to the therapeutic dose, another ECG should be performed with a serum level of the medication. This process should be repeated with each dose adjustment and with periodic monitoring for long-term use. Another concern with this class of medication is the risk of lethal overdose.

In 2004, the FDA issued a black box warning after examining the outcome of all pediatric placebo-controlled trials of antidepressant medications and finding an increased incidence of suicidal thoughts and behaviors in the medication group (4%) as compared to the placebo group (2%) (Leslie et al. 2005; U.S. Food and Drug Administration 2005). A meta-analysis by Bridge et al. (2007), which involved a larger number of pediatric clinical trials, showed in terms of suicidality and behaviors a number needed to harm (NNH) of 143 for all conditions, 140 for non-OCD anxiety disorders, and 200 for OCD. It is important for the clinician to review this information with the parents and to stress the need to contact the physician if the child experiences changes in behaviors, sleep patterns, and activity levels.

Prevention and Intervention of Adverse Effects

The best prevention and intervention for the management of medication adverse effects is the education of the parent and child about what to expect in terms of adverse effects and how the clinician plans to manage these if they should occur. As part of this education, the clinician must stress to the parent and child that although mild side effects may occur initially, the majority will usually resolve in the first several weeks of treatment.

In addition, it is important for the clinician to document baseline physical symptoms and their levels of severity prior to starting medication and review this with the child and family. Symptoms should be reviewed at each medication visit to assess change in severity or to identify the development of new symptoms. Children with anxiety disorders have somatic symptoms that may be confused with medication adverse effects. If the clinician has documented at baseline the presence of somatic symptoms, this record will assist in delineating the development of new adverse events or the worsening of previous symptoms.

For all medications, the clinician should initiate treatment at a low dose for the first 7 days and increase the dose slowly over subsequent weeks, depending on the child's clinical response to and tolerability of the medication. Unfortunately, information is limited about dosing guidelines for these medications in treating specific anxiety disorders. Once a clinically efficacious dose is achieved, it should be maintained for 8–12 weeks and then reevaluated to gauge tolerability and successful treatment of the primary anxiety target symptoms.

Practical Management Strategies

Cognitive-Behavioral Therapy

Several clinical trials have clearly demonstrated that 10- to 16-week CBT treatments (with in vivo exposure) have led to a significant reduction in anxiety symptoms in children (Barrett et al. 1996; Kendall et al. 1997). Given this information, it would be reasonable for a clinician to initially recommend treatment with CBT. However, there are several important considerations. Some families may not have access to CBT treatment because of the limited availability of pediatric therapists proficient in CBT. Also, a significant percentage of children remain symptomatic following CBT treatment. For children with comorbid diagnoses, such as major depression, the prudent approach would be to treat with a combination of CBT and an SSRI.

Combination Treatment

In this section, we review the use of combination treatment (medications plus CBT) for the various anxiety disorders. In general, medication is often considered for treating pediatric anxiety disorders when a trial of psychosocial intervention has failed and/or when anxiety symptoms are considered to be in the moderate-to-severe range, leading to functional impairment, such as poor school performance, school refusal, insomnia, and the development of comorbid diagnoses (e.g., major depression).

The scientific evidence demonstrates that both CBT and medications (SSRIs) are efficacious treatments, and some researchers have focused on the effects of combining these two treatments at the onset. For example, Bernstein et al. (2000) investigated the efficacy of imipramine plus CBT in treating school-phobic adolescents ($N = 47$) who were diagnosed with comorbid anxiety and major depressive disorders in an 8-week trial. Subjects were randomly assigned to receive imipramine (mean TDD = 182.3 mg) or placebo in combination with CBT. The results of this study indicate that school attendance improved significantly only in the imipramine plus CBT group ($z = 4.36$, $P < 0.001$) and that the imipramine plus CBT group improved at a faster rate than the placebo plus CBT group (3.6% vs. 0.9%; $z = 2.39$, $P = 0.017$), even when compared with baseline. Anxiety and depression symptoms on various measures decreased significantly for both imipramine and placebo groups, with only one measure, the Children's Depression Rating Scale—Revised (CDRS-R), favoring imipramine ($z = 2.08$; $P = 0.037$). Additionally, remission on clinical measures significantly favored imipramine plus CBT only on the school attendance variable ($\chi^2 = 7.38$, $P = 0.007$). This study supports the use of TCAs in combination with CBT in school-refusing adolescents who have a combination of anxiety and depression symptoms. As with many previous studies, there is a comorbidity factor that precludes recommending TCAs for pure anxiety disorders; nevertheless, school attendance did improve significantly.

Neziroglu et al. (2000) investigated the possible additional benefits of using a combination treatment of fluvoxamine and behavior therapy, compared with fluvoxamine alone, to treat children and adolescents with OCD ($N = 10$, ages 10–17). Subjects were eligible if they had previously failed a trial of behavior therapy lasting at least 10 sessions by not complying either inside or outside of treatment sessions. Following randomization, all subjects received 10 weeks of fluvoxamine (maximum dosage=200 mg/day) until week 5, when 20 sessions of behavior therapy were initiated with 5 of the subjects. Results showed that 8 of the 10 subjects had improved scores on the primary outcome variable, the CY-BOCS, following the initial 10 weeks of fluvoxamine treatment. At week 43, 3 of the 5 subjects in the fluvoxamine plus behavior therapy group had significantly improved scores on the CY-BOCS, and 2 remained stable; 1 of the 5 subjects in the fluvoxamine-only group significantly improved, 2 remained stable, and 2 deteriorated significantly. At week 52, the pattern was similar, and by 2-year follow-up, subjects in both treatment groups all continued to improve or remain stable.

The Pediatric OCD Treatment Study Team (2004) conducted a multisite, placebo-controlled, double-blind study assessing the efficacy of sertraline, CBT, and their combination for children and adolescents diagnosed with OCD (N=122, ages 7–17). During Phase I, subjects were randomly assigned to receive either sertraline (target dosage=200 mg/day), CBT, combination therapy, or placebo for 12 weeks. Results from intent-to-treat random regression analyses revealed that all active treatments were significantly more effective than placebo, based on change in CY-BOCS scores (CBT: P=0.003; sertraline: P=0.007; combination: P=0.001), and that combined treatment was superior to CBT alone (P=0.008) and sertraline alone (P=0.006). The results for the CBT-alone and sertraline-alone groups did not differ significantly from each other. Furthermore, the rate of clinical remission, defined as a CY-BOCS score of ≤10 in the combined treatment group, differed significantly from that of the sertraline-only (P=0.03) and placebo groups (P<0.001), but not the CBT-only group. Side effects were decreased appetite, diarrhea, enuresis, motor activity, nausea, and stomachache. Despite these reports, there were no serious adverse events or reports of suicidality. The study showed that sertraline, CBT, and their combination are effective treatments for pediatric OCD. However, because the combination and CBT-only groups showed both a higher reduction of symptoms on the CY-BOCS and a higher rate of clinical remission, the investigators recommended combination treatment or CBT alone as first-line treatment approaches.

Beidel et al. (2007) conducted a study comparing fluoxetine, pill placebo, and Social Effectiveness Therapy for Children (SET-C, a behavioral therapy combining group sessions and individualized exposure sessions) for treating social phobia in children and adolescents. The findings indicate that SET-C and fluoxetine were more effective than placebo in reducing the symptoms of social phobia, with 79% of the SET-C group and 36.4% of the fluoxetine group having a significant improvement on the CGI-I, versus 6.3% of the placebo group. The Child/Adolescent Anxiety Multimodal Study (CAMS), the most recent and largest NIMH-funded anxiety multisite study examining combination treatment to date, provides strong evidence in favor of combining CBT and an SSRI when treating non-OCD pediatric anxiety disorders. In this trial, 488 children, ages 7–17, with primary diagnoses of GAD, separation anxiety disorder, and social phobia, were randomly assigned to receive either CBT alone, CBT in combination with sertraline (up to 200 mg/day), sertraline alone, or placebo for 12 weeks (Walkup et al. 2008). The results showed that 80.7% of children assigned to the combination treatment group improved on the CGI-I ($P<0.001$), in comparison to 59.7% of those assigned to CBT ($P<0.001$) and 54.9% of those assigned to sertraline ($P<0.001$). All treatments were statistically superior to placebo ($P<0.001$), which led to only 23.7% improvement in participants. There were no significant differences in frequency of adverse events between the sertraline and placebo groups, although there were fewer reports of physical symptoms in children in the CBT group than in children in the sertraline group. The findings demonstrate that both pharmacological treatment and psychotherapy are effective in treating pediatric anxiety disorders but that their combination is most effective. A long-term follow-up study to CAMS is currently under way to examine the course of anxiety as well as the impact of treatment over time.

Conclusions

The empirical evidence supports the use of both pharmacological and psychotherapy (specifically CBT) treatments for pediatric anxiety disorders. The data suggest that several classes of medications can be used safely and lead to an efficacious outcome, although the class of SSRIs should be considered first-line treatment. In addition, for pediatric OCD, evidence suggests that a combination treatment approach or CBT alone should be considered first. Additional long-term medication studies are warranted to examine both safety and treatment outcomes.

Clinical Pearls

- Prior to initiation of medication treatment, develop a list of target anxiety symptoms to be tracked during treatment so as to determine response.
- Carefully assess for comorbid diagnoses and the severity of anxiety symptoms. Greater severity may indicate combination treatment.
- To prevent early termination from a medication trial, spend an adequate amount of time educating the child and parent about what to expect from medication treatment and about potential adverse events.
- Keep in mind that maintaining a dose that is suboptimal will frustrate the child and family, leading to treatment nonadherence and a prematurely failed trial.
- If a child's behavior change is unusual and represents a significant change from baseline, perform a careful assessment to evaluate whether medication is the cause.

References

Alessi N, Bos T: Buspirone augmentation of fluoxetine in a depressed child with obsessive-compulsive disorder. Am J Psychiatry 148:1605–1606, 1991

Allgulander C, Hackett D, Salinas E: Venlafaxine extended release (ER) in the treatment of generalized anxiety disorder: twenty-four-week placebo-controlled dose-ranging study. Br J Psychiatry 179:15–22, 2001

American Academy of Child and Adolescent Psychiatry: Practice parameters for the assessment and treatment of children and adolescents with anxiety disorders. J Am Acad Child Adolesc Psychiatry 46:267–283, 2007

American Psychiatric Association: Diagnostic and Statistical Manual: Mental Disorders. Washington, DC, American Psychiatric Association, 1952

American Psychiatric Association: Diagnostic and Statistical Manual of Mental Disorders, 2nd Edition. Washington, DC, American Psychiatric Association, 1968

American Psychiatric Association: Diagnostic and Statistical Manual of Mental Disorders, 3rd Edition. Washington, DC, American Psychiatric Association, 1980

American Psychiatric Association: Diagnostic and Statistical Manual of Mental Disorders, 4th Edition. Washington, DC, American Psychiatric Association, 1994

American Psychiatric Association: Diagnostic and Statistical Manual of Mental Disorders, 4th Edition, Text Revision. Washington, DC, American Psychiatric Association, 2000

Anderson JC, Williams S, McGee R, et al: DSM-III disorders in preadolescent children: prevalence in a large sample from the general population. Arch Gen Psychiatry 44:69–76, 1987

Aronson TA, Logue CM: On the longitudinal course of panic disorder: development history and predictors of phobic complications. Compr Psychiatry 28:344–355, 1987

Ballenger JC, Burrows GD, DuPont RL, et al: Alprazolam in panic disorder and agoraphobia: results from a multicenter trial. Arch Gen Psychiatry 45:413–422, 1988

Balon R: Buspirone in the treatment of separation anxiety in an adolescent boy. Can J Psychiatry 39:581–582, 1994

Barrett PM, Dadds MR, Rapee RM: Family treatment of childhood anxiety: a controlled trial. J Consult Clin Psychol 64:333–342, 1996

Beesdo K, Knappe S, Pine DS: Anxiety and anxiety disorders in children and adolescents: Developmental issues and implications for DSM-V. Psychiatr Clin North Am 32:483–524, 2009

Beidel DC, Fink CM, Turner SM: Stability of anxious symptomatology in children. J Abnorm Child Psychol 24:257–268, 1996

Beidel DC, Turner SM, Sallee FR, et al: SET-C versus fluoxetine in the treatment of childhood social phobia. J Am Acad Child Adolesc Psychiatry 46:1622–1632, 2007

Berney T, Kolvin I, Bhate SR, et al: School phobia: a therapeutic trial with clomipramine and short-term outcome. Br J Psychiatry 138:110–118, 1981

Bernstein GA, Shaw K: Practice parameters for the assessment and treatment of anxiety disorders. J Am Acad Child Adolesc Psychiatry 32:1089–1098, 1993

Bernstein GA, Garfinkel BD, Borchardt CM: Comparative studies of pharmacotherapy for school refusal. J Am Acad Child Adolesc Psychiatry 29:773–781, 1990

Bernstein GA, Borchadt CM, Perwien AR, et al: Imipramine plus cognitive-behavioral therapy in the treatment of school refusal. J Am Acad Child Adolesc Psychiatry 39:276–283, 2000

Biederman J: Sudden death in children treated with a tricyclic antidepressant. J Am Acad Child Adolesc Psychiatry 30:495–497, 1991

Birmaher B, Waterman GS, Ryan N, et al: Fluoxetine for childhood anxiety disorders. J Am Acad Child Adolesc Psychiatry 33:993–999, 1994

Birmaher B, Axelson DA, Monk K, et al: Fluoxetine for the treatment of childhood anxiety disorders. J Am Acad Child Adolesc Psychiatry 42:415–423, 2003

Bittner A, Egger HL, Erkanli A, et al: What do childhood anxiety disorders predict? J Child Psychol Psychiatry 48:1174–1183, 2007

Black B, Uhde TW: Elective mutism as a variant of social phobia. J Am Acad Child Adolesc Psychiatry 31:1090–1094, 1992

Black B, Uhde TW: Treatment of elective mutism with fluoxetine: a double-blind, placebo-controlled study. J Am Acad Child Adolesc Psychiatry 33:1000–1006, 1994

Bowen RC, Offord DR, Boyle MH: The prevalence of overanxious disorder and separation anxiety disorder: results from the Ontario Child Health Study. J Am Acad Child Adolesc Psychiatry 29:753–758, 1990

Brady EU, Kendall PC: Comorbidity of anxiety and depression in children and adolescents. Psychol Bull 111:244–255, 1992

Bridge JA, Iyengar S, Salary CB, et al: Clinical response and risk for reported suicidal ideation and suicide attempts in pediatric antidepressant treatment: a meta-analysis of randomized controlled trial. JAMA 297:1683–1696, 2007

Cantwell DP, Baker L: Stability and natural history of DSM-III childhood diagnoses. J Am Acad Child Adolesc Psychiatry 28:691–700, 1989

Compton SN, Grant PJ, Chrisman AK, et al: Sertraline in children and adolescents with social anxiety disorder: an open trial. J Am Acad Child Adolesc Psychiatry 40:564–571, 2001

Cook EH, Wagner KD, March JS, et al: Long-term sertraline treatment of children and adolescents with obsessive-compulsive disorder. J Am Acad Child Adolesc Psychiatry 40:1175–1181, 2001

Costello EJ: Child psychiatric disorders and their correlates: a primary care pediatric sample. J Am Acad Child Adolesc Psychiatry 28:851–855, 1989

Costello EJ, Costello AJ, Edelbrock C, et al: Psychiatric disorders in pediatric primary care: prevalence and risk factors. Arch Gen Psychiatry 45:1107–1116, 1988

Costello EJ, Angold A, Burns BJ, et al: The Great Smoky Mountains Study of Youth: Functional impairment and severe emotional disturbance. Arch Gen Psychiatry 53:1137–1143, 1996

Costello EJ, Mustillo S, Erkanli A, et al: Prevalence and development of psychiatric disorders in childhood and adolescence. Arch Gen Psychiatry 60:837–844, 2003

Costello EJ, Egger HL, Angold A: The developmental epidemiology of anxiety disorders: phenomenology, prevalence, and comorbidity. Child Adolesc Psychiatr Clin N Am 14:631–648, vii, 2005

Dadds MR, Spence SH, Holland DE, et al: Prevention and early intervention for anxiety disorders: a controlled trial. J Consult Clin Psychol 65:627–635, 1997

Davidson JRT, DuPont RL, Hedges D, et al: Efficacy, safety, and tolerability of ven-lafaxine XR extended release and buspirone in outpatients with generalized anxiety disorder. J Clin Psychiatry 60:528–535, 1999

DeVeaugh-Geiss J, Moroz G, Biederman J, et al: Clomipramine hydrochloride in child-hood and adolescent obsessive-compulsive disorder: a multicenter trial. J Am Acad Child Adolesc Psychiatry 31:45–49, 1992

Egger HL, Angold A: Common emotional and behavioral disorders in preschool chil-dren: presentation, nosology, and epidemiology. J Child Psychol Psychiatry 47:313–337, 2006

Federman EB, Costello EJ, Angold A, et al: Development of substance use and psy-chiatric comorbidity in an epidemiologic study of white and American Indian young adolescents—The Great Smoky Mountains Study. Drug Alcohol Depend 44:69–78, 1997

Feehan M, McGee R, Raja R, et al: DSM-III-R disorders in New Zealand 18 year olds. Aust N Z J Psychiatry 28:87–99, 1994

Fluvoxamine for the treatment of anxiety disorders in children and adolescents. Re-search Units on Pediatric Psychopharmacology Anxiety Study Group. N Engl J Med 344:1279–1285, 2001

Foley DL, Goldston DB, Costello EJ, et al: Proximal psychiatric risk factors for sui-cidality in youth. Arch Gen Psychiatry 63:1017–1024, 2006

Gelenberg AJ, Lydiard RB, Rudolph RL, et al: Efficacy of venlafaxine extended-release capsules in nondepressed outpatients with generalized anxiety disorder: a 6-month randomized controlled trial. JAMA 283:3082–3088, 2000

Geller DA, Hoog SL, Heiligenstein JH, et al: Fluoxetine treatment for obsessive-com-pulsive disorder in children and adolescents: a placebo-controlled clinical trial. J Am Acad Child Adolesc Psychiatry 40:773–779, 2001

Geller DA, Biederman J, Stewart SE, et al: Which SSRI? A meta-analysis of pharma-cotherapy trials in pediatric obsessive-compulsive disorder. Am J Psychiatry 160:1919–1928, 2003

Geller DA, Wagner KD, Emslie G, et al: Paroxetine treatment in children and adoles-cents with obsessive-compulsive disorder: a randomized, multicenter, double-blind, placebo-controlled trial. J Am Acad Child Adolesc Psychiatry 43:1387–1396, 2004

Gittelman-Klein R, Klein DF: Controlled imipramine treatment of school phobia. Arch Gen Psychiatry 25:204–207, 1971

Graae F, Milner J, Rizzotto L, et al: Clonazepam in childhood anxiety disorders. J Am Acad Child Adolesc Psychiatry 33:372–376, 1994

Katzelnick DJ, Kobak KA, Greist JH, et al: Sertraline for social phobia: a double-blind, placebo-controlled crossover study. Am J Psychiatry 152:1368–1371, 1995

Keller MB, Lavori PW, Wunder J, et al: Chronic course of anxiety disorders in children and adolescents. J Am Acad Child Adolesc Psychiatry 31:595–599, 1992

Kendall PC, Flannery-Schroeder E, Panichelli-Mindel SM, et al: Therapy for youths with anxiety disorders: a second randomized clinical trial. J Consult Clin Psychol 65:366–380, 1997

Klein RG, Koplewicz HS, Kanner A: Imipramine treatment of children with separation anxiety disorder. J Am Acad Child Adolesc Psychiatry 31:21–28, 1992

Kovacs M, Gatsonis C, Paulauskas SL, et al: Depressive disorders in childhood, IV: a longitudinal study of comorbidity with and risk for anxiety disorders. Arch Gen Psychiatry 46:776–782, 1989

Kranzler HR: Use of buspirone in an adolescent with overanxious disorder. J Am Acad Child Adolesc Psychiatry 27:789–790, 1988

Labellarte MJ, Walkup JT, Riddle MA: The new antidepressants: selective serotonin reuptake inhibitors. Pediatr Clin North Am 45:1137–1155, 1998

Last CG, Hersen M, Kazdin AE, et al: Comparison of DSM-III separation anxiety and overanxious disorders: demographic characteristics and patterns of comorbidity. J Am Acad Child Adolesc Psychiatry 26:527–531, 1987a

Last CG, Phillips JE, Statfeld A: Childhood anxiety disorders in mothers and their children. Child Psychiatry Hum Dev 18:103–112, 1987b

Last CG, Strauss CC, Hersen M, et al: Psychiatric illness in the mothers of anxious children. Am J Psychiatry 144:1580–1583, 1987c

Last CG, Perrin S, Hersen M, et al: A prospective study of childhood anxiety disorders. J Am Acad Child Adolesc Psychiatry 35:1502–1510, 1996

Last CG, Hansen C, Franco N: Anxious children in adulthood: a prospective study of adjustment. J Am Acad Child Adolesc Psychiatry 36:645–652, 1997

Leonard HL, Swedo SE, Rapoport JL, et al: Treatment of obsessive-compulsive disorder with clomipramine and desipramine in children and adolescents: a double-blind crossover comparison. Arch Gen Psychiatry 46:1088–1092, 1989

Leonard HL, Swedo SE, Lenane MC, et al: A double-blind desipramine substitution during long-term clomipramine treatment in children and adolescents with obsessive-compulsive disorder. Arch Gen Psychiatry 48:922–927, 1991

Leonard HL, March J, Rickler KC, et al: Pharmacology of the selective serotonin reuptake inhibitors in children and adolescents. J Am Acad Child Adolesc Psychiatry 36:725–736, 1997

Leslie LK, Newman TB, Chesney PJ, et al: The food and drug administration's deliberations on antidepressant use in pediatric patients. Pediatrics 116:195–204, 2005

Lewinsohn PM, Hops H, Roberts SE, et al: Adolescent psychopathology, I: prevalence and incidence of depression and other DSM-III-R disorders in high school students. J Abnorm Psychol 102:133–144, 1993

Liebowitz MR, Stein MB, Tancer M, et al: A randomized, double-blind, fixed-dose comparison of paroxetine and placebo in the treatment of generalized social anxiety disorder. J Clin Psychiatry 63:66–74, 2002

Livingston R, Taylor JL, Crawford SL: A study of somatic complaints and psychiatric diagnosis in children. J Am Acad Child Adolesc Psychiatry 27:185–187, 1988

March JS, Biederman J, Wolkow R, et al: Sertraline in children and adolescents with obsessive-compulsive disorder. JAMA 280:1752–1756, 1998

McGee R, Feehan M, Williams S, et al: DSM-III disorders in a large sample of adolescents. J Am Acad Child Adolesc Psychiatry 29:611–619, 1990

Meyer JS, Quenzer LQ: Psychopharmacology: Drugs, The Brain, and Behavior. Sunderland, MA, Sinauer Associates, 2005, pp 412–438

Neziroglu F, Yaryura-Tobias JA, Walz J, et al: The effect of fluvoxamine and behavior therapy on children and adolescents with obsessive-compulsive disorder. J Child Adolesc Psychopharmacol 10:295–306, 2000

Nishino S, Mignot E, Dement WC: Sedative-hypnotics, in The American Psychiatric Press Textbook of Psychopharmacology. Edited by Schatzberg AF, Nemeroff CB. Washington, DC, American Psychiatric Press, 1995, pp 405–416

Nutt D, Lawson C: Panic attacks: a neurochemical overview of models and mechanisms. Br J Psychiatry 160:165–178, 1992

Orvaschel H, Weissman M: Epidemiology of anxiety in children, in Anxiety Disorders of Childhood. Edited by Gittelman R. New York, Guilford, 1986, pp 58–72

Pediatric OCD Treatment Study (POTS) Team: Cognitive-behavior therapy, sertraline, and their combination for children and adolescents with obsessive-compulsive disorder: the Pediatric OCD Treatment Study (POTS) randomized controlled trial. JAMA 292:1969–1976, 2004

Pfeffer CR, Jiang H, Domeshek LJ: Buspirone treatment of psychiatrically hospitalized prepubertal children with symptoms of anxiety and moderately severe aggression. J Child Adolesc Psychopharmacol 7:145–155, 1997

Pigott TA: OCD: where the serotonin selectivity story begins. J Clin Psychiatry 57:11–20, 1996

Pigott TA, L'Heureux F, Hill JL, et al: A double-blind study of adjuvant buspirone hydrochloride in clomipramine-treated patients with obsessive-compulsive disorder. J Clin Psychopharmacol 12:11–18, 1991

Pine DS: Treating children and adolescents with selective serotonin reuptake inhibitors: how long is appropriate? J Child Adolesc Psychopharmacol 12:189–203, 2002

Pine DS, Grun J: Anxiety disorders, in Child Psychopharmacology. Edited by Walsh TB. Review of Psychiatry, Vol 17 (Series Editors, JM Oldham, MB Riba). Washington, DC, American Psychiatric Press, 1998, pp 115–148

Pohl RB, Wolkow RM, Clary CM: Sertraline for social phobia: a double-blind, placebo-controlled crossover study. Am J Psychiatry 155:1189–1195, 1998

Pollack MH, Zaninelli R, Goddard A, et al: Paroxetine in the treatment of generalized anxiety disorder: results of a placebo-controlled, flexible-dosage trial. J Clin Psychiatry 62:350–357, 2001

Potter WZ, Manji HK, Rudorfer MV: Tricyclic and tetracyclics, in The American Psychiatric Press Textbook of Psychopharmacology. Edited by Schatzberg AF, Nemeroff CB. Washington, DC, American Psychiatric Press, 1995, pp 141–160

Rickels K, Rynn MA: What is generalized anxiety disorder? J Clin Psychiatry 62 (suppl): 4–12, 2001

Rickels K, Csanalosi I, Greisman P, et al: A controlled clinical trial of alprazolam for the treatment of anxiety. Am J Psychiatry 140:82–85, 1983

Rickels K, Pollack MH, Sheehan DV, et al: Efficacy of venlafaxine XR extended-release capsules in nondepressed outpatients with generalized anxiety disorder. Am J Psychiatry 157:968–974, 2000

Riddle MA, Scahill L, King RA, et al: Double-blind, crossover trial of fluoxetine and placebo in children and adolescents with obsessive-compulsive disorder. J Am Acad Child Adolesc Psychiatry 31:1062–1069, 1992

Riddle MA, Geller B, Ryan N: Case study: another sudden death in a child treated with desipramine. J Am Acad Child Adolesc Psychiatry 32:792–797, 1993

Riddle MA, Reeve EA, Yaryura-Tobias JA, et al: Fluvoxamine for children and adolescents with obsessive-compulsive disorder: a randomized, controlled, multicenter trial. J Am Acad Child Adolesc Psychiatry 40:222–229, 2001

Robinson DS, Rickels K, Feighner J, et al: Clinical effects of the 5-HT$_{1A}$ partial agonists in depression: a composite analysis of buspirone in the treatment of depression. J Clin Psychopharmacol 10(suppl):67S–76S, 1990

Rockhill C, Kodish I, DiBattisto C, et al: Anxiety disorders in children and adolescents. Curr Probl Pediatr Adolesc Health Care 40:66–99, 2010

Ross SB, Renyi AL: Tricyclic antidepressant agents, I: comparison of the inhibition of the uptake of 3-H-noradrenaline and 14-C-5-hydroxytryptamine in slices and crude synaptosome preparations of the midbrain-hypothalamus region of the rat brain. Acta Pharmacol Toxicol (Copenh) 36 (suppl 5):382–394, 1975

Roy A, De Jong J, Linnoila M: Cerebrospinal fluid monoamine metabolites and suicidal behavior in depressed patients. Arch Gen Psychiatry 46:609–612, 1989

Rynn MA, Siqueland L, Rickels K: Placebo-controlled trial of sertraline in the treatment of children with generalized anxiety disorder. Am J Psychiatry 158:2008–2014, 2001

Rynn M, Yeung PP, Riddle MA, et al: Venlafaxine ER as a treatment for GAD in children and adolescents. Presented at the 157th annual meeting of the American Psychiatric Association, New York, NY, May 1–6, 2004

Rynn MA, Riddle MA, Yeung PP, et al: Efficacy and safety of extended-release venlafaxine in the treatment of generalized anxiety disorder in children and adolescents: two placebo-controlled trials. Am J Psychiatry 164:290–300, 2007

Schweizer E, Rickels K, Weiss S, et al: Maintenance drug treatment of panic disorder I: results of a prospective, placebo-controlled comparison of alprazolam and imipramine. Arch Gen Psychiatry 50:51–60, 1993

Simeon JG, Ferguson HB: Alprazolam effects in children with anxiety disorders. Can J Psychiatry 32:570–574, 1987

Simeon JG, Ferguson B, Knott V, et al: Clinical, cognitive, and neurophysiological effects of alprazolam in children and adolescents with overanxious and avoidant disorders. J Am Acad Child Adolesc Psychiatry 31:29–33, 1992

Stein MB, Liebowitz M, Lydiard RB, et al: Paroxetine treatment of generalized social phobia (social anxiety disorder): a randomized, controlled trial. JAMA 280:708–713, 1998

Strauss CC: Behavioral assessment and treatment of overanxious disorder in children and adolescents. Behav Modif 12:234–251, 1988

Tancer ME: Neurobiology of social phobia. J Clin Psychiatry 54:26–30, 1993

Thomsen PH: Child and adolescent obsessive-compulsive disorder treated with citalopram: findings from an open trial of 23 cases. J Child Adolesc Psychopharmacol 7:157–166, 1997

Thomsen PH, Mikkelson HU: The addition of buspirone to SSRI in the treatment of adolescent obsessive-compulsive disorder: a study of six cases. Eur Child Adolesc Psychiatry 8:143–148, 1999

Thomsen PH, Ebbesen C, Persson C: Long-term experience with citalopram in the treatment of adolescent OCD. J Am Acad Child Adolesc Psychiatry 40:895–902, 2001

Tourian KA, March JS, Mangano R: Venlafaxine extended release in children and adolescents with social anxiety disorder. Presented at the 157th annual meeting of the American Psychiatric Association, New York, NY, May 1–6, 2004

U.S. Food and Drug Administration: Medication guide about using antidepressants in children and teenagers. January 2005. Available at: www.fda.gov/downloads/drugs/drugsafety/informationbydrugclass/UCM161646.pdf. Accessed May 12, 2012.

Varley CK, McClellan J: Case study: two additional sudden deaths with tricyclic antidepressants. J Am Acad Child Adolesc Psychiatry 36:390–394, 1997

Vitiello B, Zuvekas SH, Norquist GS: National estimates of antidepressant medication use among U.S. children, 1997–2002. J Am Acad Child Adolesc Psychiatry 45:271–279, 2006

Wagner KD, Berard R, Stein MB, et al: A multicenter, randomized, double-blind, placebo-controlled trial of paroxetine in children and adolescents with social anxiety disorder. Arch Gen Psychiatry 61:1153–1162, 2004

Walkup J, Labellarte M, Riddle MA, et al: Treatment of pediatric anxiety disorders: an open-label extension of the research units on pediatric psychopharmacology anxiety study. Research Units on Pediatric Psychopharmacology Anxiety Study Group. J Child Adolesc Psychopharmacol 12:175–188, 2002

Walkup J, Labellarte M, Riddle MA, et al: Searching for moderators and mediators of pharmacological treatment effects in children and adolescents with anxiety disorders. Research Units on Pediatric Psychopharmacology Anxiety Study Group. J Am Acad Child Adolesc Psychiatry 42:13–21, 2003

Walkup J, Albano AM, Piacentini J, et al: Cognitive behavioral therapy, sertraline, or a combination in childhood anxiety. N Engl J Med 359:2753–2766, 2008

Waslick B: Psychopharmacology interventions for pediatric anxiety disorders: a research update. Child Adolesc Psychiatr Clin N Am 15:51–71, 2006

Weintrob N, Cohen D, Klipper-Aurbach Y, et al: Decreased growth during therapy with selective serotonin reuptake inhibitors. Arch Pediatr Adolesc Med 156:696–701, 2002

Weissman MM, Wolk S, Wickramaratne P, et al: Children with prepubertal-onset major depressive disorder and anxiety grown up. Arch Gen Psychiatry 56:794–801, 1999

Werry J: Diagnosis and assessment, in Anxiety Disorders of Childhood. Edited by Gittelman R. New York, Guilford, 1986

Witek MW, Rojas V, Alonso C, et al: Review of benzodiazepine use in children and adolescents. Psychiatr Q 76:283–296, 2005

5

Major Depressive Disorder

Boris Birmaher, M.D.

Pediatric major depressive disorder (MDD) is a familial recurrent illness associated with poor psychosocial and academic outcome, substance abuse, anxiety, psychosocial difficulties, and an increased risk of suicide and suicide attempts (Birmaher et al. 1996b, 2002; Lewinsohn et al. 1999; Pine et al. 1998; Weissman et al. 1999a, 1999b). The prevalence of MDD in children and adolescents is approximately 2% and 6%, respectively (Birmaher et al. 1996b). Because pediatric MDD is continuous into adulthood, early identification and prompt treatment at its early stages are critical.

The main aim in this chapter is to review the current pharmacological treatments for children and adolescents with MDD. Although psychotherapy interventions, including cognitive-behavioral therapy (CBT)—either alone (Brent et al. 1997) or in combination with antidepressants (Brent et al. 2009; March et al. 2004)—and interpersonal psychotherapy (Mufson et al. 2004), have also been found efficacious for the acute treatment of pediatric MDD, particularly for adolescents, treatment using only these interventions is not reviewed in this chapter.

The definitions of five terms—*response, remission, recovery, relapse,* and *recurrence*—are useful for understanding treatment outcomes. The current definitions (Birmaher et al. 2000; Emslie et al. 1997, 2002, 2008) are presented in Table 5–1.

Assessment of Treatment Response

Understanding the research definition of *treatment response* can aid clinicians in interpreting the research-based evidence for the effectiveness of each antidepressant in day-to-day practice. Treatment response has traditionally been determined by the absence of MDD criteria (e.g., no more than one DSM symptom) or, more frequently, by a significant reduction in symptom severity (usually 50%). However, when the latter criterion is used, patients, deemed *responders,* may still have considerable residual depressive symptomatology. Therefore, an absolute final score on the Beck Depression Inventory of ≤9 (Beck 1967), or on the 17-item Hamilton Rating Scale for Depression of ≤7 (Hamilton 1960), or on the Children's Depression Rating Scale, Revised (CDRS-R) of ≤28 (Poznanski et al. 1984), together with persistent improvement in patient's functioning for at least 2 weeks or longer, may better reflect a satisfactory response. *Overall improvement* has also been measured with the Improvement subscale of the Clinical Global Impression Scale (CGI-I) (Guy 1976), with scores of 1 and 2 indicating *very much* and *much improvement,* respectively. *Functional improvement* can be measured using several rating scales, such as the Global Assessment Scale (American Psychiatric Association 1994) or the Children's Global Assessment Scale (Shaffer et al. 1983).

Treatment Phases

The treatment of MDD is divided into three phases: acute, continuation, and maintenance ("Practice Guideline for the Treatment of Patients With Major Depressive Disorder [Revision]" 2000; "Practice Parameters for the Assessment and Treatment of Children and Adolescents With Depressive Disorders" 1998). The main goal of treatment during the *acute phase* is to achieve response and, more importantly, remission of the depressive symptoms. This phase usually lasts 6–12 weeks. The *continuation phase* usually lasts 4–12

Table 5–1. Definitions of treatment outcome

Response	No symptoms or a significant reduction in depressive symptoms for at least 2 weeks
Remission	A period of at least 2 weeks and less than 2 months with no or very few depressive symptoms
Recovery	Absence of symptoms of major depressive disorder for 2 months or more (e.g., can have no more than two symptoms to be considered in recovery)
Relapse	A major depressive episode during the period of remission
Recurrence	A new major depressive episode during the period of recovery

months, during which remission is consolidated to prevent relapses. The *maintenance phase* lasts 1 year or longer, and its main treatment objective is the prevention of depression recurrences. Almost all studies on children and adolescents have evaluated treatments during the acute phase. Few continuation studies (Clarke et al. 2005; Emslie et al. 2008; Goodyer et al. 2007) and no maintenance treatment studies have been reported. Therefore, recommendations regarding continuation and maintenance treatments are extrapolated from the adult literature. However, caution is warranted because youth may respond differently to continuation and maintenance interventions that thus far have only been tested on adults with MDD (Birmaher et al. 1996a).

Treatment of Major Depressive Disorder With Selective Serotonin Reuptake Inhibitors and Other Novel Antidepressants

Psychoeducation and Supportive Therapy

The optimal pharmacological management of MDD in children and adolescents should involve educative and supportive psychotherapy. In fact, at least for youth with mild-to-moderate depression, supportive management and education may be sufficient to ameliorate the symptoms of depression (Goodyer et al. 2007; Mufson et al. 2004; Renaud et al. 1998). Education of the patient and family about the disease, nature of treatment, and prognosis is critical to engagement in treatment and enhancement of compliance (Brent et al. 1993). During and after the depression remission, psychosocial scars or complications (e.g., family conflict, poor self-esteem and social skills, academic difficulties, problems with peers) need to be addressed with psychotherapy (Birmaher et al. 2000; Kovacs and Goldston 1991; Puig-Antich et al. 1985; Rao et al. 1995; Stein et al. 2000; Strober et al. 1993).

Additionally, the parents of depressed youth may also be experiencing depression and other psychiatric disorders (Klein et al. 2001; Weissman et al. 1987), and parental depression may lead to adverse outcomes in the youth. In fact, successful treatment of the parents may ameliorate or even prevent the development of psychopathology in their children (Birmaher 2011). Thus, to treat the child successfully, the clinician should assess parents and refer them for their own treatment.

Acute Phase

Studies on the acute treatment of youth with MDD have focused on the effects of tricyclic antidepressants (TCAs), selective serotonin reuptake inhibitors (SSRIs), and, more recently, serotonin-norepinephrine reuptake inhibitors (SNRIs). A few open studies have also shown that monoamine oxidase inhibitors (MAOIs) can be used safely in children and adolescents (Ryan et al. 1988b), although noncompliance with dietary requirements may present a significant problem for youth taking MAOIs. Other antidepressants, including the heterocyclics (e.g., amoxapine, maprotiline) and bupropion, have been found to be efficacious for the treatment of depressed adults ("Practice Guideline" 2000), but they have not been well studied for the treatment of MDD in children and adolescents. The TCAs have not been found to be better than placebo for the treatment of youth with MDD (Hazell et al. 2006), and they are associated with significant side effects and high risk for lethality in a case of an overdose. Therefore, this chapter mainly describes the use of SSRIs and SNRIs for youth with MDD.

Using CGI-I scores of ≤ 2 (*much improved* to *very much improved*) as indicating a positive outcome, randomized controlled trials (RCTs) using fluoxetine, citalopram, sertraline, escitalopram, and paroxetine have shown that children and adolescents with MDD responded significantly better to acute treatment with these antidepressants (50%–60%) than with placebo (30%–

50%) (Bridge et al. 2009). Of these SSRIs, fluoxetine showed the largest effect sizes, in part because of a low placebo response rate. Despite the significant rates of response, a smaller proportion of patients (30%–40%) achieved full remission (usually defined as a score of ≤28 on the CDRS-R) (Emslie et al. 1997, 2008; March et al. 2004; Wagner et al. 2004).

A possible explanation for the low rate of remission is that optimal pharmacological treatment may involve a higher dosage and/or a longer duration of treatment or that the ideal treatment for some individuals may involve a combination of pharmacological and psychosocial interventions, as suggested by the Treatment for Adolescents With Depression Study (TADS; March et al. 2004). However, in the TADS study, despite the fact that the rate of remission was higher in combination treatment (37% in combination vs. 23% in medication alone), particularly for less severely depressed subjects, the remission rate was not optimal. Moreover, other studies did not show an advantage to adding CBT to regular SSRI treatment (Clarke et al. 2005; Goodyer et al. 2007).

Several published or unpublished industry-sponsored studies with SSRIs (one each with citalopram, escitalopram, and sertraline, and two with paroxetine) did not find differences between active medication and placebo (Bridge et al. 2009). In these, as in some of the above-mentioned positive studies, subjects responded to the SSRIs (46%–63%), but the placebo response was also high (about 50%). The placebo response was associated with less depressive severity at intake and a large number of centers involved in the trial (Bridge et al. 2009).

Also, except in a large fluoxetine study (Emslie et al. 1997) in which no age differences were found, younger subjects overall have higher placebo responses than older adolescents. Mild-to-moderate depressive symptoms may have responded to supportive management offered in these studies. Also, other methodological issues may have been responsible for the lack of difference between medication and placebo. (For a review of the limitations of relatively recent pharmacological RCTs, see Cheung et al. 2005.) Table 5–2 summarizes data on SSRIs in pediatric depression.

A novel way to understand the effect of treatment is through the concept of the *number needed to treat* (NNT), which refers to the number of patients who must be treated to observe one response that it is attributable to active treatment and not placebo. Across all the published and unpublished SSRI

RCTs, patients with depression who were treated with SSRIs have had relatively good response rates (50%–70% clinically improved), but the placebo response rates have also been high (30%–60%), resulting in an overall NNT of 9 (Bridge et al. 2009; Cheung et al. 2005). Fluoxetine was the first medication to be approved by the U.S. Food and Drug Administration (FDA) for the treatment of child and adolescent depression, and it shows a larger difference between medication and placebo than do other antidepressants, with an overall NNT of 4. It is not clear whether the difference is due to actual differences in the effect of the medication, to other related properties of the medication (long half-life may lessen the impact of poor adherence to treatment), or to better design and performance of the fluoxetine studies, which may have had more severely depressed patients.

In addition to fluoxetine, escitalopram has been approved to treat major depressive disorder in adolescents, ages 12–17. Data from several escitalopram trials, in addition to safety data from studies of citalopram, led to the FDA approval of escitalopram. In the trials of escitalopram, differences in response between children under age 12 and adolescents led to the age range associated with FDA approval (Emslie et al. 2009; Wagner et al. 2004, 2006).

Few RCTs have evaluated the effects of other classes of antidepressants for the treatment of depressed youth. One unpublished study showed that nefazodone was significantly more effective than placebo for youth with MDD (Cheung et al. 2005; Mann et al. 2006). However, although the generic form of this medication is still available, the manufacturer has withdrawn Serzone from the market because of a rare but serious side effect—liver damage resulting in hepatic failure. A small RCT comparing venlafaxine with placebo showed no differences between the two (Mandoki et al. 1997). Two unpublished industry-sponsored RCTs with venlafaxine and two with mirtazapine were negative (Bridge et al. 2009; Mann et al. 2006). However, a reanalysis of the venlafaxine trials showed significant effects over placebo for adolescents but not for children. There are no reports on the use of duloxetine in youth. Although bupropion is being used clinically for the treatment of youth with MDD, no RCTs have been conducted for youth with MDD, except an open study on children with MDD and attention-deficit/hyperactivity disorder (ADHD) (Daviss et al. 2001).

Table 5–2. Selected data on selective serotonin reuptake inhibitors in pediatric depression

Medication	Study	Dosage	Randomized controlled trials Outcome	FDA approval
Citalopram	Wagner et al. 2004	20–40 mg/day	Citalopram>placebo	No
	von Knorring et al. 2006	10–40 mg/day	Did not separate from placebo	
Escitalopram	Wagner et al. 2006	10–20 mg/day	Did not separate from placebo in general population; escitalopram>placebo in adolescents	Yes; MDD ages 12–17 years
	Emslie et al. 2009	10–20 mg/day	Escitalopram>placebo	
Fluoxetine	Emslie et al. 1997	20 mg/day	Fluoxetine>placebo	Yes; MDD ages 8–18 years
	Emslie et al. 2002	20 mg/day	Fluoxetine>placebo	
	March et al. 2004	10–40 mg/day	Fluoxetine>placebo	
Paroxetine	Keller et al. 2001	20–40 mg/day	Paroxetine>placebo	No
	Berard et al. 2006	20–40 mg/day	Did not separate from placebo	
	Emslie et al. 2006	10–50 mg/day	Did not separate from placebo	
Sertraline	Wagner et al. 2003[a]	50–200 mg/day	Sertraline>placebo	No
	Donnelly et al. 2006	50–200 mg/day	Did not separate from placebo in children; sertraline>placebo in adolescents	

Note. MDD=major depressive disorder.
[a]Data pooled from two controlled trials.

Side Effects

Overall, SSRIs and other novel antidepressants have been well tolerated by both children and adolescents, with only a few short-term side effects commonly reported. It appears that the side effects of SSRIs and SNRIs are similar and dose dependent, and may subside with time (Cheung et al. 2005; Emslie et al. 1999; Leonard et al. 1997; Safer and Zito 2006). The most common side effects include gastrointestinal symptoms, restlessness, diaphoresis, headaches, akathisia, changes in appetite (increase or decrease), sleep changes (e.g., vivid dreams, nightmares, impaired sleep), and impaired sexual functioning. Approximately 3%–8% of children and adolescents taking antidepressants may show increased impulsivity, agitation, irritability, silliness, and behavioral activation (Hammad 2004; Martin et al. 2004; Wilens et al. 1998). These symptoms must be differentiated from the mania or hypomania that may appear in children and adolescents with bipolar disorder or in those who are predisposed to develop that disorder (Wilens et al. 1998).

More rarely, the use of antidepressants has been associated with serotonin syndrome (Boyer and Shannon 2005) (see later subsection "Interactions With Other Medications"), with increased suicidal behaviors (see the next subsection, "Suicidal Behaviors"), and with bruising (Lake et al. 2000). Citalopram was found to be associated with arrhythmias and prolonged QTc, particularly at dosages higher than 40 mg/day (www.fda.gov). Because of the risk of bruising, patients treated with SSRIs and SNRIs who are going to have surgery should inform their physicians, and they may wish to discontinue treatment during the preoperative period. Venlafaxine and perhaps other SNRIs may elevate blood pressure and cause tachycardia (Brent et al. 2009). Mirtazapine, a serotonin and adrenergic receptor blocker, may increase appetite, weight, and somnolence. Trazodone, a serotonin type 2A (5-HT_{2A}) receptor blocker and weak serotonin reuptake inhibitor, and mirtazapine are mainly used as adjunctive and transient treatments for insomnia. Trazodone must be used with caution in males because it can induce priapism. As noted earlier, the brand form of nefazodone (Serzone), a 5-HT_{2A} receptor blocker and weak serotonin reuptake inhibitor, was taken off the market because it may induce liver problems. The long-term side effects of antidepressants have not been systematically evaluated.

Suicidal Behaviors

Compared with pediatric patients given placebo, those taking antidepressants appear to have a small but statistically significant increase in *spontaneous* reporting of self-harm behavior and suicidal ideation. In an FDA-sponsored meta-analysis, conducted in collaboration with Columbia University (Hammad et al. 2006), of the *spontaneous* suicide adverse events (SAEs) reported in 24 RCTs (16 studies of MDD, 4 of obsessive-compulsive disorder [OCD], 2 of generalized anxiety disorder, 1 of social anxiety disorder, and 1 of ADHD) comparing several antidepressants versus placebo, the overall risk ratio (RR) for *spontaneously* reported SAEs was 1.95 (95% CI, 1.28–2.98). For only MDD studies, the overall RR was 1.66 (95% CI, 1.02–2.68). Only TADS showed a significant difference between active treatment and placebo, and among the antidepressants, only venlafaxine showed a statistically significant association with suicidality (March et al. 2004). In general, these results translate to two emergent or worsened *spontaneous reports* of suicidality for every 100 youth treated with one of the antidepressants included in the FDA meta-analysis. The study authors reported very few suicide attempts and no completions.

In contrast to the analyses of the SAEs, evaluation of the suicidality ascertained through rating scales in 17 studies did not show significant onset or worsening of suicidality ($RR \approx 0.90$) (Hammad et al. 2006). It is not clear why the FDA meta-analysis found increased rates of spontaneously reported SAEs for subjects taking drug versus placebo but no differences in suicidality on regularly assessed clinical measures. It is possible that in a subgroup of patients treated with antidepressants, particularly those already agitated and/or suicidal, treatment causes a disinhibition that leads to worsening of ideation and/or a greater tendency to make suicidal threats. Because suicidal ideation usually leads to removal of the subject from the study and a change in treatment, analyses that look at the slope of suicidal ideation will not find an effect. In addition, as measured on rating scales, suicidal ideation is highly correlated with the severity of depression, which is more likely to decline in those given drug than in those given placebo.

These results must be viewed in the context of the FDA study's limitations, which include use of the metric of relative risk (limited to trials with at least one event), inability to generalize the results to populations not included in RCTs, short-term data, failure to include all available RCTs, and multiple comparisons (Hammad et al. 2006). Also, as stated by the FDA (Hammad et al. 2006), the implications and clinical significance regarding the above-noted findings are uncertain, given that with the increase in usage of SSRIs, there has been a dramatic decline in adolescent suicide (Olfson et al. 2003). Moreover, pharmacoepidemiological studies, which are correlative rather than causal, support a positive relationship between SSRI use and the reduction in the rate of adolescent and young adult suicides (Gibbons et al. 2005; Olfson et al. 2003; Valuck et al. 2004). Moreover, a study showed increased suicide attempts only immediately *before* the SSRIs were administered (Simon et al. 2006), and later studies in several countries showed that after the FDA's black box warning for SSRIs was implemented, a surge occurred in the number of suicides (e.g., Katz et al. 2008; Libby et al. 2009).

A thorough meta-analysis extended the FDA analyses by including all existing published and unpublished antidepressant studies (13 of MDD, 6 of OCD, and 6 of anxiety disorders) (Bridge et al. 2009). This meta-analysis found comparable *overall* findings when similar statistical methods (RRs) were used rather than the methods used in the FDA study (Bridge et al. 2009)—namely, a significantly increased RR for spontaneously reported suicidality *only* for subjects with MDD. However, in pooled random-effects analyses of risk differences, which make possible an analysis of *all* the existing RCTs, a nonsignificant risk difference (drug minus placebo) was found for MDD (0.8%; 95% CI, −0.2% to 1.8%) and other disorders. The overall *number needed to harm* (NNH) (number of subjects needed to treat in order to observe one adverse event that can be attributed to the active treatment) for MDD was 125 (Bridge et al. 2009). As stated earlier in the section "Acute Phase," the overall NNT for antidepressants in pediatric depression is 9. Thus, nearly 14 times more depressed patients will respond favorably to antidepressants than will spontaneously report suicidality (although one must keep in mind the limitations of meta-analyses). The benefit-risk ratio was larger for the SSRIs (10) than for non-SSRI antidepressants (5).

In conclusion, spontaneously reported SAEs appear to be more common with antidepressant treatment than with placebo. Nevertheless, given the greater number of patients who benefit from antidepressant treatment, particularly the SSRIs, than who experience these SAEs, as well as the decline in overall suicidal ideation on rating scales, the risk-benefit ratio for SSRI use in pediatric depression appears to be favorable, with careful monitoring. Further work is required to determine if the risk-benefit ratio is indeed less favorable for children than for adolescents. Also, it remains to be clarified whether certain factors are related to increased risk for suicidality (Apter et al. 2006; Brent 2004; Hammad et al. 2006; Safer and Zito 2006)—for example, gender; subject's history of suicidality; family history of suicidality; disorder type (the effects of the disorder type appear to be more obvious in depressed youth); severity of depressive symptoms at intake; dosages; medication half-life (in terms of efficacy); type of antidepressants administered; treatment duration; poor adherence to treatment; withdrawal side effects (due to noncompliance or short medication half-life); induction of agitation, activation, or hypomania; and/or susceptibility to side effects (e.g., slow metabolizers or variations in genetic polymorphisms).

Pharmacokinetic Studies

Aside from fluoxetine, which has a half-life of 24–72 hours in children, the half-lives of most SSRIs (including paroxetine, sertraline, citalopram, and bupropion SR [sustained release]) are between 14 and 16 hours (Axelson et al. 2000a, 2000b; Clein and Riddle 1995; Daviss et al. 2005; Findling et al. 1999, 2000, 2006). One study suggested that sertraline at a dosage of 200 mg/day can be prescribed once a day (Alderman et al. 1998). Results of previously mentioned studies suggest that SSRIs, particularly when prescribed at lower dosages, may need to be given twice a day. Another option is to administer the SSRIs once a day and carefully evaluate the child for withdrawal side effects. If withdrawal side effects occur, twice-daily dosing is necessary. Otherwise, children and adolescents may experience withdrawal side effects during the evening, and these symptoms can be confused with lack of response or medication side effects. More pharmacokinetic studies conducted on the other antidepressants (i.e., SNRIs, atypical antidepressants) are necessary, because it appears that youth metabolize these medications faster than adult populations do.

Interactions With Other Medications

Careful attention to possible medication interactions is recommended, given that the antidepressants and/or their metabolites are metabolized in different degrees by the hepatic cytochrome P450 (CYP) enzymes. Of the five major CYP enzymes mediating the oxidative drug metabolism, CYP3A3/4 and

CYP2D6 are responsible for approximately 50% and 30%, respectively, of known oxidative drug metabolism. Except for citalopram/escitalopram and sertraline, the currently available SSRIs are mainly metabolized by CYP3A3/4 and/or CYP2D6 enzymes. Bupropion is mainly metabolized by the CYP2B6 enzyme, but it also inhibits the enzyme CYP2D6. Venlafaxine is metabolized by the CYP2D6 enzyme. Substantial inhibition of these enzymes converts a normal metabolizer into a slow metabolizer with regard to this specific pathway. Therefore, the clinician needs to be aware of the possibility that toxicity could result if the patient is taking other medications that are also metabolized by the CYP system; these medications include the TCAs, neuroleptics, atypical antipsychotics, antiarrhythmics, antihypertensives, theophylline, atomoxetine, benzodiazepines, carbamazepine, and warfarin. Several Web sites provide up-to-date information regarding the metabolism of SSRIs and other antidepressants by the CYP system, as well as interactions with other medications (e.g., see http://medicine.iupui.edu/flockhart, and www.pdr.net).

Interactions of the antidepressants with other serotonergic medications, in particular the MAOIs, may induce serotonin syndrome, which is marked by agitation, confusion, and hyperthermia (Boyer and Shannon 2005). MAOIs should not be given within 5 weeks after stopping fluoxetine, and for at least 2 weeks after stopping other SSRIs, because of the possibility of inducing serotonin syndrome.

Some antidepressants also have a high rate of protein binding, which can lead to increased therapeutic or toxic effects of other protein-bound medications.

Discontinuation

Especially for antidepressants with shorter half-lives (e.g., paroxetine), sudden or rapid cessation may induce withdrawal symptoms that can mimic a relapse or recurrence of a depressive episode (e.g., tiredness, irritability). Furthermore, there is the clinical impression that rapid discontinuation of antidepressants may induce relapses or recurrences of depression. Therefore, if these medications need to be discontinued, they should be tapered progressively.

Summary and Recommendations for Acute Treatment

Given that 30%–60% of children and adolescents with MDD respond to placebo (Bridge et al. 2009; Cheung et al. 2005; Mann et al. 2006) and/or very brief or supportive psychotherapy treatments (Goodyer et al. 2007; Mufson et al. 2004; Renaud et al. 1998), it is reasonable, when treating a patient with a mild depression or mild psychosocial impairment, to offer psychoeducation, support, and case management related to possible environmental stressors in the family and school. If the symptoms of mild depression worsen, or if the child has not responded after 4–6 weeks of supportive therapy, more specific forms of psychotherapy or antidepressants are warranted.

In contrast, children and adolescents who present with chronic or recurrent depression, moderate-to-severe psychosocial impairment, comorbid disorder, or a high family history of depression initially require more specific types of psychotherapies and/or antidepressants.

Independent of the treatment administered, patient and family will require education about the nature and treatment of depression, support, and management of daily problems. Problems at school, academic issues, school refusal, abuse of drugs, exposure to negative events (e.g., abuse, conflict with parents), and peer issues must be addressed. For example, family discord is associated with slower recovery and greater chance of recurrence (Birmaher et al. 2000; Rueter et al. 1999), and ongoing disappointments have been associated with chronic depression (Goodyer et al. 1998). Therefore, addressing family discord and improving the patient's coping skills are likely to improve outcome in either psychosocial or psychopharmacological treatment. Moreover, a high incidence of parental mental health problems indicates the need for evaluation and appropriate referral of parents and siblings of depressed youth, particularly because several studies have shown that a mother's depression is associated with increased risk for psychopathology in her children (Birmaher 2011). Finally, a high degree of comorbidity also emphasizes the importance of a multimodal pharmacological and psychosocial treatment approach (Hughes et al. 1999). For example, a child with MDD and ADHD may not respond to an SSRI alone, and may require either combined treatment with a stimulant plus an SSRI, or an alternative medication such as a TCA, bupropion, or venlafaxine (Daviss et al. 2001; Pliszka 2000).

Currently, the antidepressants of choice to treat children and adolescents with MDD are the SSRIs. Fluoxetine has the most consistent data showing separation from placebo, but escitalopram has shown positive findings in adolescent patients in particular. Until additional studies with better methodologies are available, other SSRIs can also be used with caution. Patients should be treated with adequate dosages for at least 6 weeks before the clinician declares a lack of response to treatment (treatment of nonresponders is described in the subsection "Treatment-Resistant Depression" later in this chapter).

The dosages of SSRIs prescribed for children and adolescents are similar to those used for adult patients (Birmaher and Brent 2007; Leonard et al. 1997) (Table 5–3), except that lower initial dosages are used to avoid unwanted effects. To avoid side effects and improve adherence to treatment, the medication should be started at a low dosage and increased slowly. Also, children might require lower dosages than adolescents, but this issue has not been well studied. During the acute phase of treatment, patients should be treated with adequate and tolerable dosages for at least 4–6 weeks. Clinical response should be assessed at 4- to 6-week intervals, and the dosage can be increased if a complete response has not been obtained. At the point of assessment, if only a partial response has been achieved, the physician may consider strategies described in the subsection "Treatment-Resistant Depression" later in this chapter. At each step, adequate time should be allowed for clinical response, and frequent, early dosage adjustments should be avoided.

Given the small but significant association between antidepressants and worsening or emergent spontaneous SAEs, all patients receiving these medications for suicidal and other symptomatology should be carefully monitored, particularly during the first weeks of treatment. The FDA recommends that subjects be seen every week for the first 4 weeks and biweekly thereafter. If weekly face-to-face appointments cannot be scheduled, evaluations should be carried out briefly by phone. However, no data are available to suggest that the face-to-face monitoring schedule proposed by the FDA or telephone calls have any impact on the risk of suicide. Although monitoring is important for all patients, it should be more carefully done for patients who have history of suicidal ideation or suicide attempts or who show behavior associated with increased risk for suicide (e.g., prior suicidality, impulsivity, substance abuse, history of sexual abuse) (Gould et al. 1996; Shaffer and Craft 1999); for patients who have become agitated, disinhibited, or irritable while using an antidepressant; and for those with family history of bipolar disorder or suicide.

Table 5–3. Dosages of antidepressants usually administered to youth with major depressive disorder

Medication group	Medication	Starting dosage (mg/day)	Dosage range (mg/day)
SSRIs	Citalopram	10	20–40[a]
	Escitalopram	10	10–40
	Fluoxetine	10	20–80
	Fluvoxamine	25	50–150
	Paroxetine	10	20–60
	Sertraline	25	50–300
SNRIs	Venlafaxine XR	37.5	75–225
Others	Bupropion SR	100	150–300
	Bupropion XL	150	150–300

Note. SNRI = serotonin-norepinephrine reuptake inhibitor; SR = sustained release; SSRI = selective serotonin reuptake inhibitor; XL = extended release; XR = extended release.
[a]Dose adjusted by U.S. Food and Drug Administration recently because of concerns about QT prolongation.

Treatment of Major Depressive Disorder Subtypes

Bipolar Depression

Many children and adolescents seeking treatment for depression are usually experiencing their first depressive episode. Because the symptoms of unipolar and bipolar depression are similar, it is difficult to decide whether a patient needs only an antidepressant or treatment with other medications or psychotherapies. Some symptoms and signs of bipolar illness, such as psychosis or psychomotor retardation, or a family history of bipolar disorder may alert the clinician to the risk that the child could develop a manic episode.

Only small negative RCTs have evaluated the effects of quetiapine for youth with bipolar depression (DelBello et al. 2009). In adults, RCTs have shown some positive effects with lithium carbonate, valproate, and some of the atypical antipsychotics such as quetiapine (either alone or in combination with mood stabilizers) (Vieta et al. 2010). Lamotrigine as monotherapy or as an adjunctive treatment appears to be efficacious to prevent relapses or recurrences of depression, although a meta-analysis showed moderate effects for the acute treatment of bipolar depression in adults (Geddes et al. 2009). A meta-analysis (Gijsman et al. 2004) showed that SSRIs are beneficial for the treatment of bipolar depression in adults, and that with the exception of the TCAs, antidepressants did not induce significantly more manic switches than placebo. Moreover, one RCT found that monotherapy with fluoxetine was better than placebo for the management of depressed adult patients with bipolar II disorder and did not induce significant increases in manic switches (Amsterdam et al. 1998). Some studies have also suggested that bupropion is less likely to induce a mania or rapid cycling (Compton and Nemeroff 2000; "Practice Guideline for the Treatment of Patients With Bipolar Disorder" 1994). Important considerations are that children and adolescents do not always respond to medications in the same way as adults, and youth may be more prone to switch to mania with antidepressants. In particular, youth with subthreshold manic symptoms or a family history of bipolar disorder may be at the greatest risk for conversion to mania with antidepressant treatment (Baumer et al. 2006; Goldsmith et al. 2011). Therefore, these recommendations must be followed with caution until controlled studies of children and adolescents are available.

Psychotic Depression

No controlled studies of psychotic depression in youth have been done. Because only 20%–40% of adults respond to antidepressant monotherapy ("Practice Guideline" 2000), recommended treatment often consists of antidepressants combined with an antipsychotic. The antipsychotics are usually tapered after remission of the depression. The newer antipsychotic medications (e.g., risperidone, olanzapine) may prove useful as monotherapy for psychotic depression, but some of them have clinically relevant metabolic effects. Electroconvulsive therapy (ECT) is particularly effective for the psychotic subtype of depression in adults ("Practice Guideline" 2000) and may be useful for depressed teens as well (Ghaziuddin et al. 2004). Treatment with antidepressants in psychotic depressed children should be conducted with caution, because the presence of psychosis is a marker for possible development of bipolar disorder (Geller et al. 1994; Strober and Carlson 1982).

Seasonal Affective Disorder

Studies in adults have shown that SSRIs and bright light therapy are beneficial for the treatment of subjects with recurrent seasonal affective disorder. One small RCT suggested that bright light therapy is efficacious for the treatment of children and adolescents with seasonal affective disorder (Swedo et al. 1997), but no studies with antidepressants have been conducted in this younger population.

Treatment-Resistant Depression

As in adults ("Practice Guideline" 2000), up to 60% of youth with MDD have a partial treatment response (moderate response on the CGI-I; presence of significant symptoms of MDD, but not the full syndrome) and 20%–30% may not respond to treatment at all (Birmaher et al. 2000; Brent et al. 2009; Emslie et al. 2008; March et al. 2004). Patients with partial response have a significantly higher rate of relapse during the first 6 months following therapy and have significantly more psychosocial, occupational, and medical problems ("Practice Guideline" 2000). Moreover, among children, chronic depressions do not usually remit spontaneously and are not responsive to placebo ("Practice Guideline" 2000; "Practice Parameters" 1998), indicating the need for aggressive treatment of patients with these conditions.

The first step in the management of patients with treatment-resistant depression is to establish the nonresponse. Several definitions of *nonresponse* have been used, including the presence of a significant number of depressive symptoms, less that 50% improvement as measured by rating scales (e.g., the CDRS-R), and no change or worsening in the CGI. After establishing that the patient has not responded, the clinician needs to try to find out why. The most common reasons for treatment failure are inappropriate diagnoses, inadequate drug dosage or length of drug trial, lack of compliance with treatment, comorbidity with other psychiatric disorders (e.g., dysthymia, anxiety, ADHD, covered substance abuse, personality disorders) or comorbid medical illnesses (e.g., hypothyroidism), and presence of bipolar disorder (Brent et al. 1998, 2009; Hughes et al. 1999; "Practice Guideline" 2000). Other factors associated with nonresponse include severe depression, suicidality, exposure to negative events (abuse, ongoing conflicts), lack of response or mild response after 2–4 weeks of treatment, and hopelessness. Carefully evaluating for subtle symptoms of hypomania is important to determine whether bipolar disorder may be the reason that the youth is not responding to treatment or even is worsening with SSRI treatment.

The Treatment of SSRI-Resistant Depression in Adolescents (TORDIA) study (Brent et al. 2008) is the only RCT of adolescents with treatment-refractory depression. This study of a large sample of adolescents with MDD indicated that the combination of CBT and an antidepressant was more efficacious than the antidepressant alone (54.8% vs. 40.5%). No differences were found among the antidepressants used in the study (fluoxetine, citalopram, venlafaxine). The expected variables were associated with poor response (e.g., more severe depression, comorbid disorder, abuse). Follow-up assessments showed continuous remission, with approximately 60% remission by 72 weeks. About 25% of the remitted subjects later experienced relapse (Emslie et al. 2010; Vitiello et al. 2011).

After noncompliance with treatment has been ruled out, the following strategies, based on the TORDIA study and the adult literature, have been recommended:

1. *Optimize initial treatments.* Although few studies have evaluated the efficacy of this strategy, initial treatment can be maximized by increasing the length of the trial or increasing the dosage.

   a. *Extend the initial medication trial.* For patients with at least partial response after receiving a therapeutic dose of antidepressant for 6 weeks, the first and simplest strategy is to extend the treatment for another 2–4 weeks, if the patient's clinical and functional status allows ("Practice Guideline" 2000; Thase and Rush 1997).

   b. *Increase the dosage.* This strategy can be used for partial responders. Occasionally, increasing the dosage in a patient with no response for another 2–3 weeks may help (Heiligenstein et al. 2006; "Practice Guideline" 2000).

2. *Switch strategies.* For patients who do not respond to a specific antidepressant medication or who do not tolerate its side effects, other antidepressants of the same class or different classes (e.g., venlafaxine for a patient who did not respond to an SSRI) can be tried. The few adult studies published to date suggest that because of the probable heterogeneity in depression mechanisms, the more efficacious approach is to switch anti-

depressant classes rather than stay within the same class. Also, severe depression appears to respond better to antidepressants with both serotonergic and adrenergic properties (e.g., venlafaxine; Poirier and Boyer 1999). MAOIs have been found beneficial for patients who have not responded to other medications ("Practice Guideline" 2000; Thase and Rush 1997). An open study suggested that adolescents with depression who had not responded to TCAs responded to MAOIs (Ryan et al. 1988b). However, these adolescents may not have responded to TCAs because this group of medications is not efficacious for the treatment of pediatric MDD (Birmaher et al. 1996a).

3. *Augment or combine strategies.* The TORDIA study (Brent et al. 2009) provided evidence that the combination of an antidepressant plus CBT is efficacious for teens with treatment-resistant MDD. However, pharmacological augmentation has not been well studied in youth. In adults, the most common augmentation or combination strategies include adding lithium carbonate at therapeutic levels for a period of 4 weeks, or L-triiodothyronine (T_3) (25–50 μg/day), or stimulants, or combining an SSRI with a TCA (Bauer et al. 2000; "Practice Guideline" 2000). In adults, the combination of lithium and antidepressants has yielded response rates of 50%–65% in studies that administered lithium at therapeutic levels for at least 4 weeks (e.g., see "Practice Guideline" 2000; Thase and Rush 1997). The interval before response to lithium augmentation has been reported to be from several days to 3 weeks ("Practice Guideline" 2000). After this period, the chance to observe improvement with lithium decreases.

In adolescents with MDD, an open-label study showed significant improvement of refractory depressive symptoms after augmentation of TCA treatment with lithium (Ryan et al. 1988a). Another open-label study, however, did not replicate this finding (Strober et al. 1992).

Case reports have suggested that adding stimulant medications or combining an SSRI with a TCA or bupropion may also be effective ("Practice Guideline" 2000), but these combinations need to be used with caution because of the possibility of interactions (as with, e.g., SSRIs and TCAs). In adolescents and adults, the combination of antidepressants and psychotherapy (CBT, interpersonal psychotherapy) for patients with severe or treatment-resistant depression has also been found useful (Keller et al. 2000; March et al. 2004).

4. *Consider electroconvulsive therapy.* ECT is one of the most efficacious treatments for adults with nonresistant MDD (70% response) and resistant MDD (50% response) (Ghaziuddin et al. 2004; "Practice Guideline" 2000). However, because of the invasiveness of this treatment, it remains the treatment of choice only for the most severe, incapacitating forms of resistant depression. No controlled studies have been conducted in adolescents, although anecdotal reports suggest that adolescents with refractory depression may respond to ECT without significant side effects (Ghaziuddin et al. 2004; Rey and Walter 1997). Approximately 60% of adult patients who are treated successfully with ECT tend to relapse after 6 months ("Practice Guideline" 2000). Therefore, they also have to receive maintenance treatment with antidepressants and sometimes maintenance ECT. However, maintenance ECT has never been reported in adolescents.

5. *Try other biological treatments.* Other innovative treatments, such as intravenous clomipramine, transcranial magnetic stimulation, and vagal nerve stimulation, have been used for the treatment of depressed adults who have not responded to standard treatment. In adolescents, intravenous clomipramine has been shown to be efficacious for patients who have failed to respond to other antidepressant treatment (Sallee et al. 1997), but no studies using transcranial magnetic stimulation or vagal nerve stimulation have been conducted in depressed youth.

All of the strategies listed above require implementation in a systematic fashion (for reviews, see "Practice Guideline" 2000; "Practice Parameters" 1998; Thase and Rush 1997). Comparing these strategies with other treatments of medical disorders can be useful to help patients and their families understand the medication plan and to improve compliance with and tolerance of treatment. The example of hypertension is appropriate: diuretics may be used alone, or combined with other antihypertensives in different trials, according to response. Psychoeducation for the patient and family is also required to avoid the development of hopelessness in the patient and family, as well as in the clinician.

Treatment of Comorbid Conditions and Suicidality

Comorbid disorders may influence the onset, maintenance, and recurrence of depression (Birmaher et al. 1996a, 1996b; Emslie et al. 2010; Vitiello et al. 2011). Therefore, in addition to treating the depressive symptoms, the clinician should treat the comorbid conditions that frequently accompany the depressive disorders (Hughes et al. 1999).

For example, depressed adolescents with comorbid ADHD respond less well to treatment than do adolescents with depression only (Emslie et al. 1997; Hamilton and Bridge 1999). For patients with depression and ADHD, recommendations are that the ADHD should be treated first; then, if the depressive symptoms continue after stabilization of the ADHD, an SSRI should be added (Hughes et al. 1999; Pliszka 2000). This strategy, however, has not been validated. An open study using bupropion suggested that this medication can be efficacious to treat both MDD and ADHD (Daviss et al. 2001), although the effect of bupropion on ADHD is not as impressive as that obtained by treatment with stimulants (Conners et al. 1996).

Treatment of comorbid anxiety, which more often precedes depression than vice versa, is essential insofar as it contributes to improvement, and because the anxiety, if left untreated, may predispose the individual to future depressive episodes (Hayward et al. 2000; Kovacs et al. 1989). Fortunately, similar pharmacotherapy and psychotherapy treatments found useful for the treatment of MDD have also been found beneficial for the treatment of youth with anxiety disorders (Birmaher et al. 2003; "Fluvoxamine for the Treatment of Anxiety Disorders in Children and Adolescents" 2001; Kendall 1994).

Other comorbid conditions, such as OCD, conduct disorder, eating disorders, and posttraumatic stress disorder, have also been found to affect treatment response. These conditions must be addressed if treatment of depressed youth is to be successful (Birmaher et al. 1996b; Brent et al. 1998; Goodyer et al. 1997).

Suicidal ideation and behavior are common symptoms accompanying major depression and are more likely to occur in the face of comorbid disruptive disorders, substance abuse, physical or sexual abuse, impulsive behaviors, prior suicide attempts, and family history of suicidal behavior (e.g., Gould et al. 1996). Assessment of suicidality, the securing of any lethal agents (e.g., medications, firearms), and the development of safety plans with the patient and family are essential components of the management of the suicidal, depressed patient. Patients who cannot agree to a no-suicide contract may require inpatient hospitalization. Treatment of the underlying depression may be necessary but not sufficient to prevent recurrent attempts. Other contributors to suicidality, such as sexual abuse, drug and alcohol use, ADHD, conduct problems, impulsivity and aggression, personality disorders, and family discord, must be assessed and targeted (Brent et al. 1999).

An important consideration is that in TADS, the combination of CBT plus fluoxetine was associated with lower risk for suicidality (March et al. 2007). However, not all studies have found the protective effect of CBT (e.g., TORDIA; Spirito et al. 2011).

Continuation Therapy

Naturalistic longitudinal studies and open follow-up studies after acute RCTs have shown that the rate of MDD relapse is very high (Birmaher et al. 2002; Kennard et al. 2009a, 2009b; Vitiello et al. 2011). A fluoxetine discontinuation RCT showed that compared with a switch to placebo, continued treatment with fluoxetine was associated with a much lower rate of relapse (Emslie et al. 2008). Similar results have been reported in adults with MDD ("Practice Guideline" 2000). Therefore, until further research results are available, to consolidate the response and prevent relapse of symptoms, clinicians should offer all patients continuation treatment for 6–12 months after complete symptom remission. During this phase, patients should be seen biweekly or monthly depending on the patient's clinical status, functioning, support systems, environmental stressors, motivation for treatment, and other psychiatric or medical disorders. The patient and his or her family should be taught to recognize early signs of relapse.

During the continuation phase, antidepressants must be maintained at the same dosage used to attain remission of acute symptoms, provided that the medication causes no significant side effects or dose-related negative effects on the patient's compliance ("Practice Guideline" 2000). At the end of the continuation phase, if a decision is made to discontinue the antidepressant, the medication should be tapered gradually (e.g., over a period of

6 weeks) to avoid withdrawal effects (e.g., sleep disturbance, irritability, gastrointestinal symptoms) that may lead the clinician to misinterpret the need for continued medication treatment. In addition, clinical practice has suggested that rapid discontinuation of antidepressants may precipitate a relapse or recurrence of depression. Ideally, treatment discontinuation should occur while children and adolescents are on extended vacation, rather than during the school year.

If relapse occurs, the clinician should first determine whether the patient has been compliant. If the patient has not been compliant, the antidepressant medication should be resumed. If the patient has been compliant and had been previously responding to the medication (without significant side effects), the clinician should consider the presence of ongoing stressors (e.g., conflict, abuse), comorbid psychiatric disorders (anxiety disorders, ADHD inattentive or combined type, substance abuse, dysthymia, bipolar II disorder, eating disorder), and medical illnesses. Depending on the circumstances, an increase in the medication dosage, a change to another medication, augmentation strategies, or psychotherapy may be indicated. For patients receiving only psychotherapy, the clinician should consider adding medications and/or utilizing new psychotherapeutic strategies.

Maintenance Therapy

After the patient has been asymptomatic for approximately 6–12 months (continuation phase), the clinician has to decide whether the patient should receive maintenance therapy, which therapy to use, and for how long. The main goal of the maintenance phase is to prevent recurrences. This phase may last from 1 year to much longer and is typically conducted with a visit frequency of every 1–3 months depending on the patient's clinical status, functioning, support systems, environmental stressors, motivation for treatment, and other psychiatric or medical disorders.

Determining Who Should Receive Maintenance Therapy

The recommendation for maintenance therapy depends on several factors, such as severity of the initial depressive episode (e.g., suicidality, psychosis, functional impairment), number and severity of prior depressive episodes, chronicity, comorbid disorders, family psychopathology, presence of support, patient and family willingness to adhere to the treatment program, and contraindications to treatment.

Factors associated with increased risk for recurrence in naturalistic studies and open follow-ups after acute RCTs of depressed children and adolescents may serve as a guide for the clinician in deciding who needs maintenance treatment. These factors include history of prior depressive episodes, female sex, late onset, suicidality, double depression, subsyndromal symptoms, poor functioning, comorbid disorders, personality disorders, exposure to negative events (e.g., abuse, conflicts), and family history of recurrence (≥2 MDD) (Birmaher et al. 1996a, 1996b; Goodyer et al. 1998; Kennard et al. 2009a, 2009b; Klein et al. 2001; Rao et al. 1999; Rueter et al. 1999; Vitiello et al. 2011; Wagner et al. 2004; Weissman et al. 1999a, 1999b).

No maintenance RCTs in depressed children and adolescents have been reported. Among depressed adults, those who have had only a single uncomplicated episode of depression, mild episodes, or lengthy intervals between episodes (e.g., 5 years) probably should not start maintenance treatment ("Practice Guideline" 2000), whereas those who have had three or more depressive episodes (especially if they occur in a short period of time and have deleterious consequences) and chronic depressions should have maintenance treatment.

Controversy exists regarding whether to treat patients who have had two previous episodes using maintenance treatment. Overall, maintenance treatment has been recommended for adult depressed patients who have had two depressive episodes and who meet one or more of the following criteria (Depression Guideline Panel 1993): 1) the family has a history of bipolar disorder or recurrent depression, 2) the first depressive episode occurred before age 20, and 3) both episodes were severe or life threatening and occurred during the previous 3 years. Given that depression in youth has similar clinical presentation, sequelae, and natural course as in adults, these guidelines should probably also be applied for youth who have experienced two previous major depressive episodes.

Deciding Which Treatment to Use

For practical reasons, unless there is any contraindication (e.g., medication side effects), the treatment that was efficacious in the induction of remission of the acute episode should be used for maintenance therapy. However, patients being maintained with medications should also be offered psychotherapy to help them cope with the psychosocial scars induced by the depression. Furthermore, many depressed youth live in environments charged with stressful situations, and their parents usually have psychiatric disorders; therefore, multimodal treatments are ideal.

In selecting medication for maintenance therapy, the clinician should consider the side-effect profile and the way the side effects may affect the patient's compliance. For example, dry mouth, weight gain, increased sweating, sexual dysfunction, and polyuria (if the patient is taking lithium) may be very troublesome and may induce discontinuation of treatment. In addition, in children and adolescents, the long-term consequences of using antidepressant medications (e.g., chronic inhibition of the serotonin reuptake by the SSRI) are not known.

Other factors, such as a patient's embarrassment with friends, uneasiness about the idea of having his or her mind "controlled by a medication," view of treatment with medications as a sign of "weakness," and uncertainty about the risk of relapse in spite of doing well while taking medications, should all be addressed with both patient and parents.

Determining How Long the Maintenance Phase Should Last

Adult patients with second episodes, who fulfill the criteria for maintenance therapy noted earlier in this section, should be maintained for several years (up to 5 years in adult studies) with the same antidepressant dosage used to achieve clinical remission during the acute treatment phase. However, patients with three or more episodes and patients with second episodes associated with psychosis, severe impairment, and severe suicidality who proved very difficult to treat should be considered for longer periods of treatment or even lifelong treatment ("Practice Parameters" 1998).

TCAs, SSRIs, and lithium have been found to be efficacious for the prevention of depressive recurrences in adults ("Practice Guideline" 2000). However, given the apparent lack of efficacy of TCAs in youth, as well as the advantages of SSRIs and their efficacy in the acute treatment of MDD, the SSRIs are considered first-line medications in maintenance therapy in youth.

Antidepressant medication, unless it is not tolerated, should be continued at the full dosage used to exert the initial therapeutic effect.

For most children and adolescents, multimodal therapies are recommended. However, if antidepressant medications are used alone, psychosocial maintenance strategies should be implemented to help the patient's inner and interpersonal conflicts, improve coping and social skills, deal with the psychosocial and personal scars left by the depression, and improve academic and social functioning. The reduction of family stress, promotion of a supportive environment, and effective treatment of parents and siblings with psychiatric disorders may also help diminish the risk for recurrence.

Clinical Pearls

- Inform patients and families that the treatment of MDD includes three phases: acute, continuation, and maintenance.
- Consider the goal of treatment to be achieving response, remission, and good psychosocial functioning.
- Offer education and support to depressed youth and their families during all phases of treatment. Some mildly depressed youth may respond well to short-term management with education and support.
- Depending on the severity and chronicity of the youth's depression and other factors, use antidepressants (SSRIs) and/or psychotherapy (CBT and interpersonal psychotherapy) during the acute phase.
- Question youth and families about side effects, because children and adolescents treated with SSRIs may show onset or worsening of suicidal ideation and, more rarely, suicide attempts.
- After successful acute treatment, offer all youth continuation treatment with SSRIs and/or psychotherapy for 6–12 months to prevent relapses.
- After the continuation phase, provide maintenance treatment with SSRIs and/or psychotherapy for at least 1 year or more to prevent recurrences for some depressed youth, especially those with severe depressions or frequent recurrences.

- Consider using special treatments such as bright light therapy, antipsychotics, and mood stabilizers for the treatment of seasonal, psychotic, and bipolar depression, respectively.
- Manage comorbid disorders, ongoing conflicts, and family psychopathology to achieve remission in the youth.
- In managing resistant depressions, take into account factors associated with poor response to treatment, such as poor treatment adherence, misdiagnoses, ongoing negative life events, and presence of comorbid disorders.

References

Alderman J, Wolkow R, Chung M, et al: Sertraline treatment of children and adolescents with obsessive-compulsive disorder or depression: pharmacokinetics, tolerability, and efficacy. J Am Acad Child Adolesc Psychiatry 37:386–394, 1998

American Psychiatric Association: Diagnostic and Statistical Manual of Mental Disorders, 4th Edition. Washington, DC, American Psychiatric Association, 1994

Amsterdam JD, Garcia-Espana F, Fawcett J, et al: Efficacy and safety of fluoxetine in treating bipolar II major depressive episode. J Clin Psychopharmacol 18:435–440, 1998

Apter A, Lipschitz A, Fong R, et al: Evaluation of suicidal thoughts and behaviors in children and adolescents taking paroxetine. J Child Adolesc Psychopharmacol 16:77–90, 2006

Axelson D, Perel, J, Rudolph G, et al: Sertraline pediatric/adolescent PK-PD parameters: dose/plasma level ranging for depression (abstract). Clin Pharmacol Ther 67:169, 2000a

Axelson D, Perel J, Rudolph G, et al: Significant differences in pharmacokinetics/dynamics of citalopram between adolescents and adults: implications for clinical dosing (abstract). Proceedings of the 39th Annual Meeting of the American College of Neuropsychopharmacology, San Juan, Puerto Rico, 2000b, p 122

Bauer M, Bschor T, Kunz D, et al: Double-blind, placebo-controlled trial of the use of lithium to augment antidepressant medication in continuation treatment of unipolar major depression. Am J Psychiatry 157:1429–1435, 2000

Baumer FM, Howe M, Gallelli K, et al: A pilot study of antidepressant-induced mania in pediatric bipolar disorder: characteristics, risk factors, and the serotonin transporter gene. Biol Psychiatry 60:1005–1012, 2006

Beck AT: Depression: Clinical, Experimental and Theoretical Aspects. New York, Harper & Row, 1967

Berard R, Fong R, Carpenter DJ, et al: An international, multicenter, placebo-controlled trial of paroxetine in adolescents with major depressive disorder. J Child Adolesc Psychopharmacol 16:59–75, 2006

Birmaher B: Remission of a mother's depression is associated with her child's mental health. Am J Psychiatry 168:563–565, 2011

Birmaher B, Brent DA: Practice parameter for the assessment and treatment of children and adolescents with depressive disorders. J Am Acad Child Adolesc Psychiatry 46:1503–1526, 2007

Birmaher B, Ryan ND, Williamson D, et al: Childhood and adolescent depression: a review of the past 10 years, part I. J Am Acad Child Adolesc Psychiatry 35:1427–1439, 1996a

Birmaher B, Ryan ND, Williamson DE, et al: Childhood and adolescent depression: a review of the past 10 years, part II. J Am Acad Child Adolesc Psychiatry 35:1575–1583, 1996b

Birmaher B, Brent DA, Kolko D, et al: Clinical outcome after short-term psychotherapy for adolescents with major depressive disorder. Arch Gen Psychiatry 57:29–36, 2000

Birmaher B, Arbelaez C, Brent D: Course and outcome of child and adolescent major depressive disorder. Child Adolesc Psychiatr Clin N Am 11:619–637, 2002

Birmaher B, Axelson DA, Monk K, et al: Fluoxetine for the treatment of childhood anxiety disorders. J Am Acad Child Adolesc Psychiatry 42:415–423, 2003

Boyer EW, Shannon M: The serotonin syndrome. N Engl J Med 352:1112–1120, 2005

Brent DA: Antidepressants and pediatric depression—the risk of doing nothing. N Engl J Med 351:1598–601, 2004

Brent DA, Poling K, McCain B, et al: A psychoeducational program for families of affectively ill children and adolescents. J Am Acad Child Adolesc Psychiatry 32:770–774, 1993

Brent DA, Holder D, Birmaher B, et al: A clinical psychotherapy trial for adolescent depression comparing cognitive, family, and supportive therapy. Arch Gen Psychiatry 54:877–885, 1997

Brent DA, Kolko D, Birmaher B, et al: Predictors of treatment efficacy in a clinical trial of three psychosocial treatments for adolescent depression. J Am Acad Child Adolesc Psychiatry 37:906–914, 1998

Brent DA, Kolko D, Birmaher, et al: A clinical trial for adolescent depression: predictors of additional treatment in the acute and follow-up phases of the trial. J Am Acad Child Adolesc Psychiatry 38:263–270, 1999

Brent DA, Emslie G, Clarke G, et al: Switching to another SSRI or to venlafaxine with or without cognitive behavioral therapy for adolescents with SSRI-resistant depression: the TORDIA randomized controlled trial. JAMA 299:901–913, 2008

Brent DA, Emslie GJ, Clarke GN, et al: Predictors of spontaneous and systematically assessed suicidal adverse events in the treatment of SSRI-resistant depression in adolescents (TORDIA) study. Am J Psychiatry 166:418–426, 2009

Bridge JA, Birmaher B, Iyengar S, et al: Placebo response in randomized controlled trials of antidepressants for pediatric major depressive disorder. Am J Psychiatry 166:42–49, 2009

Cheung AH, Emslie GJ, Mayes TL: Review of the efficacy and safety of antidepressants in youth depression. J Child Psychol Psychiatry 46:735–754, 2005

Clarke G, Debar L, Lynch F, et al: A randomized effectiveness trial of brief cognitive-behavioral therapy for depressed adolescents receiving antidepressant medication. J Am Acad Child Adolesc Psychiatry 44:888–898, 2005

Clein PD, Riddle MA: Pharmacokinetics in children and adolescents. Child Adolesc Psychiatr Clin N Am 4:59–75, 1995

Compton MT, Nemeroff CB: The treatment of bipolar depression. J Clin Psychiatry 61:57–67, 2000

Conners CK, Casat CD, Gualtieri CT, et al: Bupropion hydrochloride in attention deficit disorder with hyperactivity. J Am Acad Child Adolesc Psychiatry 35:1314–1321, 1996

Daviss WB, Bentivogli P, Racusin R, et al: Bupropion sustained release in adolescents with comorbid attention deficit hyperactivity. J Am Acad Child Adolesc Psychiatry 40:307–314, 2001

Daviss WB, Perel JM, Rudolph GR, et al: Steady-state pharmacokinetics of bupropion SR in juvenile patients. J Am Acad Child Adolesc Psychiatry 44:349–357, 2005

DelBello MP, Chang K, Welge JA, et al: A double-blind, placebo-controlled pilot study of quetiapine for depressed adolescents with bipolar disorder. Bipolar Disord 11:483–493, 2009

Depression Guideline Panel: Depression in Primary Care, Vol 2: Treatment of Major Depression (Clinical Practice Guideline No 5). AHCPR Publication No 93-0551. Rockville, MD, U.S. Department of Health and Human Services, Public Health Service, Agency for Health Care Policy and Research, April 1993

Donnelly CL, Wagner KD, Rynn M, et al: Sertraline in children and adolescents with major depressive disorder. J Am Acad Child Adolesc Psychiatry 45:1162–1170, 2006

Emslie GJ, Rush AJ, Weinberg WA, et al: A double-blind, randomized, placebo-controlled trial of fluoxetine in children and adolescents with depression. Arch Gen Psychiatry 54:1031–1037, 1997

Emslie GJ, Walkup JT, Pliszka SR, et al: Nontricyclic antidepressants: current trends in children and adolescents. J Am Acad Child Adolesc Psychiatry 38:517–528, 1999

Emslie GJ, Heiligenstein JH, Wagner KD, et al: Fluoxetine for acute treatment of depression in children and adolescents: a placebo-controlled, randomized clinical trial. J Am Acad Child Adolesc Psychiatry 41:1205–1215, 2002

Emslie GJ, Wagner KD, Kutcher S, et al: Paroxetine treatment in children and adolescents with major depressive disorder: a randomized, double-blind, placebo-controlled trial. J Am Acad Child Adolesc Psychiatry 45:709–719, 2006

Emslie GJ, Kennard BD, Mayes TL, et al: Fluoxetine versus placebo in preventing relapse of major depression in children and adolescents. Am J Psychiatry 165:459–467, 2008

Emslie GJ, Ventura D, Korotzer A, et al: Escitalopram in the treatment of adolescent depression: a randomized placebo-controlled multisite trial. J Am Acad Child Adolesc Psychiatry 48721–729, 2009

Emslie GJ, Mayes T, Porta G, et al: Treatment of Resistant Depression in Adolescents (TORDIA): week 24 outcomes. Am J Psychiatry 167:782–791, 2010

Findling RL, Reed MD, Myers C, et al: Paroxetine pharmacokinetics in depressed children and adolescents. J Am Acad Child Adolesc Psychiatry 38:952–959, 1999

Findling RL, Preskorn SH, Marcus RN, et al: Nefazodone pharmacokinetics in depressed children and adolescents. J Am Acad Child Adolesc Psychiatry 39:1008–1016, 2000

Findling RL, McNamara NK, Stansbrey RJ, et al: The relevance of pharmacokinetic studies in designing efficacy trials in juvenile major depression. J Child Adolesc Psychopharmacol 16:131–145, 2006

Fluvoxamine for the treatment of anxiety disorders in children and adolescents. Research Units on Pediatric Psychopharmacology Anxiety Study Group. N Engl J Med 344:1279–1285, 2001

Geddes JR, Calabrese JR, Goodwin GM: Lamotrigine for treatment of bipolar depression: independent meta-analysis and meta-regression of individual patient data from five randomised trials. Br J Psychiatry 194:4–9, 2009

Geller B, Fox LW, Clark KA: Rate and predictors of prepubertal bipolarity during follow-up of 6- to 12-year-old depressed children. J Am Acad Child Adolesc Psychiatry 33:461–468, 1994

Ghaziuddin N, Kutcher SP, Knapp P, et al; Work Group on Quality Issues; AACAP: Practice parameter for use of electroconvulsive therapy with adolescents. J Am Acad Child Adolesc Psychiatry 43:1521–1539, 2004

Gibbons RD, Hur K, Bhaumik DK, et al: The relationship between antidepressant medication use and rate of suicide. Arch Gen Psychiatry 62:165–172, 2005

Gijsman HJ, Geddes JR, Rendell JM, et al: Antidepressants for bipolar depression: a systematic review of randomized, controlled trials. Am J Psychiatry 161:1537–1547, 2004

Goldsmith M, Singh M, Chang K: Antidepressants and psychostimulants in pediatric populations: is there an association with mania? Pediatr Drugs 13:225–243, 2011

Goodyer IM, Herbert J, Secher SM, et al: Short-term outcome of major depression, I: comorbidity and severity at presentation as predictors of persistent disorder. J Am Acad Child Adolesc Psychiatry 36:179–187, 1997

Goodyer IM, Herbert J, Altham PM: Adrenal, steroid secretion and major depression in 8- to 16-year-olds, III: influence of cortisol/DHEA ratio at presentation on subsequent rates of disappointing life events and persistent major depression. Psychol Med 28:265–273, 1998

Goodyer I, Dubicka B, Wilkinson P, et al: Selective serotonin reuptake inhibitors (SSRIs) and routine specialist care with and without cognitive behaviour therapy in adolescents with major depression: randomised controlled trial. BMJ 335:142, 2007

Gould MS, Fisher P, Parides M, et al: Psychosocial risk factors of child and adolescent completed suicide. Arch Gen Psychiatry 53:1155–1162, 1996

Guy W: Clinical Global Impressions, in ECDEU Assessment Manual for Psychopharmacology, Revised (NIMH Publ No 76-338). Rockville, MD, National Institute of Mental Health, 1976, pp 218–222

Hamilton JD, Bridge J: Outcome at 6 months of 50 adolescents with major depression treated in a health maintenance organization. J Am Acad Child Adolesc Psychiatry 38:1340–1346, 1999

Hamilton M: A rating scale for depression. J Neurol Neurosurg Psychiatry 23:56–61, 1960

Hammad TA: Review and Evaluation of Clinical Data: Relationship Between Psychotropic Drugs and Pediatric Suicidality. Rockville, MD, U.S. Food and Drug Administration. 2004. Available at: www.fda.gov/ohrms/dockets/ac/04/briefing/2004-4065b1-10-TAB08-Hammads-Review.pdf. Accessed May 12, 2012.

Hammad TA, Laughren T, Racoosin J: Suicidality in pediatric patients treated with antidepressant drugs. Arch Gen Psychiatry 63:332–333, 2006

Hayward C, Killen JD, Kraemer HC, et al: Predictors of panic attacks in adolescents. J Am Acad Child Adolesc Psychiatry 39:207–214, 2000

Hazell P, O'Connell D, Heathcote D, et al: Tricyclic drugs for depression in children and adolescents. Cochrane Database of Systematic Reviews, 2006, Issue 2. Art No: CD002317. DOI: 10.1002/14651858.CD002317.

Heiligenstein JH, Hoog SL, Wagner KD, et al: Fluoxetine 40–60 mg versus fluoxetine 20 mg in the treatment of children and adolescents with a less-than-complete response to nine-week treatment with fluoxetine 10–20 mg: a pilot study. J Child Adolesc Psychopharmacol 16:207–217, 2006

Hughes CW, Emslie GJ, Crismon ML, et al: The Texas Childhood Medication Algorithm Project: update from the Texas Consensus Conference Panel on Medication Treatment of Childhood Major Depressive Disorder. J Am Acad Child Adolesc Psychiatry 38:1442–1454, 1999

Katz LY, Kozyrskyj AL, Prior HJ, et al: Effect of regulatory warnings on antidepressant prescription rates, use of health services and outcomes among children, adolescents and young adults. CMAJ 178:1005–1011, 2008

Keller MB, McCullough JP, Klein DN, et al: A comparison of nefazodone, the cognitive behavioral-analysis system of psychotherapy, and their combination for the treatment of chronic depression. N Engl J Med 342:1462–1470, 2000

Keller MB, Ryan ND, Strober M, et al: Efficacy of paroxetine in the treatment of adolescent major depression: a randomized, controlled trial. J Am Acad Child Adolesc Psychiatry 40:762–772, 2001

Kendall PC: Treating anxiety disorders in children: results of a randomized clinical trial. J Consult Clin Psychol 62:100–110, 1994

Kennard BD, Silva SG, Mayes TL, et al: Assessment of safety and long-term outcomes of initial treatment with placebo in TADS. Am J Psychiatry 166:337–344, 2009a

Kennard BD, Silva SG, Tonev S, et al: Remission and recovery in the Treatment for Adolescents with Depression Study (TADS): acute and long-term outcomes. J Am Acad Child Adolesc Psychiatry 48:186–195, 2009b

Klein DN, Lewinsohn PM, Seeley JR, et al: A family study of major depressive disorder in a community sample of adolescents. Arch Gen Psychiatry 58:13–20, 2001

Kovacs M, Goldston D: Cognitive and social cognitive development of depressed children and adolescents. J Am Acad Child Adolesc Psychiatry 30:388–392, 1991

Kovacs M, Gatsonis C, Paulauskas SL, et al: Depressive disorders in childhood, IV: a longitudinal study of comorbidity with and risk for anxiety disorders. Arch Gen Psychiatry 46:776–782, 1989

Lake MB, Birmaher B, Wassick S, et al: Bleeding and selective serotonin reuptake inhibitors in childhood and adolescence. J Child Adolesc Psychopharmacol 10:35–38, 2000

Leonard HL, March J, Rickler KC, et al: Pharmacology of the selective serotonin reuptake inhibitors in children and adolescents. J Am Acad Child Adolesc Psychiatry 36:725–736, 1997

Lewinsohn PM, Allen NB, Seeley JR, et al: First onset versus recurrence of depression: differential processes of psychosocial risk. J Abnorm Psychol 108:483–489, 1999

Libby AM, Orton HD, Valuck RJ: Persisting decline in depression treatment after FDA warnings. Arch Gen Psychiatry 66:633–639, 2009

Mandoki MW, Tapia MR, Tapia MA, et al: Venlafaxine in the treatment of children and adolescents with major depression. Psychopharmacol Bull 33:149–154, 1997

Mann JJ, Emslie G, Baldessarini RJ, et al: ACNP Task Force report on SSRIs and suicidal behavior in youth. Neuropsychopharmacology 31:473–492, 2006

March J, Silva S, Petrycki S, et al: Fluoxetine, cognitive-behavioral therapy, and their combination for adolescents with depression: Treatment for Adolescents With Depression Study (TADS) randomized controlled trial. JAMA 292:807–820, 2004

March JS, Silva S, Petrycki S, et al: The Treatment for Adolescents With Depression Study (TADS): long-term effectiveness and safety outcomes. Arch Gen Psychiatry 64:1132–1143, 2007

Martin A, Young C, Leckman JF, et al: Age effects on antidepressant-induced manic conversion. Arch Pediatr Adolesc Med 158:773–780, 2004

Mufson L, Dorta KP, Wickramaratne P, et al: A randomized effectiveness trial of interpersonal psychotherapy for depressed adolescents. Arch Gen Psychiatry 61:577–584, 2004

Olfson M, Shaffer D, Marcus SC, et al: Relationship between antidepressant medication treatment and suicide in adolescents. Arch Gen Psychiatry 60:978–982, 2003

Pine DS, Cohen P, Gurley D, et al: The risk for early adulthood anxiety and depressive disorders in adolescents with anxiety and depressive disorders. Arch Gen Psychiatry 55:56–64, 1998

Pliszka S: Patterns of psychiatric comorbidity with attention-deficit hyperactivity disorder. Child Adolesc Psychiatr Clin N Am 9:525–540, 2000

Poirier MF, Boyer P: Venlafaxine and paroxetine in treatment-resistant depression: double blind, randomized comparison. Br J Psychiatry 175:12–16, 1999

Poznanski EO, Freeman LN, Mokros HB: Children's Depression Rating Scale–Revised. Psychopharmacol Bull 21:979–989, 1984

Practice guideline for the treatment of patients with bipolar disorder. American Psychiatric Association. Am J Psychiatry 151:1–36, 1994

Practice guideline for the treatment of patients with major depressive disorder (revision). American Psychiatric Association. Am J Psychiatry 157:1–45, 2000

Practice parameters for the assessment and treatment of children and adolescents with depressive disorders. AACAP. J Am Acad Child Adolesc Psychiatry 37:63S–83S, 1998

Puig-Antich J, Lukens E, Davies M, et al: Psychosocial functioning in prepubertal depressive disorders, II: interpersonal relationships after sustained recovery from the affective episode. Arch Gen Psychiatry 42:511–517, 1985

Rao U, Dahl RE, Ryan ND, et al: Unipolar depression in adolescents: clinical outcome in adulthood. J Am Acad Child Adolesc Psychiatry 34:566–578, 1995

Rao U, Hammen C, Daley SE: Continuity of depression during the transition to adulthood: a 5-year longitudinal study of young women. J Am Acad Child Adolesc Psychiatry 38:908–915, 1999

Renaud J, Brent D, Baugher MA, et al: Rapid response to psychosocial treatment for adolescent depression: a 2-year follow-up. J Am Acad Child Adolesc Psychiatry 37:1184–1190, 1998

Rey JM, Walter G: Half a century of ECT use in young people. Am J Psychiatry 154:595–602, 1997

Rueter MA, Scaramella L, Wallace LE, et al: First onset of depressive or anxiety disorders predicted by the longitudinal course of internalizing symptoms and parent-adolescent disagreements. Arch Gen Psychiatry 56:726–732, 1999

Ryan N, Meyer V, Dachille S, et al: Lithium antidepressant augmentation in TCA-refractory depression in adolescents. J Am Acad Child Adolesc Psychiatry 27:371–376, 1988a

Ryan N, Puig-Antich J, Rabinovich H, et al: MAOIs in adolescent major depression unresponsive to tricyclic antidepressant. J Am Acad Child Adolesc Psychiatry 27:755–758, 1988b

Safer DJ, Zito JM: Treatment-emergent adverse events from selective serotonin reuptake inhibitors by age group: children versus adolescents. J Child Adolesc Psychopharmacol 16:159–169, 2006

Sallee FR, Vrindavanam NS, Deas-Nesmith D, et al: Pulse intravenous clomipramine for depressed adolescents: a double-blind, controlled trial. Am J Psychiatry 154:668–673, 1997

Shaffer D, Craft L: Methods of adolescent suicide prevention. J Clin Psychiatry 60 (suppl):70–74, discussion 75–76, 113–116, 1999

Shaffer D, Gould MS, Brasic J, et al: A Children's Global Assessment Scale (CGAS). Arch Gen Psychiatry 40:1228–1231, 1983

Simon GE, Savarino J, Operskalski B, et al: Suicide risk during antidepressant treatment. Am J Psychiatry 163:41–47, 2006

Spirito A, Esposito-Smythers C, Wolff J, et al: Cognitive-behavioral therapy for adolescent depression and suicidality. Child Adolesc Psychiatr Clin N Am 20:191–204, 2011

Stein D, Williamson DE, Birmaher B, et al: Parent-child bonding and family functioning in depressed children and children at high-risk and low risk for future depression. J Am Acad Child Adolesc Psychiatry 39:1220–1226, 2000

Strober M, Carlson G: Bipolar illness in adolescents with major depression: clinical, genetic, and psychopharmacologic predictors in a three-to four-year prospective follow-up investigation. Arch Gen Psychiatry 39:549–555, 1982

Strober M, Freeman R, Rigali J, et al: The pharmacotherapy of depressive illness in adolescence, II: effects of lithium augmentation in nonresponders to imipramine. J Am Acad Child Adolesc Psychiatry 31:16–20, 1992

Strober M, Lampert C, Schmidt S, et al: The course of major depressive disorder in adolescents, I: recovery and risk of manic switching in a follow-up of psychotic and nonpsychotic subtypes. J Am Acad Child Adolesc Psychiatry 32:34–42, 1993

Swedo S, Allen AJ, Glod CA, et al: A controlled trial of light therapy for the treatment of pediatric seasonal affective disorder. J Am Acad Child Adolesc Psychiatry 36:816–821, 1997

Thase ME, Rush AJ: When at first you don't succeed: sequential strategies for antidepressant nonresponders. J Clin Psychiatry 58:23–29, 1997

Valuck RJ, Libby AM, Sills MR, et al: Antidepressant treatment and risk of suicide attempt by adolescents with major depressive disorder: a propensity-adjusted retrospective cohort study. CNS Drugs 18:1119–1132, 2004

Vieta E, Locklear J, Gunther O, et al: Treatment options for bipolar depression: a systematic review of randomized, controlled trials. J Clin Psychopharmacol 30:579–590, 2010

Vitiello B, Emslie G, Clarke G, et al: Long-term outcome of adolescent depression initially resistant to selective serotonin reuptake inhibitor treatment: a follow-up study of the TORDIA sample. J Clin Psychiatry 72:388–996, 2011

von Knorring AL, Olsson GI, Thomsen PH, et al: A randomised double-blind placebo-controlled study of citalopram in adolescents with major depressive disorder. J Clin Psychopharmacol 26:311–315, 2006

Wagner KD, Ambrosini P, Rynn M, et al: Efficacy of sertraline in the treatment of children and adolescents with major depressive disorder: two randomized controlled trials. JAMA 290:1033–1041, 2003

Wagner KD, Robb AS, Findling RL, et al: A randomized, placebo-controlled trial of citalopram for the treatment of major depression in children and adolescents. Am J Psychiatry 161:1079–1083, 2004

Wagner KD, Jonas J, Findling RL, et al: A double-blind, randomized, placebo-controlled trial of escitalopram in the treatment of pediatric depression. J Am Acad Child Adolesc Psychiatry 45:280–288, 2006

Weissman MM, Gammon GD, John K, et al: Children of depressed parents: increased psychopathology and early onset of major depression. Arch Gen Psychiatry 44:847–853, 1987

Weissman MM, Wolk S, Goldstein RB, et al: Depressed adolescents grown up. JAMA 281–1707–1713, 1999a

Weissman MM, Wolk S, Wickramaratne PJ, et al: Children with prepubertal-onset major depressive disorder and anxiety grown up. Arch Gen Psychiatry 56:794–801, 1999b

Wilens TE, Wyatt D, Spencer TJ: Disentangling disinhibition. J Am Acad Child Adolesc Psychiatry 37:1225–1227, 1998

6

Bipolar Disorders

Tiffany Thomas, M.D.

Kevin W. Kuich, M.D.

Robert L. Findling, M.D., M.B.A.

Research over the past 10 years has helped better define the phenomenology and course of bipolar disorder in children and adolescents. Pediatric bipolar disorder (PBD) has been shown to have a chronic course with little interepisode recovery, and therefore can lead to substantive psychosocial dysfunction (Biederman et al. 2004; Findling et al. 2001; Geller et al. 2004). For these reasons, effective treatments are needed for youth with PBD. The purpose of this chapter is to present a rational, practical, and commonsense approach to the pharmacotherapeutic management of bipolar disorder in children and adolescents.

When thinking about the pharmacotherapy of PBD, one should begin by considering which agent or agents might be prescribed. The question of initiating treatment with either monotherapy or combination therapy often depends on symptom presentation and a careful, meticulous review of past medication response. Strong consideration should be given to restarting agents that have been helpful in the past. Similarly, agents that have been problematic or ineffective during prior therapeutic trials should generally be avoided.

Many medications used to treat bipolar illness may be associated with substantial risks, have a narrow therapeutic index, and/or require monitoring of drug levels and other laboratory parameters. For this reason, the clinician should carefully review medication treatment options with the patient and caregivers, and consider anticipated barriers to medication or monitoring adherence. Possible adherence barriers can include medication cost, lack of nearby laboratory facilities, and social factors that may interfere with adherence to the regular administration of medications.

Pharmacotherapy guidelines and practice parameters for treating PBD have been published (Kowatch et al. 2005; McClellan et al. 2007). The authors of these guidelines based their recommendations on the available scientific literature and current clinical practice. The guidelines also provide useful algorithms that may assist in medication selection. Briefly, use of lithium, an anticonvulsant, or an atypical antipsychotic as monotherapy is suggested in the initial treatment of manic or mixed bipolar presentations in outpatients without psychosis. It is recommended that partial response to monotherapy with a given agent may be addressed by adding another drug from a different class of compounds to the preexisting pharmacological regimen. A rational approach to patients who do not respond at all to a given agent might be to treat the youth with a medication from a different drug class.

In this chapter, we review individual medications that have been studied in the treatment of pediatric bipolar illness and summarize the extant evidence for combination pharmacotherapy.

Lithium

Lithium has been widely used in the acute treatment of mania in adults. In addition, research has demonstrated that lithium also has efficacy as a maintenance therapy for bipolar disorder in adults and may be helpful in treating the depressed phase of bipolar illness.

Lithium was the first medication that was approved by the U.S. Food and Drug Administration (FDA) for use in treating bipolar disorder in children and adolescents ages 12 years and older. However, this indication had been given based on the results of adult research. Although multiple open-label trials of lithium in PBD had shown favorable effects, definitive studies of lithium in the acute and maintenance treatment of pediatric mania were lacking. In 2006, however, the Collaborative Lithium Trials (CoLT) group began the definitive testing of lithium in juvenile mania under the auspices of a National Institute of Child Health and Human Development contract. These innovative studies will provide data to inform the labeling of lithium for children and adolescents with bipolar disorder. In addition, it will enhance the clinical decision making regarding the use of lithium in these patients. The CoLT trials are currently under way and will provide definitive data that will 1) establish evidence-based dosing strategies for lithium, 2) characterize the pharmacokinetic and biodisposition of lithium in pediatric patients, 3) examine the acute efficacy of lithium in pediatric bipolar illness, 4) investigate the long-term effectiveness of lithium treatment, and 5) characterize the short- and long-term safety of lithium (Findling et al. 2008).

Supporting Studies in Youth

Although much of the published literature on lithium consists of case reports and studies lacking methodological rigor, some prospective studies have provided evidence to suggest that lithium is both effective and reasonably well tolerated in the treatment of PBD. In an open-label monotherapy study, Kowatch et al. (2000) described lithium as being effective in the short-term treatment of pediatric mania. In a short-term, double-blind trial, Geller et al. (1998) found lithium helpful in reducing substance abuse and improving global functioning in a dually diagnosed adolescent population. Yet another prospective trial found that lithium combined with divalproex was effective and tolerated in treating severe manic symptoms (Findling et al. 2003). Other studies that have found lithium to be useful involved treatment of young patients with both lithium and antipsychotics (Kafantaris et al. 2003; Pavuluri et al. 2004). As for maintenance studies, one 18-month study evaluating the effectiveness of lithium monotherapy in PBD found it to be as useful as divalproex monotherapy (Findling et al. 2005). However, the National Institute of Mental Health (NIMH) sponsored a double-blind comparison study of lithium, divalproex, or placebo over an 8-week period. Divalproex was found to be superior to placebo at the completion of the study. Although there was a trend toward efficacy for lithium, the results were not statistically significant for lithium compared with placebo (Kowatch et al. 2007).

Findling et al. (2011) investigated evidence-based dosing strategies for lithium in children and adolescents with bipolar I disorder. Sixty-one youths ages 7–17 years with bipolar I disorder were eligible for 8 weeks of open-label treatment with lithium in one of three dosing arms. In Arm I, participants began treatment at a lithium dose of 300 mg bid. The starting dose of lithium in Arms II and III was 300 mg tid. Patients in Arms I and II could have their dose increased by 300 mg/day, depending on clinical response and blood levels, at weekly visits. Patients in Arm III also had midweek telephone interviews, after which they could have their dose increased by 300 mg/day. All three treatment arms resulted in similar effectiveness, side-effect profiles, and tolerability of lithium. Most patients had a ≥50% improvement in Young Mania Rating Scale score, and more than half of the patients (58%) achieved response. However, as reported with many other drug monotherapy studies, remission was not achieved in most patients.

In summary, although lithium can be a complicated medication to use, some evidence supports its effectiveness. However, definitive efficacy trials must still be performed.

Formulations

Lithium is available in tablets, liquid, and long-acting formulations. Lithium carbonate is perhaps the most widely used formulation and comes in generic tablets at strengths of 150 mg, 300 mg, and 600 mg. Lithobid, a sustained-release preparation in film-coated dissolving tablets, is available in 300-mg strength. Lithium citrate is an oral solution of lithium with a concentration of 300 mg/teaspoon (8 mEq/5 mL).

Preliminary Evaluation

Prior to initiating any medication regimen, thoughtful consideration should be given to the target symptoms and their severity, anticipated barriers to medication adherence, and the patient's ability to swallow pills. Before lithium treatment is initiated, a careful medical history should be obtained. Particular attention should be paid to reviewing organ systems known to be affected by lithium administration: renal, endocrinological, neurological, and cardiovascular. Given that lithium is known to be a teratogen, increasing the likelihood of Ebstein's anomaly, especially during the first trimester of pregnancy, a pregnancy test should be completed for females of childbearing capacity prior to initiating treatment. Discussions with females of childbearing potential should also be considered both before and throughout treatment to assess whether these patients are sexually active or intend to become pregnant. Baseline laboratories, including blood urea nitrogen (BUN)/creatinine, electrolytes, and thyrotropin (thyroid-stimulating hormone [TSH]), should be obtained to evaluate for the possibility of any preexisting renal impairment, electrolyte imbalances, or hypothyroidism that may lead the clinician to eschew prescribing lithium to an individual patient. We also recommend that a pretreatment electrocardiogram (ECG) be obtained for each patient to rule out any cardiac conduction abnormalities.

Medication Dosing

Lithium has a narrow therapeutic index. Therefore, identifying the correct dosage of lithium for a given patient is important to maximize therapeutic effectiveness while minimizing untoward side effects. Fortunately, new data are available to guide clinicians about how to initiate lithium dosing in children and teenagers. Weight-based approaches suggest that the initial dosing of lithium can be made based on a milligram-per-kilogram (mg/kg) basis, with lithium doses subsequently titrated based on clinical response and serum level (Weller et al. 1986). Another approach that has been described includes the administration of an initial test dose of lithium and the use of a nomogram. Serum levels are then measured at the 24-hour time point, with daily dosing prescribed according to the nomogram (Cooper et al. 1973; Geller and Fetner 1989). Head-to-head comparison of the two methods in a small inpatient sample indicated that the methods were equally effective (Hagino et al. 1998).

As described above in "Supporting Studies in Youth," Findling et al. (2011) studied dosing strategies for lithium monotherapy in children and adolescents with bipolar I disorder in an 8-week, open-label trial. Based on their results, a dosing paradigm in which patients begin treatment with lithium at a dose of 300 mg tid, followed by 300-mg weekly increases (with an additional 300-mg increase during the first week) until a priori stopping criteria are met, will be used in an upcoming randomized, placebo-controlled trial. In this trial, the maximum allowable lithium serum concentration above which further dosage increases cannot occur will be 1.4 mEq/L.

We recommend following the dosing guidelines as studied by Findling et al. (2011). We try to avoid single doses greater than 900 mg because we have found that such high single doses are generally not well tolerated. Lithium can be increased by 300 mg every 4–5 days, based on clinical response and serum levels. Serum levels should be taken approximately 12 hours after the last dose and repeated every 4–5 days as the dosage is being adjusted. The therapeutic range for lithium appears to be between 0.6 and 1.4 mEq/L in pediatric patients, similar to what has been reported in adults.

Findling et al. (2010) investigated the first-dose pharmacokinetics of oral doses of lithium carbonate in children and adolescents ages 7–17 years after administration of immediate-release capsules of 600 mg or 900 mg. Lithium plasma concentrations were followed over 48–72 hours in 39 subjects. Lithium clearances did not vary systematically with age, dose, sex, or creatinine clearances. Allometrically scaled clearance and volume of distribution from the population analysis were within the range reported in adults. Single-dose profiles of lithium in these young patients did show marked variability. This indicates that ongoing serum monitoring is needed during continued lithium therapy. Serum levels at the higher end of this therapeutic range appear to be associated with better symptom amelioration but are associated with greater side effects. When the lithium dosage is stable, we recommend that screening laboratories be repeated. Subsequently, lithium levels, TSH, and renal function (BUN/creatinine or creatinine clearance) should be evaluated every 3 months, or more frequently if necessary.

Side Effects

Adverse effects from lithium are common and involve the central nervous system (CNS) and the renal, dermatological, endocrine, and gastrointestinal (GI) systems (Table 6–1). Although side effects during lithium treatment are common, they generally do not lead to lithium discontinuation. It appears that GI symptoms (stomachache, nausea, vomiting, and diarrhea) are the most common side effects noted. Often, GI side effects can be addressed by recommending that the patient take lithium with food, dividing the doses more frequently throughout the course of the day, or administering lithium in the liquid citrate formulation. Notably, persistent nausea, vomiting, and diarrhea (as well as other side effects noted below) may all signal the presence of lithium toxicity. For this reason, careful inquiry and reassessment of serum lithium levels should be considered for patients presenting with these concerns. If the lithium level is indeed high, lithium doses may be stopped for 24 hours while the level is rechecked and reinitiation at a lower dose is considered.

Other side effects appear to be less common. CNS side effects that have been reported include tremor, ataxia, and slowed mentation. Tremor is usually mild and can be aided by dose reduction. Although the use of propranolol has been described as a treatment for lithium-related tremor in adults, this management strategy is not one we generally recommend for youth. Renal side effects include polyuria, polydipsia, and possible morphological changes to the kidney after long-term use. Unfortunately, insufficient data are available regarding the long-term renal effects of lithium in young patients. Dermatologically, an acne-like rash can be a troubling side effect for adolescents, and education concerning this possibility is suggested. Rash and hair loss have been infrequently described in relation to lithium therapy. Lastly, endocrine side effects can include weight gain and hypothyroidism.

Drug Interactions and Cautions

Lithium is excreted by the kidney. Thus, drug-drug interactions may occur as a result of modification of renal excretion by other agents. Concomitant use of other drugs or substances may either increase or decrease lithium levels. For example, nonsteroidal anti-inflammatory drugs (NSAIDs) can increase lithium levels by reducing renal excretion. Although use of NSAIDs is not necessarily contraindicated for patients prescribed lithium, care should be given if NSAIDs are taken during lithium therapy, with particular attention to symptoms of lithium toxicity. Thiazide diuretics, though not commonly used in young people, may substantively increase lithium levels. On the other hand, theophylline and caffeine may decrease lithium levels by enhancing renal excretion. Because sodium chloride can also affect the renal excretion of lithium, excessive intake of salty snack foods or salt-repleting sports drinks can lower the lithium level. Discussion about these drug-drug interactions, dietary considerations, and adequate hydration, especially during summer months and during vigorous physical activities, is recommended.

Table 6–1.   Management of common lithium side effects

System	Side effect	Suggested intervention
Gastrointestinal	Nausea, emesis, diarrhea	Reduce dose or split dose Take with food Change to citrate formulation
CNS	Tremor, ataxia, slowed mentation	Reduce or split dose
Renal	Polyuria, changes in renal function	Allow for bathroom breaks Monitor kidney function every 3 months
Dermatological	Acne, rash	Provide education about side effects
Endocrine	Weight gain, thyroid abnormalities	Educate patient about appropriate diet and exercise Monitor thyroid function every 3–6 months

In summary, lithium use in PBD is supported by numerous case studies and open-label reports, but data from randomized controlled trials (RCTs) are only emerging. However, lithium is an agent that has a great deal of support in the adult literature for use in bipolar disorder. At present, lithium is one of the available FDA-approved treatments for PBD. Although use of lithium does have substantive burdens in terms of monitoring and its side-effect profile, its potential for significant benefit allows it to remain a first-line agent in treating PBD.

Anticonvulsants

Although anticonvulsants appear to be widely used in treating PBD, no anticonvulsants are FDA approved for treating acute mania or as a maintenance therapy for bipolar disorder in children and adolescents. In adults, divalproex sodium, lamotrigine, and extended-release carbamazepine have approved uses for bipolar disorder. Carbamazepine, oxcarbazepine, divalproex sodium, lamotrigine, and topiramate have all been investigated in youth with bipolar illness. Other, newer agents, such as zonisamide, levetiracetam, and tiagabine, have not received rigorous testing to date in children and adolescents with bipolar disorder.

Carbamazepine

Carbamazepine was the first anticonvulsant extensively studied as a potential treatment for bipolar disorder in adults. However, carbamazepine is not commonly used in the treatment of bipolar disorder in youth. This lack of use is most likely due to a paucity of clinical trials data for carbamazepine in this patient population when compared with lithium or divalproex sodium. Another possible contributing factor is that challenges associated with the administration of carbamazepine might complicate its use. These challenges include the possibility of drug-drug interactions, concerns regarding aplastic anemia and agranulocytosis, and metabolic autoinduction.

Supporting Studies in Youth

The limited data that exist regarding the use of carbamazepine in PBD suggest that carbamazepine may be useful in the treatment of youth. In an open-label trial comparing carbamazepine, lithium, and divalproex sodium, 5 of 13 children, ages 6–18 years, with bipolar I or II disorder achieved a 50% reduction in manic symptoms within 6 weeks of initiation of carbamazepine therapy (Kowatch et al. 2003). The reported serum level that led to these results was 7.11 ± 1.79 µg/mL. Nausea and sedation were noted as adverse effects in the carbamazepine-treated subjects. In addition, case studies have suggested that carbamazepine may be useful in treating symptoms of mania in children as young as age 5 years, and in those who might be unresponsive to lithium (Craven and Murphy 2000; Tuzun et al. 2002; Woolston 1999). One prospective, 8-week, open-label trial investigated the use of extended-release carbamazepine monotherapy in 27 participants ages 6–12 years with bipolar disorder. Extended-release carbamazepine was initiated at 200 mg qd, and the dose was increased by 100 mg in the first 2 weeks and 200 mg weekly thereafter per clinician judgment based on tolerability and response. The maximum dosage used in the study was 1,200 mg/day (not to exceed 35 mg/kg body weight or serum concentrations > 12 µg /mL). In this trial, extended-release carbamazepine was found to have modest antimanic effects and a somewhat better antidepressive and antipsychotic response. Although the medication was well tolerated in this trial, high dropout rates occurred, predominantly due to lack of response (Joshi et al. 2010).

Formulations

Carbamazepine is available in several forms. Generic carbamazepine is available as 100-mg chewable tablets, 200-mg tablets, and an oral solution of 100-mg/5 mL strength. These forms of carbamazepine are generally dosed thrice daily or four times daily. An extended-release formulation of carbamazepine (Carbatrol) is also available in 100-mg, 200-mg, and 300-mg capsule form, which allows twice-daily dosing. The contents of a Carbatrol capsule may be sprinkled over food, such as applesauce. This form is similar to the extended-release formulation, Equetro, which is available in sprinkle capsules of strengths of 100 mg, 200 mg, and 300 mg. The tablet version of extended-release carbamazepine, Tegretol-XR, is available in strengths of 100 mg, 200 mg, and 400 mg.

Preliminary Evaluation

A thorough medical history should be obtained before prescribing carbamazepine. Particular attention should be paid to any history of hepatic dysfunction, hematological abnormalities, cardiac conduction problems, or immunological concerns. Laboratory work should include a complete blood count (CBC) with differential and platelets, electrolytes, BUN/creatinine, transaminases, and a urine pregnancy test, if applicable. Careful discussion regarding the teratogenic potential of carbamazepine should occur with all women of childbearing capacity, both prior to the initiation of treatment and throughout maintenance therapy. Because carbamazepine can autoinduce its metabolism, blood levels should be monitored carefully and dose adjustments made accordingly (Kudriakova et al. 1992). In addition, carbamazepine can significantly affect the metabolism of numerous other medications, so a complete assessment of concomitant medications is recommended.

Medication Dosing

Carbamazepine use in the child and adolescent population has been extensively studied in the pediatric neurology literature, and the following recommendations are based on those studies. In children younger than age 6 years, carbamazepine should be initiated at 10–20 mg/kg/day bid or tid, and the dosage should be titrated at weekly intervals to symptom resolution or dose-limiting side effects. As noted earlier (see "Formulations"), the carbamazepine oral solution should be administered in a thrice-daily or four-times-daily dosing regimen to minimize any side effects from the higher peak serum levels seen with this formulation. In children ages 6–12 years, carbamazepine may be initiated at 100 mg bid and increased weekly by 100 mg, with the total daily dose not to exceed 1 g. For individuals older than 12 years, the carbamazepine can be initiated at 200 mg bid and titrated by 200 mg weekly. Adequate serum levels in individuals older than 12 years are generally achieved at dosages similar to those used in adults (800–1,200 mg/day). Of note, in the open-label study to compare carbamazepine, lithium, and divalproex sodium in children and adolescents with bipolar disorder, all of the subjects in the carbamazepine arm had carbamazepine initiated at a dosage of 15 mg/kg/day (Kowatch et al. 2000). Joshi et al. (2010) studied extended-release carbamazepine in an open-label trial mentioned previously (see "Supporting Studies in Youth"). In this study, extended-release carbamazepine was initiated at 200 mg qd, and the dose was increased by 100 mg in the first 2 weeks and 200 mg weekly thereafter. The maximum dosage used in the study was 1,200 mg/day (not to exceed 35 mg/kg body weight or serum concentrations >12 µg /mL).

We have generally found that initiating carbamazepine at a dosage of approximately 15 mg/kg/day is reasonably well tolerated. The therapeutic serum level range is 4–12 µg/mL, with 7–10 µg/mL being a common maintenance drug level. Because autoinduction may occur during carbamazepine therapy, dosages that were initially found to be therapeutic may subsequently be inadequate. For this reason, careful laboratory and symptom monitoring are indicated. We recommend that drug levels, CBC with differential and platelets, and liver enzyme measurements be completed at least every other week during the first 2 months of treatment, then at least every 3 months thereafter.

Side Effects

Common side effects of carbamazepine affect both the GI system and the CNS (Table 6–2). Nausea and sedation are commonly experienced and can often be minimized with gradual titration of treatment and divided dosing. Blurred vision and ataxia can also be noted.

Hematological, dermatological, and hepatic side effects seem to be less common. Mild leukopenia and thrombocytopenia may occur in some individuals. Rarely, some patients develop aplastic anemia or agranulocytosis. Transient skin rashes may occur. Stevens-Johnson syndrome may occur very

Table 6–2.   Management of common carbamazepine side effects

System	Side effect	Suggested intervention
Gastrointestinal	Nausea	Reduce dose or split dose Take with food Change formulation used
CNS	Blurred vision, ataxia, sedation	Reduce or split dose
Hematological	Leukopenia, thrombocytopenia, agranulocytosis, aplastic anemia	Advise patients to immediately notify clinician if flu symptoms or signs of infection occur Monitor laboratory values regularly Agranulocytosis/aplastic anemia: Immediately discontinue drug and consider medical hospitalization
Hepatic	Elevated transaminases	Monitor laboratory values regularly Educate patient on symptoms of hepatic failure (jaundice, fatigue)
Dermatological	Skin rash	Carefully monitor and consider discontinuation

rarely with carbamazepine use as well. Transaminase levels may become mildly elevated with carbamazepine administration. Hyponatremia has been reported, in addition to abnormal renal function, in some individuals. Weight gain does not appear to be a substantive problem with this drug.

Drug Interactions and Cautions

Carbamazepine is metabolized through the cytochrome P450 (CYP) 3A3 and 3A4 systems and therefore has the potential to interact with many commonly used medications. A partial listing of drugs that can *increase* carbamazepine levels includes fluoxetine, fluvoxamine, valproate, tricyclic antidepressants, prednisolone, and macrolide antibiotics (erythromycin). Use of carbamazepine may *decrease* the blood levels of oral contraceptives, benzodiazepines, theophylline, sertraline, and neuroleptics, among other medications. Carbamazepine has been associated with fetal abnormalities when used by pregnant women in the first trimester.

In summary, carbamazepine has limited data on its effectiveness in treating pediatric mania. No randomized, double-blind trials currently exist to support the routine use of carbamazepine. In addition, the numerous risks related to carbamazepine use and its extensive interactions with other concomitant medications suggest it should be considered a second-line or adjunctive agent in treating PBD until further studies are performed.

Divalproex Sodium

Divalproex sodium received FDA approval for treatment of mania in adults in 1994. It appears that valproate, unlike carbamazepine, is commonly prescribed to children and adolescents with bipolar disorder.

Supporting Studies in Youth

Acute treatment of manic, hypomanic, and mixed mania symptoms in children and adolescents has been evaluated in open-label trials of up to 8 weeks in length (Papatheodorou et al. 1995; Scheffer et al. 2005; Wagner et al. 2002). These studies suggest that divalproex may be effective in the treatment of bipolar disorder in young patients. Headache, GI complaints, and sedation were commonly observed side effects in these reports.

Two published studies have evaluated the longer-term use of divalproex sodium in PBD. In a 6-month, prospective, open-label trial by Pavuluri et al. (2005), treatment with divalproex sodium was started at a dose of 250–500 mg the first night, and the dosage was then adjusted to 15–20 mg/kg/day given in divided doses. Children and adolescents, ages 5–18 years, achieved a response rate of 73.5% and a remission rate of 52.9% during the study period, while weight gain and transient transaminase elevations were noted. Findling et al. (2005) reported on an 18-month, double-blind, maintenance comparison of lithium and divalproex sodium in youth ages 5–18 years with bipolar disorder. Divalproex was initiated in divided doses and gradually increased to a target dosage of 20 mg/kg/day. In this trial, lithium and divalproex treatment appeared to have similar effectiveness as maintenance treatments. GI complaints, tremor, and headache were commonly reported side effects.

As mentioned earlier in the section on lithium, the NIMH funded a double-blind comparison study of lithium, divalproex, and placebo over an 8-week period. In that trial, divalproex was found to be superior to placebo (Kowatch et. al 2007). However, in a randomized, double-blind, industry-sponsored study investigating the use of extended-release divalproex in youth with bipolar disorder (N=150), no statistically significant improvement in acute manic symptoms was found for those taking divalproex rather than placebo (Wagner et al. 2009). An explanation for the discrepant results between these two studies may be related to between-site variability. The NIMH-supported study was conducted at substantially fewer sites than the industry-sponsored trial; therefore, intersite variability may have contributed to the results of the industry-supported trial. Furthermore, combination pharmacotherapy studies have suggested that divalproex may be beneficial when coadministered with lithium, quetiapine, or risperidone (Findling et al. 2003; Kowatch et al. 2003).

Formulations

Standard valproic acid without enteric coating is available in the form of Depakene in 250-mg capsules; Depakene is also available as an elixir of 250 mg/5 mL. Enteric-coated valproic acid (divalproex sodium) is available as Depakote in 125-mg, 250-mg, and 500-mg tablets. Depakote Sprinkle Capsules are available in 125-mg strength. The beaded contents of the capsules can be sprinkled over applesauce for children who have difficulty swallowing pills. Depakote ER is available in 250-mg and 500-mg tablets, and once-daily dosing may be possible with this form. A delayed-release soft gel capsule (Stavzor) containing valproate is available in strengths of 125 mg, 250 mg, and 500 mg. These capsules are smaller than Depakote tablets and may be easier to swallow, especially for younger patients.

Preliminary Evaluation

A detailed medical history is recommended prior to initiating treatment with valproate. Particular attention should be paid to any history of hepatic and/or hematological dysfunction. Concomitant medications that are hepatically metabolized should also be reviewed. The teratogenic potential for neural tube defects has been well established with valproate therapy, and urine pregnancy testing and documentation of education regarding this possibility is suggested for females of childbearing potential. Concerns regarding polycystic ovary syndrome (PCOS) have prompted some clinicians to document pretreatment menstrual patterns to facilitate the identification of any changes in menses that might occur during valproate therapy. Baseline laboratory work should include a CBC with differential and platelets, as well as an assessment of liver function (e.g., transaminases, bilirubin). Because treatment with divalproex may lead to weight gain, monitoring of weight and height prior to and during valproate treatment is also recommended.

Medication Dosing

Enteric-coated preparations are generally preferred over generic valproic acid for the treatment of pediatric patients with bipolar illness, given that enteric-coated formulations are associated with a reduced risk for GI side effects such as dyspepsia and abdominal pain. For outpatients, we generally recommend initiating divalproex sodium at a dosage of approximately 10–15 mg/kg/day (in divided doses). Then, based on the results of serum levels and clinical response, dosage increases in 250-mg to 500-mg increments may be considered. Serum levels of valproic acid should be obtained shortly after initiation of treatment, during dose titration periods, or as clinically indicated. Adequate serum levels have been reported in the 50- to 125-μg/mL range, and the total daily dose should not exceed 60 mg/kg. After dosage stabilization, liver function tests, CBC with differential and platelets, and serum levels should be obtained at least every 6 months, or when clinical symptoms change.

Side Effects

Side effects reported to be associated with divalproex pharmacotherapy in the pediatric bipolar population have included GI, CNS, hematological, and hepatic events (Table 6–3). Weight gain was noted in 59% of the sample treated by Pavuluri et al. (2005). CNS effects that have been reported include cognitive dulling, headaches, tremor, and somnolence. Although the enteric-coated divalproex sodium preparations can minimize GI symptoms, patients taking these formulations have reported nausea, stomach pain, diarrhea, and emesis. Rare cases of hepatic failure and potentially fatal pancreatitis have also been observed. Therefore, we routinely advise patients to notify their physician about new-onset symptoms of nausea, lethargy, jaundice, or anorexia. Thrombocytopenia also may occur, so monitoring for bleeding or easy bruising is suggested.

The issue surrounding PCOS has received renewed interest in the past decade. PCOS is a syndrome of hyperandrogenism (menstrual irregularities, hirsutism, acne, and alopecia). Small studies have failed to consistently show a relationship between PCOS and valproate use among patients without seizure disorders (H. Joffe et al. 2003; R.T. Joffe et al. 2003). However, Qin et

Table 6–3. Management of divalproex sodium–related side effects

System	Side effect	Suggested intervention
Gastrointestinal	Nausea, emesis, stomach pain, diarrhea	Take with food Switch to Depakote formulation Consider checking serum level for toxicity
CNS	Tremor, headache, sedation, cognitive dulling	Reduce or split dose
Hematological	Leukopenia, thrombocytopenia	Consider hematology consultation Consider medication discontinuation
Hepatic	Elevated transaminases/ pancreatic enzymes	Consider rechecking of laboratory values Consider medication discontinuation
Endocrine	Menstrual irregularities, hyperandrogenism	Consider referral to an endocrinologist Consider switching mood-stabilizing agents
General	Weight gain	Educate patient about appropriate diet and exercise Consider nutrition consultation

al. (2006) identified a functional polymorphism, SNP-71G, that may contribute to the creation of excessive testosterone production. Furthermore, valproate has been shown to potentiate this gene's expression in ovarian cells (Nelson-DeGrave et al. 2004; Wood et al. 2005). In sum, valproate treatment may play a role in the potentiation of PCOS in certain patients, so careful monitoring may be indicated until a clearer picture of the association between valproate administration and PCOS is available.

Drug Interactions and Cautions

Like many other psychotropic agents, valproate is metabolized in the liver. Because of the possibility of drug-drug interactions, care should be used when valproate is prescribed with concomitant medications. Commonly used agents that can *increase* valproate levels include erythromycin, fluoxetine, aspirin, and ibuprofen. Similarly, carbamazepine is a medication that may *decrease* valproate levels during concomitant use. In addition, valproate can lead to substantive increases in lamotrigine levels when both agents are used together. This elevation in lamotrigine concentrations may result in serious dermatological reactions. Therefore, dosing of lamotrigine should be modified when prescribed concomitantly with valproate.

Other Anticonvulsants

Evidence for the use of other, newer anticonvulsants in treating PBD is sparse. For this reason, we generally do not prescribe these compounds to patients unless other agents with more extensive empirical support do not provide adequate therapeutic benefit.

Lamotrigine is indicated for the maintenance treatment of adults with bipolar disorder, although its acute management of mood episodes in adults is not well established. Open-label studies indicate that lamotrigine may provide benefit for adolescents experiencing mixed or manic states of bipolar disorder (Pavuluri et al. 2009). Further RCTs are needed.

One methodologically stringent clinical trial examined the use of topiramate. In that study, DelBello et al. (2005) conducted a double-blind, placebo-controlled trial of topiramate in children ages 6–17 years with bipolar I disorder. In this pediatric trial, topiramate appeared to be trending toward indeed having some therapeutic efficacy, but the trial was ended before the entire planned sample was ascertained because results of concurrent adult mania studies failed to demonstrate efficacy for the compound. However, definitive conclusions about the short-term efficacy of topiramate cannot be made on the basis of the results of this trial, because this pediatric study had a limited sample size, and therefore reduced statistical power to detect a difference between drug and placebo.

Similar to what had been suggested in adults (Benedetti et al. 2004; Hummel et al. 2002), oxcarbazepine was described in two separate case reports as possibly being beneficial in the treatment of PBD (Davanzo et al. 2004; Teitelbaum 2001). However, in a large, multisite, randomized, double-blind, placebo-controlled study in children and adolescents, treatment with oxcarbazepine was found not to be superior to treatment with placebo (Wagner et al. 2006).

Although some reports have considered zonisamide, levetiracetam, and tiagabine in the adult literature, these published studies were not placebo controlled and generally lacked methodological rigor. At present, we do not prescribe these three agents to youth, given the lack of data to support their use in the management of PBD.

Atypical Antipsychotics

At present, the atypical antipsychotic agents that are available to clinicians in the United States include aripiprazole, clozapine, olanzapine, paliperidone (the active metabolite of risperidone), quetiapine, risperidone, and ziprasidone. In addition, at this point, asenapine, iloperidone, and lurasidone have been marketed in the United States but remain unstudied in children and adolescents (www.fda.gov). The mood-stabilizing properties of atypical antipsychotic medications have received significant attention in the literature on adult bipolar disorder over the past several years. In the adult literature, atypical antipsychotic monotherapy has been shown to provide similar benefits to traditional mood-stabilizer monotherapy for acute mania. Researchers in pediatric bipolar illness have also begun to explore the usefulness of atypical antipsychotics as a monotherapy and as an adjunctive therapy in this often difficult-to-treat population.

General Evaluation and Monitoring

Before any atypical antipsychotic medication is prescribed, care must be taken to obtain an accurate psychiatric, medical, and family history. Particular attention should be paid to a medical history, family history, and physical examination that consider weight/obesity, endocrine and cardiovascular system issues, as well as neurological status and movement disorders. We recommend that when prescribing any psychotropic medication to children and adolescents, the clinician should review the potential for short-term and long-term side effects with both the patient and the patient's guardians. In addition to considerations that pertain to this entire class of drugs, some issues are specific to individual agents. These drug-specific topics are discussed as each agent is considered individually below.

One of the key aspects that confers *atypicality* to this class of drugs is their reduced propensity to cause extrapyramidal side effects (EPS) when compared with the older, *typical* antipsychotics. However, neurological side effects such as dystonia, parkinsonism, and tardive dyskinesia have been reported with these agents. The potential for these risks should be reviewed with patients and their guardians. In addition, we recommend that extra care be paid to the assessment of extrapyramidal symptoms prior to and during the course of treatment with this group of drugs. In addition, because tardive dyskinesia is a possibly irreversible side effect, we recommend carefully evaluating and monitoring for this possibility. A commonly used instrument that can facilitate this process is the Abnormal Involuntary Movement Scale (National Institute of Mental Health 1985).

Much discussion has occurred concerning the potential for metabolic/endocrinological and cardiovascular complications in patients taking atypical antipsychotics. Although the adult literature has data to support the assertion that atypical antipsychotics are effective and reasonably well-tolerated medications for the acute treatment of symptoms of psychosis and mania, concerns over adverse lipid-profile changes, dramatic weight increases, and the development of glucose intolerance during longer-term treatment with these drugs have been notable. Consensus guidelines (based on adult data) to assist clinicians with suggested monitoring strategies that address these concerns regarding treatment with atypical antipsychotics are available (American Diabetes Association et al. 2004).

Avoiding drug interactions with atypical antipsychotics generally involves avoiding specific concomitant therapies. Because atypical antipsychotic medications can be sedating, caution should be used when combining these medications with other CNS depressants. In addition, medications that affect cardiac conduction by lengthening the QT interval should be avoided. Concomitant use of medications affecting hepatic metabolism can reduce (e.g., carbamazepine) or increase (e.g., fluvoxamine, atomoxetine) blood levels of certain atypical antipsychotics.

Aripiprazole

Aripiprazole has recently been determined to be an effective monotherapy in adult bipolar disorder (Keck et al. 2003). Of the atypical antipsychotics, it is distinct in that it acts as a partial dopamine agonist. Aripiprazole is currently approved by the FDA for the acute and maintenance treatment of manic and mixed episodes associated with bipolar I disorder in patients ages 10–17 years.

Supporting Studies

One randomized, double-blind, placebo-controlled study of 296 patients ages 10–17 years with bipolar I disorder showed that aripiprazole, at dosages of 10 and 30 mg/day, was superior to placebo in the acute treatment of manic and·mixed episodes (Findling et al. 2009).

Formulations

Aripiprazole (Abilify) is available in both tablet and liquid forms. Tablets are available in 2-, 5-, 10-, 15-, 20-, and 30-mg strengths. The liquid preparation is available as a 1-mg/mL elixir. An orally disintegrating tablet formulation is available in strengths of 10 mg and 15 mg. Aripiprazole is also available in an injectable form that has not yet been studied in children.

Medication Dosing

With its long half-life, aripiprazole is routinely prescribed in once-daily dosing. On the basis of our clinical experience, we generally recommend initiating aripiprazole at a dose of 2 mg or 5 mg at bedtime and titrating by 2- to 5-mg increments every 2–3 days to maximize salutary effects while minimizing side effects. We do not recommend exceeding the FDA-approved maximum dose of 30 mg/day.

Side Effects

Common side effects that have been reported with aripiprazole in youth include sedation, motoric activation, nausea, and emesis (Table 6–4). Studies in adults suggest that aripiprazole may have a reduced propensity for inducing weight gain compared with some of the other atypical agents. However, aripiprazole treatment does appear to be associated with weight gain in youth. Clinically significant electrocardiographic changes appear not to be common with aripiprazole. In addition, because of aripiprazole's distinct partial dopamine agonism mechanism of action, prolactin levels seem to decrease during therapy with this medication.

Clozapine

Whereas the other atypical antipsychotic agents are considered to be first-line agents, clozapine is generally reserved for patients who fail to respond to other forms of therapy and appears to be used only rarely in pediatric patients with

Table 6–4. Management of aripiprazole side effects

System	Side effect	Suggested intervention
Gastrointestinal	Nausea, emesis	Take with food Titrate more slowly Reduce dose
CNS	Headache, sedation, activation, akathisia	Reduce or split dose Change time of daily administration
General	Weight gain	Educate patient about appropriate diet and exercise Consider nutrition consultation Switch to another treatment

bipolar illness. This is due to clozapine's associated risk for potentially fatal agranulocytosis. Also, clozapine can lower the seizure threshold and lead to both electroencephalographic changes as well as overt seizures in youth who take this drug.

Some evidence suggests that clozapine may be of benefit to adolescents with treatment-resistant bipolar illness (Masi et al. 2002). Unfortunately, no prospective RCTs have been reported of clozapine in youth with bipolar illness.

Olanzapine

Olanzapine, which was introduced in the United States in 1996, is approved for use in adults for the treatment of schizophrenia and mania in bipolar disorder. Olanzapine is also FDA approved for the acute treatment of manic or mixed episodes associated with bipolar I disorder in adolescents ages 13–17 years. Concerns over weight gain and endocrine abnormalities (diabetes, dyslipidemias) associated with olanzapine therapy have received attention in adults. These issues are of important clinical concern for children and adolescents, who may be at greater risk for antipsychotic-related weight gain.

Supporting Studies

One of the first publications to suggest that olanzapine might be effective in youth was a case series involving patients ages 12–17 years with acute mania (Soutullo et al. 1999). Frazier et al. (2001) subsequently conducted an open-label olanzapine monotherapy trial. Over the course of the 8-week study, treatment with olanzapine was effective in reducing symptoms of mania in patients ages 5–14 years. Biederman et al. (2005) described the treatment of children ages 4–6 with bipolar disorder who were administered olanzapine (1.25–10 mg) or risperidone (0.25–2 mg). The authors noted that both medications appeared to be effective.

Of particular note are the results of a 3-week double-blind, randomized, placebo-controlled trial (Tohen et al. 2007). In that study, adolescent patients with mania ages 13–17 years were given olanzapine ($n=107$) or placebo ($n=54$) at dosages ranging from 2.5 to 20 mg/day. The investigators found that compared with placebo, treatment with olanzapine was associated with greater reductions in manic symptoms. Patients randomly assigned to receive olanzapine gained more weight (3.7 kg) than did those given placebo (0.3 kg). Furthermore, the olanzapine-treated group showed significantly greater changes in levels of prolactin, fasting glucose, fasting total cholesterol, uric acid, and the hepatic enzymes aspartate transaminase and alanine transaminase. These results suggest that the benefits of olanzapine for the treatment of PBD should be considered within the context of its safety profile and may lead clinicians to consider this medication after other atypical antipsychotics have been tried first.

Formulations

Olanzapine (Zyprexa) is available as tablets, as an intramuscular preparation, and as the dissolving formulation Zydis. Tablets are available in strengths of 2.5 mg, 5 mg, 7.5 mg, 10 mg, 15 mg, and 20 mg. Zydis orally disintegrating tablets, available in strengths of 5 mg, 10 mg, 15 mg, and 20 mg, may be useful for children who are unable to swallow tablets. The injectable form of olanzapine is generally reserved for management of emergencies and potentially dangerous situations.

Preliminary Evaluation

Given that olanzapine therapy may be associated with weight gain and endocrine dysfunction, care should be exercised to establish any history of endocrine dysfunction or obesity both in the child or adolescent and in his or her biological family prior to therapy. Discussions with patients and their families should include both short-term risks noted in acute pediatric trials and long-term risks seen in adult studies. Active participation of the patient and family in monitoring side effects is also suggested.

Table 6–5. Management of olanzapine side effects

System	Side effect	Suggested intervention
Endocrine	Glucose intolerance	Monitor fasting glucose and hemoglobin A_{1C} at least annually Consider nutrition consultation
CNS	Headache, sedation	Reduce or split dose Administer dose at bedtime
General	Weight gain	Educate patient about appropriate diet and exercise Consider nutrition consultation Switch to another atypical antipsychotic Consider addition of metformin or topiramate

Medication Dosing

In the Biederman et al. (2005) olanzapine study of children ages 4–6 years, olanzapine was initiated at 1.25 mg at bedtime, and the dosage was increased weekly to a maximum of 10 mg/day. In the open-label study of Frazier et al. (1999), olanzapine was initiated at 2.5 mg as a single evening dose, and the dosage was increased by that same amount every 3 days, as tolerated. The FDA-approved dosing guidelines recommend that oral olanzapine be initiated at doses of 2.5 or 5 mg, with a target dosage of 10 mg/day. Dosing adjustments in increments of 2.5 or 5 mg are recommended. Dosages above 20 mg/day have not been clinically evaluated in the pediatric population.

Side Effects

Side effects reported to be associated with olanzapine include glucose intolerance, headache, sedation, and weight gain (Table 6–5). Weight gain has been noted in the published pediatric bipolar trials. Although sedation is commonly reported with olanzapine use, GI problems appear to be relatively uncommon. Unfortunately, methodologically stringent long-term studies of olanzapine in this patient group are lacking. Therefore, the magnitude of weight gain associated with long-term olanzapine therapy in the pediatric population has yet to be adequately characterized.

Quetiapine

Quetiapine monotherapy is FDA approved in adults for the treatment of schizophrenia, acute mania in bipolar disorder, and depressive episodes associated with bipolar disorder. In addition, quetiapine is FDA approved for the acute treatment of manic episodes in pediatric patients ages 10–17 years with bipolar I disorder. Quetiapine was introduced in the U.S. market in 1997.

Supporting Studies

In a retrospective chart review, the response rate for youth receiving quetiapine monotherapy to treat a bipolar spectrum illness was 78.6% (Marchand et al. 2004). In addition, in one prospective study, 50 patients ages 12–18 years with mania were randomly assigned to receive treatment with either quetiapine, at dosages ranging from 400 to 600 mg/day, or divalproex, at dosages necessary to achieve serum levels of 80–120 µg/mL, for up to 4 weeks. The authors found both medications to be equally effective in symptom amelioration of mania and both agents to be reasonably well tolerated (DelBello et al. 2006). Another randomized, placebo-controlled trial of 277 patients ages 10–17 years found that quetiapine, at dosages of 400 and 600 mg/day, was more effective than placebo in treating acute manic symptoms in PBD (DelBello et al. 2007).

Other studies have evaluated the usefulness of quetiapine as an adjunctive treatment in PBD. These clinical trials are considered in the section "Combination Pharmacotherapy" later in this chapter.

Formulations

Quetiapine (Seroquel) is available in strengths of 25 mg, 50 mg, 100 mg, 200 mg, 300 mg, and 400 mg. In addition, a long-acting formulation of quetiapine, Seroquel XR, is available in strengths of 50 mg, 150 mg, 200 mg, 300 mg, and 400 mg, although the XR formulation has not been studied in the pediatric population to date.

Medication Dosing

In a quetiapine-adjunctive inpatient study by DelBello et al. (2002), quetiapine was initiated at 25 mg bid, and the dosage was titrated to 150 mg tid over the course of 1 week. Our clinical practice has suggested that upward dosage increments of 50–100 mg/day are generally well tolerated in adolescents, and that increases of 25–50 mg/day are reasonably well tolerated in younger patients. Sedation is the dose-limiting side effect that we observe most frequently during

Table 6–6. Management of quetiapine side effects

System	Side effect	Suggested intervention
Cardiovascular	Elevated blood pressure (both systolic and diastolic)	Monitor blood pressure closely in patients taking quetiapine, adjust dosage as necessary to minimize blood pressure changes
CNS	Sedation, orthostasis	Reduce or split dosage to thrice daily, with larger dose at night Caution patient to be careful when getting out of bed or standing up
Visual	Cataracts	Educate patient about possible changes in eyesight Recommend regular ophthalmological evaluation
General	Weight gain	Educate patient about appropriate diet and exercise Consider nutrition consultation Consider switch to another agent

dosing increases. As with adults, we generally administer quetiapine in twice-daily doses that are equal in size. For adolescents, the FDA recommends that the total daily dose for the initial 5 days of therapy should be 50 mg (day 1), 100 mg (day 2), 200 mg (day 3), 300 mg (day 4), and 400 mg (day 5). After day 5, the dosage should be adjusted within the recommended range of 400–600 mg/day based on response and tolerability. Dosage adjustments should be in increments no greater than 100 mg/day. No additional benefit has been shown in dosing above 600 mg/day in adolescents. It is recommended that the dosing schedule be twice daily, or three times daily as necessary.

Side Effects/Preliminary Evaluation

The management of common side effects of quetiapine is described in Table 6–6. The adult literature notes blood pressure elevation, sedation, and orthostatic hypotension as common adverse effects that occur with quetiapine treatment. Although we have observed weight gain with quetiapine in our clinical practice, weight gain appears to be less than that noted with olanzapine and clozapine treatment. The risk of EPS may be relatively modest with quetiapine when compared with the other atypical agents.

Cataract formation has been noted in laboratory animals administered quetiapine. Although a relationship between quetiapine use and cataract formation has not been established in humans, in addition to the previously noted evaluations that might be considered prior to beginning atypical antipsychotic therapy (see "General Evaluation and Monitoring"), the clinician may consider recommending ophthalmological examinations for patients prescribed this drug.

Risperidone

Like other atypical antipsychotics, risperidone is FDA approved as a monotherapy for schizophrenia and acute mania in adults with bipolar disorder. In addition, risperidone was the first atypical antipsychotic to receive FDA approval for the treatment of acute mania or mixed episodes associated with bipolar I disorder in youth ages 10–17 years.

Supporting Studies

Frazier et al. (1999), in one of the first communications regarding the use of risperidone in pediatric bipolarity, reported that with risperidone at an average dosage of 1.7 mg/day, youth ages 4–17 years demonstrated substantive improvement in symptoms of mania and aggression over the treatment period. Biederman et al. (2005) compared risperidone with olanzapine monotherapy in preschool children ages 4–6 years with bipolar disorder. At dosages of up to 2 mg/day, risperidone was found to be generally beneficial. In another study from the same research group (Biederman et al. 2005c), 30 patients ages 6–17 years were treated in a prospective 8-week, open-label study. The authors found that treatment with risperidone at a mean dosage of 1.25 mg/day was associated with symptom amelioration and was reasonably well tolerated.

Haas et al. (2009) conducted a randomized study of risperidone versus placebo in the acute treatment of manic or mixed episodes in 169 patients ages 10–17 years. Risperidone was found to be superior to placebo and was relatively well tolerated at dosages as low as 0.5–2.5 mg/day.

Formulations

Risperidone (Risperdal) is available in tablet, liquid, disintegrating tablet, and long-acting injectable forms. The tablets are available in strengths of 0.25 mg, 0.5 mg, 1 mg, 2 mg, 3 mg, and 4 mg. The concentration of the liquid formulation is 1 mg/mL. The orally disintegrating form, Risperdal M-Tab, is available in strengths of 0.5 mg, 1 mg, 2 mg, 3 mg, and 4 mg. Neither injectable Risperdal Consta nor long-acting oral paliperidone (Invega) has been studied in the pediatric population.

Preliminary Evaluation

As recommended before any atypical antipsychotic initiation, the clinician should obtain an accurate psychiatric, medical, and family history (see earlier section "General Evaluation and Monitoring"). Risperidone, compared with other atypical antipsychotics, appears to have a greater propensity to increase prolactin concentrations. Because in our experience prolactin-related side effects are not often problematic, we generally do not monitor prolactin concentrations over time. However, we do recommend that a pretreatment prolactin level be obtained for youth prior to risperidone initiation. Then, if side effects that might be attributable to prolactin (e.g., irregular menses/amenorrhea, galactorrhea, breast enlargement) develop de novo, and a prolactin measurement is subsequently obtained, the clinician has a baseline level for comparison.

Medication Dosing

The FDA recommends initiating dosing of risperidone in youth with bipolar disorder at 0.5 mg/day, administered as a single daily dose in either the morning or evening. Dosage adjustments, if indicated, should occur at intervals of not less than 24 hours, in increments of 0.5 or 1 mg/day, as tolerated, to a recommended dosage of 2.5 mg/day. Although efficacy has been demonstrated in studies of pediatric patients with bipolar mania at dosages between 0.5 and 6 mg/day, no additional benefit was seen above 2.5 mg/day, and higher dosages were associated with more adverse events. Dosages higher than 6 mg/day have not been studied. In our experience, dose-limiting side effects during risperidone titration are sedation and EPS.

For younger children, we generally suggest starting at 0.25 mg/day, with titration every 2–3 days, to a total dosage that does not exceed 2 mg/day. This total daily dosage is typically administered in two relatively equal doses. For older children and adolescents (typically weighing more than 40 kg), we generally consider a similar dosing strategy that employs 0.5-mg dosing increments and a total dosage that does not exceed 4 mg/day.

Table 6–7. Management of risperidone side effects

System	Side effect	Suggested intervention
CNS	Sedation, headache	Reduce the total dose Administer more of the daily dose at night
Endocrine	Glucose intolerance; prolactin elevation	Monitor fasting glucose Monitor for changes in menses, galactorrhea, or gynecomastia
General	Weight gain	Educate patient about appropriate diet and exercise Consider switching to another agent

Side Effects

The most commonly reported side effects during risperidone treatment include weight gain, headache, and sedation (Table 6–7). A more rapid rate of dose titration, as well as higher final total daily dosages, seems to increase the risk of EPS during pediatric risperidone therapy. As noted earlier (see "Preliminary Evaluation"), the rates of hyperprolactinemia seem higher with risperidone than with other atypical antipsychotics.

Ziprasidone

Ziprasidone has been marketed in the United States since 2000 and has been approved by the FDA as monotherapy for schizophrenia and acute mania in adults. It does not appear to cause weight gain in adults. Ziprasidone does have a generally modest effect on intracardiac conduction. The risks associated with this effect in adults appear to be modest (Daniel 2003). Although concerns have been raised (Blair et al. 2005), the effects of ziprasidone on cardiac electrophysiology have not yet been well characterized in children or adolescents. To date, the FDA has not approved ziprasidone for any pediatric indication.

Supporting Studies

Literature supporting the use of ziprasidone in the pediatric population is somewhat limited. One case series described subjects receiving concomitant medications along with ziprasidone (Barnett 2004). All subjects seem to have received some benefit at dosages ≤80 mg/day. One randomized, placebo-controlled trial of 238 patients ages 10–17 years with bipolar disorder found that ziprasidone at dosages of 80–160 mg/day was effective and generally well tolerated for the treatment of mania (DelBello et al. 2008).

Formulations

Ziprasidone, marketed in the United States as Geodon, is available in capsules and as an intramuscular injection. Capsules are available in strengths of 20 mg, 40 mg, 60 mg, and 80 mg. The injectable form is reserved for acute agitation, and although its use has been described in case reports (Hazaray et al. 2004; Staller 2004), this formulation has not been examined in methodologically stringent research in the pediatric population.

Preliminary Evaluation

The evaluation prior to initiating ziprasidone therapy is similar to that mentioned previously for the other atypical antipsychotic medications (see earlier section "General Evaluation and Monitoring"). Particular attention should be paid to inquiring about any individual or family history of cardiac conduction problems or symptoms associated with cardiac disease (e.g., syncope, arrhythmias, or family history of sudden cardiac death). In the absence of adequate data to characterize ziprasidone's effects on intracardiac conduction, we recommend that ECGs be obtained prior to and during the course of ziprasidone therapy (see subsection "Side Effects" below).

Medication Dosing

Considering the paucity of published literature, it is not surprising that no definitive guidelines exist about the dosing of ziprasidone in pediatric bipolar patients. Our experience suggests that in teenagers, optimal final dosages of ziprasidone are similar to those reported to be beneficial to adults. Lower dosages appear to be effective in younger children (putatively attributable to their smaller size). On the basis of the available data, we recommend that ziprasidone be administered twice daily in divided doses. Because ingestion of ziprasidone with food increases this agent's bioavailability, we generally recommend that patients take their ziprasidone consistently with food to achieve predictable drug exposure.

Side Effects

Sedation, akathisia, and elevated heart rates have been noted when ziprasidone is prescribed to youth (Barnett 2004) (Table 6–8). Unlike with many of

Table 6–8. Management of ziprasidone side effects

System	Side effect	Suggested intervention
CNS	Sedation, akathisia, extrapyramidal side effects	Reduce the daily dose Administer the total daily dose in thrice-daily rather than twice-daily divided doses Administer a larger proportion of the total daily dose at bedtime
Cardiovascular	QTc prolongation, elevated heart rates	Monitor for any syncopal events or dizziness Consider electrocardiographic monitoring at baseline and during upward dose titration Consider electrocardiographic monitoring when optimal dosage achieved, then periodically, or if symptoms change

the other atypical agents, substantive weight increases and dyslipidemias do not appear to be associated with ziprasidone therapy in adults. In the absence of definitive information regarding the magnitude of QTc prolongation that may occur in youth, no definitive recommendations about electrocardiographic monitoring in youth treated with ziprasidone can be made. However, in our practice, in addition to a baseline ECG, we generally suggest that an ECG be repeated after every 40- to 60-mg/day increase in dosage.

Also worthy of note is that ziprasidone-associated mania has been described (Keating et al. 2005). The mechanism for this action and the frequency of this occurrence in young people remain empirical questions for which further research is needed.

Maintenance Therapy

Bipolar illness is a chronic, long-term condition. However, most pharmacotherapy studies in the pediatric bipolar literature have been no longer than 8 weeks. Limited studies are available to provide physicians with long-term efficacy and safety information.

Although the pediatric neurology literature provides some insights into the long-term safety of several of the anticonvulsants, data are limited regarding the long-term effectiveness and use of these medications in children and adolescents with bipolar illness. One 18-month study compared the efficacy of lithium with that of divalproex sodium as maintenance therapy. Results indicated that both drugs were generally well tolerated and showed equal effectiveness in preventing relapse over the 18-month trial period (Findling et al. 2005). One study evaluated the long-term efficacy of aripiprazole in the treatment of 296 youth ages 10–17 years with bipolar mania. Participants were randomized to receive aripiprazole 10 mg, aripiprazole 30 mg, or placebo in a 4-week, double-blind trial. Subjects then continued their randomly assigned treatments in a 26-week extension phase. Both dosages of aripiprazole were found to be superior to placebo at 4 weeks and again at 30 weeks (Wagner et al. 2007). Safety and tolerability data demonstrated that adverse events were mild to moderate and appeared to be dose related. In addition, no significant changes in weight or lipid or glucose values were observed (Correll et al. 2007).

Another study investigated the long-term efficacy of aripiprazole versus placebo in children with bipolar disorders. In this study, outpatients ages 4–9 years who met criteria for a bipolar disorder were eligible to receive up to 16 weeks of open-label treatment with aripiprazole (Phase I). Patients were randomized into a 72-week, double-blind phase of the study once they met a priori response criteria for stabilization (Phase II). During Phase II, patients either remained on their current aripiprazole regimen or began a double-blind taper in which they were switched from aripiprazole to placebo. The primary outcome measure for Phase II was time to discontinuation due to a mood event. Thirty patients were randomly assigned to continue aripiprazole, and 30 were randomly assigned to placebo. Despite the random assignment, both the aripiprazole and placebo groups showed high rates of discontinuation from the study over the initial 4 weeks (50% for aripiprazole; 90% for placebo). These results may indicate a possible nocebo effect (knowledge of possibly switching from active medication to placebo increasing concern for relapse). Despite the possible nocebo effect, the study results indicated that compared with placebo, aripiprazole may be superior in the long-term treatment of children with bipolar disorder (Findling et al. 2012).

Clearly, more studies are needed to address the long-term effectiveness and safety of maintenance medication options in the pediatric bipolar population.

Treatment of Pediatric Bipolar Depression

Although children and adolescents with bipolar disorder are known to experience depressive symptoms (Chang 2009), studies on treatment options for pediatric bipolar depression are limited. Some evidence supports the use of lithium for the management of the depressive phase in adults with bipolar disorder; however, its effectiveness in the pediatric population for bipolar depression in not well known. In 2006, Patel et al. conducted a 6-week, open-label study of 27 subjects ages 12–18 years with a history of bipolar disorder who were currently experiencing acute depressive symptoms. The subjects received lithium at dosages adjusted to achieve therapeutic levels of 1.0–1.2 mEq/L. In this study, lithium was associated with significant improvement in depressive symptoms. This study indicates that lithium may offer promise in treating pediatric bipolar depression; however, more evidence-based trials are necessary.

Lamotrigine has been considered in a case series of adolescents ages 14–18 years taking concomitant medications (Carandang et al. 2003) and in one small open-label study in adolescents with bipolar depression (Chang et al. 2006). The adjunctive use of lamotrigine in the depressed phase of adolescent bipolar disorder was also considered in a five-subject case report (Soutullo et al. 2006). These data provide the basis for a possible role for lamotrigine in young people with bipolar illness, but clinical trials are needed.

Quetiapine has evidence supporting its use in adult bipolar depression. DelBello et al. (2009) published the first double-blind, placebo-controlled trial investigating the treatment of pediatric bipolar depression. In this study, 32 subjects ages 12–18 years were randomized to receive quetiapine at dosages of 300–600 mg/day or placebo over an 8-week period. Contrary to findings among adult studies, quetiapine was not found to be superior to placebo in treating depressive symptoms in this trial. However, the results indicated a high rate of placebo response that may have played a role in the failure of quetiapine to separate statistically from placebo.

Antidepressant use in adults with bipolar disorder may be associated with the potential to induce mania; however, less is known about this phenomenon in the pediatric population (Joseph et al. 2009). No randomized trials of antidepressant treatment in PBD have been reported. Therefore, treatment recommendations generally advise avoiding antidepressant monotherapy in youth with bipolar disorder (Kowatch et al. 2005).

Studies investigating the treatment of pediatric bipolar depression are lacking and are necessary in the future to provide safe and effective treatment options.

Combination Pharmacotherapy

Much of the recent treatment research into PBD suggests that lithium, mood stabilizers, or atypical antipsychotics may be effective as drug monotherapy in treating this illness. Increasing evidence suggests that combination pharmacotherapy, consisting of more than one agent, also might be appropriate for some patients, including inpatients, youth with psychosis, and patients who have only a partial response to one class of medications. It appears that most clinicians opt to treat pediatric mania with psychosis using either lithium or divalproex sodium in combination with an atypical antipsychotic.

Combining lithium with divalproex sodium also has demonstrated effectiveness in treating pediatric mania (Findling et al. 2003). Other data suggest that lithium in combination with other antipsychotics may also be a rational therapeutic strategy (Kafantaris et al. 2001). Similarly, adjunctive administration of quetiapine with divalproex has been found to be an effective approach in adolescent mania (DelBello et al. 2002). In addition, risperidone administered concomitantly with either lithium or divalproex sodium has been noted to be an effective combination treatment for pediatric mania (Pavuluri et al. 2004).

Despite the fact that combination pharmacotherapy may be a reasonable mood-stabilizing strategy for some patients, clinicians should not infer that all patients should be treated with more than one thymoleptic. Unfortunately, at present, identifying which patients will or will not respond to drug monotherapy prior to treatment initiation is not possible. For this reason, with the exception of mania accompanied by psychosis, and mania of the severity requiring inpatient hospitalization, we generally recommend that mood-stabilizer pharmacotherapy for children with bipolar disorder begin with one agent.

A significant number of young patients with bipolar illness are being treated with multiple medications (sometimes in excess of five psychotropic agents) concurrently (Kowatch et al. 2005). Because of the inherent risks of such combinations, this degree of polypharmacy should be avoided, if at all possible. Clinicians should remember that incremental benefits should be seen when a new medication is added to an existing pharmacological regimen that has been partially effective. If improvement is not clearly observed with the addition of a new drug, the clinician should not simply add more medications to a youth's pharmacological regimen. Rather, the clinician should assess the potential benefit and risk of each agent and consider discontinuing one or more of the agents to help achieve mood stabilization.

Because psychiatric comorbidity is the rule, not the exception, in PBD, the clinician should pay careful attention to discerning whether other psychiatric conditions are present when faced with a young patient with bipolarity. Unfortunately, very few data are available about how to treat psychiatric comorbidities in PBD.

The best evidence available regarding psychiatric comorbidities in PBD pertains to the treatment of comorbid attention-deficit/hyperactivity disorder (ADHD). Scheffer et al. (2005) demonstrated that addition of mixed amphetamine salts was effective in treating ADHD symptoms following mood stabilization with divalproex monotherapy. Similarly, in youth who had achieved a stable mood with lithium and/or divalproex sodium, those treated with stimulants did not have an increased risk of relapse when compared with those who were not treated with a psychostimulant (Findling et al. 2005).

Another study investigated the short-term efficacy of methylphenidate in 16 youths with bipolar disorder and ADHD who were euthymic when taking at least one mood stabilizer but continued to experience clinically significant symptoms of ADHD. Study participants received 1 week each of placebo, methylphenidate 5 mg bid, methylphenidate 10 mg bid, and methylphenidate 15 mg bid in a crossover design. Findings demonstrated that treatment with methylphenidate was superior to placebo in treating ADHD symptoms, and its administration was not associated with mood destabilization (Findling et al. 2007).

Conclusions

Quite a bit of progress has occurred over the past 10 years in the pharmacological treatment of PBD. Clinicians are now better able to recognize and more effectively treat this condition. Continued research into the phenomenology, longitudinal course, genetics, and therapeutics of this spectrum of illnesses will eventually provide insights into the pathophysiology of PBD. Those insights, in turn, should contribute to the development of a broader, evidence-based foundation for the identification and management of PBD. As research into those domains continues, and as a better appreciation and understanding of the development and course of the illness develops, it is possible that these avenues of research may eventually lead to useful preventive strategies for this chronic, debilitating illness.

Clinical Pearls

- Be sure the diagnosis is correct. Because pediatric bipolar disorder can be difficult to diagnose, it is important to be sure the right patients are receiving the correct interventions.
- Select a medication regimen that is based on scientific data from pediatric populations.
- Use the right dosage of medication. Some medicines require therapeutic drug concentration monitoring. In addition, many agents will be less effective if underdosed or may be less safe if prescribed at too high a dosage.
- Continue the medication trial for an adequate period of time. Some drugs do not provide noteworthy salutary effects until after several weeks of treatment at an appropriate dosage.
- Be aware of any psychiatric comorbidities, which might contribute to what seemingly is "treatment nonresponse."
- Carefully assess for side effects because the medications used in the treatment of pediatric bipolarity may be associated with substantive risks.
- Remove agents that might be exacerbating the illness. Some medications can worsen the course of illness in some patients.

References

American Diabetes Association, American Psychiatric Association, American Association of Clinical Endocrinologists, North American Association for the Study of Obesity: Consensus and development conference on antipsychotic drugs and obesity and diabetes. J Clin Psychiatry 65:267–272, 2004

Barnett MS: Ziprasidone monotherapy in pediatric bipolar disorder. J Child Adolesc Psychopharmacol 14:471–477, 2004

Benedetti A, Lattanzi L, Pini S, et al: Oxcarbazepine as add-on treatment in patients with bipolar manic, mixed or depressive episodes. J Affect Disord 79:273–277, 2004

Biederman J, Mick E, Faraone SV, et al: A prospective follow-up study of pediatric bipolar disorder in boys with attention-deficit/hyperactivity disorder. J Affect Disord 82(suppl):S17–S23, 2004

Biederman J, Mick E, Hammerness P, et al: Open-label, 8-week trial of olanzapine and risperidone for the treatment of bipolar disorder in preschool-age children. Biol Psychiatry 58:589–594, 2005

Biederman J, Mick E, Wozniak J, et al: An open-label trial of risperidone in children and adolescents with bipolar disorder. J Child Adolesc Psychopharmacol 15:311–317, 2005c

Blair J, Scahill L, State M, et al: Electrocardiographic changes in children and adolescents treated with ziprasidone: a prospective study. J Am Acad Child Adolesc Psychiatry 44:73–79, 2005

Carandang CG, Maxwell DJ, Robbins DR, et al: Lamotrigine in adolescent mood disorders. J Am Acad Child Adolesc Psychiatry 42:750–751, 2003

Chang K: Challenges in the diagnosis and treatment of pediatric bipolar depression. Dialogues Clin Neurosci 11:73–80, 2009

Chang K, Saxena K, Howe M: An open-label study of lamotrigine adjunct or monotherapy for the treatment of adolescents with bipolar depression. J Am Acad Child Adolesc Psychiatry 45:298–304, 2006

Cooper TB, Bergner PE, Simpson GM: The 24-hour serum lithium level as a prognosticator of dosage requirements. Am J Psychiatry 130:601–602, 1973

Correll CU, Nyilas M, Aurang C, et al: Safety and tolerability of aripiprazole in children (10–17) with mania. Poster presented at the annual meeting of the American Academy of Child and Adolescent Psychiatry. Boston, MA, October 23–28, 2007

Craven C, Murphy M: Carbamazepine treatment of bipolar disorder in an adolescent with cerebral palsy. J Am Acad Child Adolesc Psychiatry 39:680–681, 2000

Daniel DG: Tolerability of ziprasidone: an expanding perspective. J Clin Psychiatry 64(suppl):40–49, 2003

Davanzo P, Nikore V, Yehya N, et al: Oxcarbazepine treatment of juvenile-onset bipolar disorder. J Child Adolesc Psychopharmacol 14:344–345, 2004

DelBello MP, Schwiers ML, Rosenberg HL, et al: A double-blind, randomized, placebo-controlled study of quetiapine as adjunctive treatment for adolescent mania. J Am Acad Child Adolesc Psychiatry 41:1216–1223, 2002

DelBello MP, Findling RL, Kushner S, et al: A pilot controlled trial of topiramate for mania in children and adolescents with bipolar disorder. J Am Acad Child Adolesc Psychiatry 44:539–547, 2005

DelBello MP, Kowatch RA, Adler CM, et al: A double-blind randomized pilot study comparing quetiapine and divalproex for adolescent mania. J Am Acad Child Adolesc Psychiatry 45:305–313, 2006

DelBello MP, Findling RL, Earley WR, et al: Efficacy of quetiapine in children and adolescents with bipolar mania: a 3-week, double-blind, randomized, placebo-controlled trial. Poster presented at the annual meeting of the American Academy of Child and Adolescent Psychiatry. Boston, MA, October 23–28, 2007

DelBello MP, Findling RL, Wang PP et al: Efficacy and safety of ziprasidone in pediatric bipolar disorder. Poster presented at the 161st annual meeting of American Psychiatric Association, Washington, DC, May 3–8, 2008

DelBello MP, Chang K, Welge JA, et al: A double-blind, placebo-controlled pilot study of quetiapine for depressed adolescents with bipolar disorder. Bipolar Disord 11:483–493, 2009

Findling RL, Gracious BL, McNamara NK, et al: Rapid, continuous cycling and psychiatric comorbidity in pediatric bipolar I disorder. Bipolar Disord 3:202–210, 2001

Findling RL, McNamara NK, Gracious B, et al: Combination lithium and divalproex sodium in pediatric bipolarity. J Am Acad Child Adolesc Psychiatry 42:895–901, 2003

Findling RL, McNamara NK, Youngstrom EA, et al: Double-blind 18-month trial of lithium versus divalproex maintenance treatment in pediatric bipolar disorder. J Am Acad Child Adolesc Psychiatry 44:409–417, 2005

Findling RL, Short EJ, McNamara NK, et al: Methylphenidate in the treatment of children and adolescents with bipolar disorder and attention-deficit/hyperactivity disorder. J Am Acad Child Adolesc Psychiatry 46:1445–1453, 2007

Findling RL, Frazier JA, et al: The Collaborative Lithium Trials (CoLT): specific aims, methods, and implementation. Child Adolesc Psychiatry Ment Health 2:21, 2008

Findling RL, Nyilas M, Forbes RA, et al: Acute treatment of pediatric bipolar I disorder, manic or mixed episode, with aripiprazole: a randomized, double-blind, placebo-controlled study. J Clin Psychiatry 70:1441–1451, 2009

Findling RL, Landersdorfer CB, Kafantaris V, et al: First-dose pharmacokinetics of lithium carbonate in children and adolescents. J Clin Psychopharmacol 30:404–410, 2010

Findling RL, Kafantaris V, Pavuluri M, et al: Dosing strategies for lithium monotherapy in children and adolescents with bipolar I disorder. J Child Adolescent Psychopharmacol 21:195–205, 2011

Findling RL, Youngstrom EA, McNamara NK, et al: Double-blind, randomized, placebo-controlled long-term maintenance study of aripiprazole in children with bipolar disorder. J Clinical Psychiatry 73:57–63, 2012

Frazier JA, Meyer MC, Biederman J, et al: Risperidone treatment for juvenile bipolar disorder: a retrospective chart review. J Am Acad Child Adolesc Psychiatry 38:960–965, 1999

Frazier JA, Biederman J, Tohen M, et al: A prospective open-label treatment trial of olanzapine monotherapy in children and adolescents with bipolar disorder. J Child Adolesc Psychopharmacol 11:239–250, 2001

Geller B, Fetner HH: Children's 24-hour serum lithium level after a single dose of predicts initial dose and steady-state plasma levels. J Clin Psychopharmacol 9:155, 1989

Geller B, William M, Zimerman D, et al: Prepubertal and early adolescent bipolarity differentiate from ADHD by manic symptoms, grandiose delusions, ultra-rapid or ultradian cycling. J Affect Disord 51:81–91, 1998

Geller B, Tillman R, Craney JL, et al: Four-year prospective outcome and natural history of mania in children with a prepubertal and early adolescent bipolar phenotype. Arch Gen Psychiatry 61:459–467, 2004

Haas M, DelBello MP, Pandina G, et al: Risperidone for the treatment of acute mania in children and adolescents with bipolar disorder: a randomized, double-blind, placebo-controlled study. Bipolar Disord 11:687–700, 2009

Hagino OR, Weller EB, Weller RA, et al: Comparison of lithium dosage methods for preschool and early school-age children. J Am Acad Child Adolesc Psychiatry 37:60–65, 1998

Hazaray E, Ehret J, Posey DJ, et al: Intramuscular ziprasidone for acute agitation in adolescents. J Child Adolesc Psychopharmacol 14:464–470, 2004

Hummel B, Walden J, Stamper R, et al: Acute antimanic efficacy and safety of oxcarbazepine in an open-label trial with an on-off-on design. Bipolar Disord 4:412–417, 2002

Joffe H, Hall JE, Cohen LS, et al: A putative relationship between valproic acid and polycystic ovarian syndrome: implications for treatment of women with seizure and bipolar disorders. Harv Rev Psychiatry 11:99–108, 2003

Joffe RT, Brasch JS, MacQueen GM: Psychiatric aspects of endocrine disorders in women. Psychiatric Clin North Am 26:683–691, 2003

Joseph M, Youngstrom EA, Soares JC: Antidepressant-coincident mania in children and adolescents treated with selective serotonin reuptake inhibitors. Future Neurol 4:87–102, 2009

Joshi G, Wozniak J, Mick E, et al: A prospective open-label trial of extended-release carbamazepine monotherapy in children with bipolar disorder. J Child Adolesc Psychopharmacol 20:7–14, 2010

Kafantaris V, Coletti DJ, Dicker R, et al: Adjunctive antipsychotic treatment of adolescents with bipolar psychosis. J Am Acad Child Adolesc Psychiatry 40:1448–1456, 2001

Kafantaris V, Coletti DJ, Dicker R, et al: Lithium treatment of acute mania in adolescents: a large open trial. J Am Acad Child Adolesc Psychiatry 42:1038–1045, 2003

Keating AM, Aoun SL, Dean CE: Ziprasidone-associated mania: a review and report of 2 additional cases. Clin Neuropharmacol 28:83–86, 2005

Keck PE Jr, Marcus R, Tourkodimitris S, et al: A placebo-controlled, double-blind study of the efficacy and safety of aripiprazole in patients with acute bipolar mania. Am J Psychiatry 160:1651–1658, 2003

Kowatch RA, Suppes T, Carmody TJ, et al: Effect size of lithium, divalproex sodium, and carbamazepine in children and adolescents with bipolar disorder. J Am Acad Child Adolesc Psychiatry 39:713–720, 2000

Kowatch RA, Sethuraman G, Hume JH, et al: Combination pharmacotherapy in children and adolescents with bipolar disorder. Biol Psychiatry 53:978–984, 2003

Kowatch RA, Fristad M, Birmaher B, et al: Treatment guidelines for children and adolescents with bipolar disorder. J Child Adolesc Psychopharmacol 44:213–235, 2005

Kowatch RA, Findling RL, Scheffer RE, et al: Pediatric bipolar collaborative mood stabilizer trial. Poster presented at the annual meeting of the American Academy of Child and Adolescent Psychiatry. Boston, MA, October 23–28, 2007

Kudriakova TB, Sirtoa LA, Rozova GI, et al: Autoinduction and steady-state pharmacokinetics of carbamazepine and its major metabolites. Br J Clin Pharmacol 33:611–615, 1992

Marchand WR, Wirth L, Simon C: Quetiapine adjunctive monotherapy for pediatric bipolar disorder: a retrospective chart review. J Child Adolesc Psychopharmacol 14:405–411, 2004

Masi G, Mucci M, Millepiedi S: Clozapine in adolescent inpatients with acute mania. J Child Adolesc Psychopharmacol 12:93–99, 2002

McClellan J, Kowatch R, Findling RL: Practice parameter for the assessment and treatment of children and adolescents with bipolar disorder. J Am Acad Child Adolesc Psychiatry 46:107–125, 2007

National Institute of Mental Health: Abnormal Involuntary Movement Scale (AIMS). Psychopharmacol Bull 21:1077–1080, 1985

Nelson-DeGrave VL, Wickenheisser JK, Cockrell JE, et al: Valproate potentiates androgen biosynthesis in human ovarian theca cells. Endocrinology 145:799–808, 2004

Papatheodorou G, Kutcher SP, Katic M, et al: The efficacy and safety of divalproex sodium in the treatment of acute mania in adolescents and young adults: an open clinical trial. J Clin Psychopharmacol 15:110–116, 1995

Patel NC, DelBello MP, Bryan HS, et al: Open-label lithium for the treatment of adolescents with bipolar depression. J Am Acad Child Adolesc Psychiatry 45:289–297, 2006

Pavuluri MN, Henry DB, Carbray JA, et al: Open-label prospective trial of risperidone in combination with lithium or divalproex sodium in pediatric mania. J Affect Disord 82(suppl):S103–S111, 2004

Pavuluri MN, Henry DB, Carbray JA, et al: Divalproex sodium for pediatric mixed mania: a 6-month prospective trial. Bipolar Disord 7:266–273, 2005

Pavuluri MN, Henry DB, Moss M, et al: Effectiveness of lamotrigine in maintaining symptom control in pediatric bipolar disorder. J Child Adolesc Psychopharmacol 19:75–82, 2009

Qin K, Ehrmann DA, Cox N, et al: Identification of a functional polymorphism of the human type 5 17beta-hydroxysteroid dehydrogenase gene associated with polycystic ovarian syndrome. J Clin Endocrinol Metab 91:270–276, 2006

Scheffer RE, Kowatch RA, Carmody T, et al: Randomized, placebo-controlled trial of mixed amphetamine salts for symptoms of comorbid ADHD in pediatric bipolar disorder after mood stabilization with divalproex sodium. Am J Psychiatry 162:58–64, 2005

Soutullo CA, Sorter MT, Foster KD, et al: Olanzapine in the treatment of adolescent acute mania: a report of seven cases. J Affect Disord 53:279–283, 1999

Soutullo CA, Díez-Suárez A, Figueroa-Quintana A: Adjunctive lamotrigine treatment for adolescents with bipolar disorder: retrospective report of five cases. J Child Adolesc Psychopharmacol 16:357–364, 2006

Staller JA: Intramuscular ziprasidone in youth: a retrospective chart review. J Child Adolesc Psychopharmacol 14:590–592, 2004

Teitelbaum M: Oxcarbazepine in bipolar disorder. J Am Acad Child Adolesc Psychiatry 40:993–994, 2001

Tohen M, Kryzhanovskaya L, Carlson G, et al: Olanzapine versus placebo in the treatment of adolescents with bipolar mania. Am J Psychiatry 164:1547–1556, 2007

Tuzun U, Zoroglu SS, Savas HA: A 5-year-old boy with recurrent mania successfully treated with carbamazepine. Psychiatry Clin Neurosci 56:589–591, 2002

Wagner KD, Weller EB, Carlson GE, et al: An open-label trial of divalproex in children and adolescents with bipolar disorder. J Am Acad Child Adolesc Psychiatry 41:1224–1230, 2002

Wagner KD, Kowatch RA, Emslie GJ, et al: A double-blind, randomized, placebo-controlled trial of oxcarbazepine in the treatment of bipolar disorder in children and adolescents. Am J Psychiatry 163:1179–1186, 2006

Wagner KD, Nyilas M, Johnson B, et al: Long-term efficacy of aripiprazole in children (10–17 years old) with mania. Poster presented at the annual meeting of the American Academy of Child and Adolescent Psychiatry. Boston, MA, October 23–28, 2007

Wagner KD, Redden L, Kowatch RA, et al: A double-blind, randomized, placebo-controlled trial of divalproex extended-release in the treatment of bipolar disorder in children and adolescents. J Am Acad Child Adolesc Psychiatry 48:519–532, 2009

Weller EB, Weller RA, Fristad MA: Lithium dosage guide for prepubertal children: a preliminary report. J Am Acad Child Adolesc Psychiatry 25:92–95, 1986

Wood JR, Nelson-DeGrave VL, Jansen E, et al: Valproate-induced alterations in human theca gene expression: clues to the association between valproate use and metabolic side effects. Physiol Genomics 20:233–243, 2005

Woolston JL: Case study: carbamazepine treatment of juvenile-onset bipolar disorder. J Am Acad Child Adolesc Psychiatry 38:335–338, 1999

7

Autism and Other Pervasive Developmental Disorders

Kimberly A. Stigler, M.D.

Craig A. Erickson, M.D.

Christopher J. McDougle, M.D.

In 1943, Leo Kanner presented 11 case histories illustrating a syndrome in which the "pathognomonic, fundamental disorder is the children's inability to relate themselves in the ordinary way to people and situations from the beginning of life" (p. 242). He described several common characteristics, such

This work was supported in part by a Research Units on Pediatric Psychopharmacology Psychosocial Intervention grant (U10-MH66766) from the National Institute of Mental Health (NIMH) to Indiana University (Drs. McDougle, Stigler), a Daniel X. Freedman Psychiatric Research Fellowship Award (Dr. Stigler), and a Research Career Development Award (K23-MH082119) from the NIMH (Dr. Stigler).

as an autistic aloneness, impaired language development, stereotypies, literalness, and a need for sameness. In this compelling article, Kanner illustrated the clinical entity known today as *autistic disorder*. Thirty-seven years later, the publication of DSM-III (American Psychiatric Association 1980) heralded the inclusion of infantile autism among its formal diagnoses. Many of Kanner's initial findings were reflected in the criteria in DSM-III, as well as in subsequent revisions. The pervasive developmental disorders (PDDs), presently classified in DSM-IV-TR (American Psychiatric Association 2000), include autistic disorder (autism), Asperger disorder, Rett disorder, childhood disintegrative disorder, and pervasive developmental disorder not otherwise specified (PDD NOS). Similar to Kanner's observations, current criteria include severe impairments in social interaction and communication, as well as restricted interests and activities. In this chapter, we focus on the pharmacotherapy of the most commonly diagnosed PDDs: autism, Asperger disorder, and PDD NOS.

The therapeutic approach to the management of autism and related disorders is multimodal. Because approximately 75% of persons affected with autism are believed to have some degree of mental retardation, educational interventions are particularly important. In addition, many exhibit delays in language development, thus making speech therapy essential to improving outcome. Occupational therapy, social skills training, and physical therapy are also frequently necessary. Educating caregivers in behavioral management techniques can be very useful and may decrease the use of pharmacotherapy in this population.

In addition to nonpharmacological approaches, medication is often required to diminish severe maladaptive behaviors. The decision to prescribe medication to youth with PDDs can significantly impact their ability to benefit from behavioral and educational interventions. To date, risperidone and aripiprazole are the only drugs approved for autism by the U.S. Food and Drug Administration (FDA). Although no other medications have obtained FDA approval for use in treatment of PDDs, a variety of drugs are used to treat interfering target symptoms in this population. In this chapter, we present current evidence regarding the pharmacotherapy of PDDs (Table 7–1), review the adverse effects of the medications used, and outline practical management strategies.

Atypical Antipsychotics

Research into the pharmacotherapy of PDDs began in the 1960s with the typical antipsychotics. Because of significant adverse effects associated with the low-potency antipsychotics, the high-potency antipsychotic haloperidol was systematically investigated in numerous well-designed studies (Anderson et al. 1989; Campbell et al. 1978; Cohen et al. 1980). However, haloperidol's potent dopamine D_2 receptor antagonism frequently led to acute dystonic reactions, as well as drug-induced and withdrawal-related dyskinesias (Campbell et al. 1997). Currently, the typical antipsychotics as a whole are reserved for individuals with severe treatment-resistant symptoms.

Concerns regarding the typical antipsychotics directed researchers toward the development of the atypical antipsychotics. These drugs, with their profile of potent antagonism at serotonin (5-HT) and dopamine receptors, have a purported decreased risk of acute extrapyramidal side effects (EPS) and tardive dyskinesia (TD).

Clozapine

Clozapine is an antagonist at the serotonin 5-HT_{2A}, 5-HT_{2C}, and 5-HT_3 receptors and the dopamine D_1, D_2, D_3, and D_4 receptors (Baldessarini and Frankenburg 1991). Four case reports, as well as one small retrospective study, have been published on the use of this drug for irritability (defined as severe tantrums, aggression, and self-injury) in autism (Beherec et al. 2011; Chen et al. 2001; Gobbi and Pulvirenti 2001; Lambrey et al. 2010; Zuddas et al. 1996). Overall, the lack of research on clozapine in patients with PDDs is largely due to the drug's adverse-effect profile. The propensity of clozapine to lower the seizure threshold is troubling, particularly in a patient population predisposed to develop seizures. In addition, individuals with cognitive limitations and an impaired ability to communicate would have difficulty conveying information on symptoms associated with agranulocytosis and tolerating frequent venipuncture.

Risperidone

Risperidone has been approved by the FDA for the treatment of irritability in children and adolescents with autism, ages 5–16 years. Risperidone has negligible affinities for muscarinic receptors and high affinities for serotonin 5-HT_{1D},

Table 7–1. Selected published double-blind, placebo-controlled trials in pervasive developmental disorders

Drug	Study	Subjects		Design	Results
		N	Age		
Antipsychotics					
Aripiprazole	Marcus et al. 2009	218	6–17 years	8 weeks, parallel groups	Aripiprazole>placebo (29/52 [56%] responders)
Aripiprazole	Owen et al. 2009	98	6–17 years	8 weeks, parallel groups	Aripiprazole>placebo (24/46 [52%] responders)
Haloperidol	Anderson et al. 1989	45	2–7 years	12 weeks, crossover	Haloperidol>placebo
Risperidone	McDougle et al. 1998b	31	Adults	12 weeks, parallel groups	Risperidone>placebo (8/14 [57%] responders)
Risperidone	RUPP Autism Network 2002	101	5–17 years	8 weeks, parallel groups	Risperidone>placebo (34/49 [69%] responders)
Risperidone	Shea et al. 2004	79	5–12 years	8 weeks, parallel groups	Risperidone>placebo (35/40 [87%] responders)
Serotonin reuptake inhibitors					
Citalopram	King et al. 2009	149	5–17 years	12 weeks, parallel groups	Citalopram=placebo

Table 7–1. Selected published double-blind, placebo-controlled trials in pervasive developmental disorders (*continued*)

Drug	Study	Subjects		Design	Results
		N	Age		
Clomipramine	Gordon et al. 1993	24	6–23 years	10 weeks, crossover	Clomipramine>placebo Clomipramine>desipramine (19/28 [68%] responders)
Clomipramine	Remington et al. 2001	36	10–36 years	7 weeks, crossover	Clomipramine>placebo
Fluoxetine	Hollander et al. 2005	39	5–16 years	20 weeks, crossover	Fluoxetine>placebo
Fluoxetine	Autism Speaks 2009	158	5–17 years	14 weeks, parallel groups	Fluoxetine=placebo
Fluvoxamine	McDougle et al. 1996a	30	Adults	12 weeks, parallel groups	Fluvoxamine>placebo (8/15 [53%] responders)
Fluvoxamine	McDougle et al. 2000	34	5–18 years	12 weeks, parallel groups	Fluvoxetine=placebo
Fluvoxamine	Sugie et al. 2005	18	3–8 years	12 weeks, parallel groups	Fluvoxamine>placebo (10/18 [55%] responders)

Table 7–1. Selected published double-blind, placebo-controlled trials in pervasive developmental disorders (*continued*)

Drug	Study	Subjects		Design	Results
		N	Age		
Alpha₂-adrenergic agonists					
Clonidine	Jaselskis et al. 1992	8	5–13 years	14 weeks, crossover	Clonidine>placebo by teacher and parent, but not clinician, ratings (6/8 [75%] responders)
Clonidine (transdermal)	Fankhauser et al. 1992	9	5–33 years	10 weeks, crossover	Clonidine>placebo (6/9 [67%] responders)
Psychostimulants					
Methylphenidate	Quintana et al. 1995	10	7–11 years	4 weeks, crossover	Methylphenidate>placebo
Methylphenidate	Handen et al. 2000	13	5–11 years	3 weeks, crossover	Methylphenidate>placebo (8/13 [62%] responders)
Methylphenidate	RUPP Autism Network 2005a	72	5–14 years	4 weeks, crossover	Methylphenidate>placebo (35/72 [49%] responders)

Note. RUPP=Research Units on Pediatric Psychopharmacology.

5-HT$_{2A}$, and 5-HT$_{2C}$ receptors; dopamine D$_2$, D$_3$, and D$_4$ receptors; α_1-adrenergic receptors; and H$_1$-histaminic receptors (Leysen et al. 1988). Several open-label studies have demonstrated that risperidone effectively targets core and related symptoms of PDDs (Findling et al. 1997; Masi et al. 2001a; McDougle et al. 1997; Nicolson et al. 1998). The efficacy of risperidone was considered in a 12-week, double-blind, placebo-controlled study of adults with autism ($n=17$) or PDD NOS ($n=14$) (McDougle et al. 1998b). Eight (57%) of 14 subjects randomly assigned to risperidone (mean dosage = 2.9 mg/day), versus none in the placebo group, were deemed responders as measured by the Improvement subscale of the Clinical Global Impression Scale (CGI-I). The most common adverse effect was transient somnolence. Weight gain was reported in only two of the subjects in the risperidone group.

The first double-blind, placebo-controlled study of risperidone in youth was conducted by the Research Units on Pediatric Psychopharmacology (RUPP) Autism Network (2002). In this 8-week study, 101 children and adolescents (mean age = 8.8 years) with target symptoms of tantrums, aggression, or self-injurious behavior were treated with risperidone or placebo. Risperidone treatment at a mean dosage of 1.8 mg/day (range = 0.5–3.5 mg/day) was found to reduce the Aberrant Behavior Checklist (ABC) Irritability subscale score by 56.9%, compared with a 14.1% reduction with placebo. Overall, 69% of risperidone-treated subjects were judged responders, compared with only 12% of those given placebo. Adverse effects of risperidone included weight gain (mean 2.7 kg vs. 0.8 kg with placebo), increased appetite, sedation, dizziness, and sialorrhea. Further analyses revealed the drug to be significantly more effective for reducing interfering stereotypic and repetitive behaviors (McDougle et al. 2005).

The RUPP Autism Network subsequently published results of an open-label extension study to the aforementioned short-term study (Research Units on Pediatric Psychopharmacology Autism Network 2005b). This 16-week study involved 63 of the subjects who responded to risperidone in the 8-week trial. The mean risperidone dosage remained stable. Subjects in this study continued to gain weight (mean = 5.1 kg over 24 weeks). Overall, only 8% discontinued the drug because of loss of efficacy; one subject discontinued the drug because of adverse effects (constipation). At the end of this phase, 32 subjects who were considered responders were then randomly assigned to receive continued risperidone versus gradual substitution with placebo over a duration of

4 weeks. A statistically significant difference in relapse rate was reported, with 10 (62.5%) of 16 subjects gradually switched to placebo relapsing versus 2 (12.5%) of 16 who continued taking risperidone.

In a second double-blind, placebo-controlled study of risperidone in children and adolescents with PDDs, Shea et al. (2004) randomly assigned 79 youth, ages 5–12 years, to receive risperidone at a mean dosage of 1.2 mg/day or placebo over a duration of 8 weeks. Overall, 87% of risperidone-treated subjects improved compared with 40% of the subjects given placebo. In addition, there was a 64% reduction on the ABC Irritability subscale score for children given risperidone versus a 31% reduction for those given placebo. In regard to adverse effects, weight gain was more common in the risperidone group (2.7 kg) than in the placebo group (1.0 kg), as was increased sedation, heart rate, and systolic blood pressure.

Olanzapine

Olanzapine has high affinity for dopamine D_1, D_2, and D_4 receptors; serotonin 5-HT_{2A}, 5-HT_{2C}, and 5-HT_3 receptors; α_1-adrenergic receptors; H_1-histaminic receptors; and muscarinic receptors (Bymaster et al. 1996). Olanzapine has been found to be beneficial in PDDs in case reports, open-label trials, and a small double-blind, placebo-controlled trial (Hollander et al. 2004; Malone et al. 2001; Potenza et al. 1999). However, significant weight gain, along with its possible associated metabolic sequelae, has restricted its use in this population. A small 8-week, double-blind, placebo-controlled trial evaluated the use of olanzapine in 11 youths, ages 6–14 years, with PDD (Hollander et al. 2004). At a mean dosage of 10 mg/day (range = 7.5–12.5 mg/day), 3 (50%) of 6 subjects in the olanzapine group, versus 1 (20%) of 5 subjects in the placebo group, were considered responders based on the CGI-I scale. Olanzapine treatment was associated with sedation and increased appetite, as well as with considerable weight gain (olanzapine = 3.4±2.2 kg; placebo = 0.68±0.68 kg).

Quetiapine

Quetiapine has affinity for dopamine D_1 and D_2 receptors, serotonin 5-HT_{2A} and 5-HT_{1A} receptors, and H_1-histaminic receptors (Arnt and Skarsfeldt 1998). The drug has been investigated in an uncontrolled fashion, with mixed findings. A retrospective review of quetiapine was conducted of all patients in an outpatient PDD clinic (Corson et al. 2004). Twenty patients, ages 5–28 years (mean age = 12.1 years), were included in the study and received a quetiapine trial (mean dosage = 248.7 mg/day, range = 25–600 mg/day) over a mean duration of 59.8 weeks (range = 4–180 weeks). Of the 20 patients, 8 (40%) were considered responders to quetiapine. Adverse effects were reported in 50% of the patients, and 15% subsequently discontinued the drug.

A 16-week, open-label trial of quetiapine was conducted with six subjects (mean age = 10.9 years) (Martin et al. 1999). Two subjects who completed the trial were considered responders. Three withdrew because of sedation and lack of effectiveness, and one dropped out after a possible seizure. Overall, no statistically significant improvement was reported. Findling et al. (2004) conducted a 12-week, open-label study of quetiapine (mean dosage = 292 mg/day, range = 100–400 mg/day) in nine children, ages 12–17 years (mean age = 14.6±2.3 years), with autism. Two (22%) of the patients responded to the treatment, as assessed by the CGI-I. The most common adverse effects included sedation, weight gain, and increased agitation.

Ziprasidone

Ziprasidone is a potent antagonist at dopamine D_1 and D_2 receptors and serotonin 5-HT_{2A} and 5-HT_{2C} receptors (Tandon et al. 1997). In addition, it is a 5-HT_{1A} receptor agonist that also inhibits serotonin and norepinephrine reuptake. A case series of ziprasidone in 12 patients, ages 8–20 years (mean age = 11.6 ±4.4 years), with autism (n = 9) or PDD NOS (n = 3) has been published (McDougle et al. 2002). Six (50%) of the patients responded to the drug, as assessed by the CGI-I, at a mean dosage of 59.2 mg/day (range = 20–120 mg/day) over a duration of at least 6 weeks. Treatment with ziprasidone resulted in improvement in symptoms of aggression, agitation, and irritability. The most common adverse effect was transient sedation. Mean weight change was −5.8 pounds (range from −35.5 to +6.0 pounds). No cardiovascular adverse effects were reported. Malone et al. (2007) conducted a 6-week, open-label study of ziprasidone for irritability in 12 adolescents (mean age = 14.5 years, range = 12–18 years) with autism. Nine (75%) of the participants were judged treatment responders as determined by the CGI-I. The drug was associated with mild-to-moderate sedation, and dystonic reactions occurred in two subjects. The authors reported that ziprasidone treatment was weight neutral. Although the mean QTc increased by 14.7 msec during the study, the clinical significance of this finding was unclear.

Aripiprazole

Aripiprazole is approved by the FDA for the treatment of irritability in youth with autism, ages 6–17 years. The drug is a partial dopamine D_2 and serotonin 5-HT$_{1A}$ agonist, as well as a serotonin 5-HT$_{2A}$ antagonist (Burris et al. 2002). A 14-week, prospective, open-label study of aripiprazole for irritability was conducted in 25 children and adolescents with PDD NOS and Asperger disorder (mean age=8.6 years, range=5–17 years) (Stigler et al. 2009). Twenty-two (88%) of 25 subjects were considered responders to the drug at a mean dosage of 7.8 mg/day (range=2.5–15 mg/day), as assessed by the CGI-I and ABC Irritability subscale. Aripiprazole was well tolerated, with tiredness and weight gain among the more commonly recorded adverse effects.

Two larger-scale controlled studies of aripiprazole have subsequently been conducted in youth with autism and associated irritability (Marcus et al. 2009; Owen et al. 2009). The study by Marcus et al. (2009) was an 8-week, double-blind, placebo-controlled, fixed-dose study of aripiprazole in 218 youths ages 6–17 years. Subjects were randomized to placebo or aripiprazole (5, 10, or 15 mg/day). Improvement in irritability was demonstrated on the ABC Irritability subscale at all doses of the drug. Adverse effects included sedation, weight gain, and EPS, among others. The other study by Owen et al. (2009) was an 8-week, double-blind, placebo-controlled trial of flexibly dosed aripiprazole (2–15 mg/day) in 98 children and adolescents with autism, ages 6–17 years. The authors reported significant improvement in irritability, as demonstrated by the CGI-I and ABC Irritability subscale. Weight gain, drooling, tremor, vomiting, and sedation were among the adverse effects recorded.

The long-term safety and tolerability of aripiprazole (range=2–15 mg/day) for irritability in children and adolescents, ages 6–17 years, with autism was recently investigated in a 52-week, open-label, flexibly dosed study (Marcus et al. 2011b). In addition to de novo subjects, participants of the aforementioned studies by Marcus et al. (2009) and Owen et al. (2009) were eligible to enroll in this study. A total of 199 (60%) of 300 subjects completed

52 weeks of treatment. Common adverse effects included weight increase, vomiting, and increased appetite, among others. Evaluation of efficacy, a secondary objective after evaluation of safety and tolerability in this study, was conducted using the CGI-I and ABC Irritability subscale (Marcus et al. 2011a). Concomitant psychotropic medications were permitted during the study (except α_2-adrenergic agonists, carbamazepine, oxcarbazepine, and other antipsychotics). At endpoint, the majority of subjects had a CGI-I score of *much* or *very much improved*. The authors concluded that aripiprazole reduced symptoms of irritability associated with autism in pediatric subjects ages 6–17 years who were studied for up to 1 year.

Paliperidone

Paliperidone, 9-hydroxy-risperidone, has received FDA approval for schizophrenia in adolescents ages 12–17 years. Stigler et al. (2012) evaluated the effectiveness and tolerability of paliperidone for irritability in autism. In this 8-week, prospective, open-label study, 21 (84%) of 25 subjects with autism (mean age=15.3 years, range=12–21 years) were considered responders to paliperidone (mean dosage=7.1 mg/day, range=3–12 mg/day), based on the CGI-I and ABC Irritability subscale. Mean serum prolactin increased from 5.3 (baseline) to 41.4 ng/mL (endpoint); however, there were no observed or reported signs or symptoms associated with hyperprolactinemia. Weight gain, sedation, and EPS were among the adverse effects reported.

Serotonin Reuptake Inhibitors

Research into the pathophysiology of autism has often focused on the serotonergic system. Schain and Freedman (1961) first reported on elevated whole blood levels of serotonin in children with autism compared with control children. Additional reports have pointed to the possibility of abnormal maturational processes of the serotonergic system in subjects with autism, as exhibited by a lack of age-related serotonin decline in blood seen in normally developing subjects (Anderson et al. 1987; Leboyer et al. 1999).

Research investigating the genetic basis of a potential serotonergic abnormality in autism has yielded mixed results. Four studies have noted nominally significant excess transmission of alleles of the serotonin transporter gene, whereas three studies have reported no excess transmission (Conroy et al. 2004).

Other evidence suggesting the potential utility of drugs affecting serotonin in patients with PDDs comes from findings of an exacerbation of behavioral symptoms in drug-free autistic adults undergoing acute dietary depletion of the serotonin precursor tryptophan (McDougle et al. 1996b).

Clomipramine

Clomipramine is a tricyclic antidepressant that potently inhibits serotonin reuptake and also affects norepinephrine and dopamine reuptake (Greist et al. 1995). Clomipramine is FDA approved for obsessive-compulsive disorder (OCD) in youth ages 10–17 years.

One open-label and two controlled studies have evaluated clomipramine in patients with PDDs. In a 12-week open-label trial of clomipramine (mean dosage = 139.4±50.4 mg/day) in 35 adults with PDDs, 18 (55%) of the 33 patients who completed the trial were judged, on the basis of the CGI-I, to have responded to treatment (Brodkin et al. 1997). Improvement was recorded in aggression, self-injurious behavior, repetitive phenomena, and social relatedness. Thirteen (39%) of the patients experienced significant adverse effects, including seizures (three patients), weight gain, constipation, sedation, and agitation.

Clomipramine (mean dosage = 152±56 mg/day) was found superior to the relatively selective norepinephrine reuptake inhibitor desipramine (mean dosage = 127±52 mg/day) and placebo in a 10-week, randomized, crossover study of 24 children with autism (mean age = 9.6 years) (Gordon et al. 1993). Improvement with clomipramine was associated with decreased anger and obsessive-compulsive symptoms. Adverse effects included tachycardia, prolongation of the QTc interval, and grand mal seizure. Similar tolerability issues were noted by Remington et al. (2001) in their report on a 7-week, double-blind, placebo-controlled trial of clomipramine (mean dosage = 128 mg/day), haloperidol (mean dosage = 1.3 mg/day), and placebo in 36 patients with autism, ages 10–36 years. Among patients who completed this trial, clomipramine and haloperidol were similarly effective in reducing irritability and stereotypy. However, significantly fewer individuals receiving clomipramine versus haloperidol were able to complete the trial (37.5% vs. 69.7%).

Reasons for leaving the trial that were associated with clomipramine included lack of efficacy and the emergence of adverse effects, among which sedation and tremor were most prevalent. Because of tolerability issues, the use of clomipramine in patients with PDDs remains limited.

Fluvoxamine

Fluvoxamine is a selective serotonin reuptake inhibitor (SSRI) approved by the FDA for use in children and adolescents, ages 8–17 years, with OCD. Fluvoxamine (mean dosage = 276.7 mg/day) reduced repetitive and maladaptive behavior in 8 (53%) of 30 adults with autism enrolled in a double-blind, placebo-controlled study (McDougle et al. 1996a). In these adults, fluvoxamine was generally well tolerated, with adverse effects including sedation and nausea. A double-blind, placebo-controlled study did not find fluvoxamine (mean dose = 107 mg/day) effective in 34 children and adolescents with PDDs (McDougle et al. 2000). In these younger patients, fluvoxamine was poorly tolerated, with 14 patients experiencing adverse effects, including hyperactivity, insomnia, aggression, and agitation. In an open-label report of 18 children (mean age = 11.3±3.6 years) with PDDs who received low-dose fluvoxamine (1.5 mg/kg/day) for 10 weeks, fluvoxamine was similarly not associated with a significant treatment response (Martin et al. 2003). In a 12-week, double-blind, placebo-controlled, crossover study of fluvoxamine in 18 children with autism, Sugie et al. (2005) noted that 10 children (55%) had at least a mild treatment response, with 5 (28%) showing an *excellent* drug response. In this report, fluvoxamine was generally well tolerated. Three children (17%) had to exit the study due to behavioral activation. Overall, although the findings are mixed, fluvoxamine appears to be better tolerated in adults than in children with PDDs.

Fluoxetine

Fluoxetine is an SSRI approved in youth for the treatment of OCD (ages 7–17 years) and major depressive disorder (ages 8–17 years). Two open-label trials and two small placebo-controlled, crossover trials of fluoxetine suggested that the drug may be effective for repetitive symptoms in individuals with PDDs (Buchsbaum et al. 2001; DeLong et al. 2002; Fatemi et al. 1998; Hollander et al. 2005). The trial by Hollander et al. (2005) was a 20-week, placebo-controlled, crossover study of fluoxetine (mean dosage = 9.9 mg/day, range = 2.4–20 mg/day) in 39 children (mean age = 8.2 years) with PDDs. The investigators found the drug significantly better than placebo in reducing repetitive behaviors. No improvement on measures of speech or social interaction was noted, and adverse effects were not significantly different between fluoxetine and placebo. Although these initial trials were promising, a recent large-scale, 14-week, double-blind, placebo-controlled study of fluoxetine (2–18 mg/day) in 158 youths (5–17 years) with autism found the drug no more effective than placebo for repetitive behavior (Autism Speaks 2009).

Sertraline

Only open-label trials have described the use of the SSRI sertraline in treatment of PDDs. Sertraline is approved for the treatment of OCD in children ages 6–17 years. McDougle et al. (1998a) found sertraline (mean dosage= 122 mg/day) effective at reducing aggression and repetitive behavior in a 12-week, open-label study of 42 adults with PDDs. Subjects with autism and PDD NOS showed significantly more improvement than those with Asperger disorder. The authors attributed this response to the possibility that the patients with Asperger disorder were less symptomatic at baseline. Three patients (7%) dropped out of the study because of worsening agitation and anxiety. An open-label trial of sertraline (25–50 mg/day for 2–8 weeks) was conducted in nine children with autism, ages 6–12 years (Steingard et al. 1997). Eight children (88%) showed improvement during the trial, manifesting reduced irritability, anxiety, and need for sameness.

Paroxetine

The SSRI paroxetine has been the subject of a few uncontrolled reports on PDDs. Two case reports have noted decreased irritable behavior associated with paroxetine use in a 15-year-old boy with autism (Snead et al. 1994) and a 7-year-old boy with autism (Posey et al. 1999). In a heterogeneous sample, 15 adults with mental retardation with or without a concomitant PDD received 16 weeks of open-label treatment with paroxetine (20–50 mg/day) (Davanzo et al. 1998). The drug was associated with reduced aggression after 1 month but not at the 4-month follow-up.

Citalopram

Two retrospective studies have evaluated the SSRI citalopram in individuals with PDDs. In a retrospective case series, 17 youths with PDDs, ages 4–15 years, received citalopram (mean dosage = 19.7±7.8 mg/day) over a mean duration of 7.4 months. Ten patients (59%) were responders as determined by the CGI-I (Couturier and Nicolson 2002). No improvements in social interaction or communication were noted. Four patients (24%) discontinued the drug due to adverse effects, including agitation, tics, and insomnia.

A retrospective review of citalopram (mean dosage = 16.9±12.1 mg/day) in 15 children and adolescents, ages 6–16 years, with PDDs was completed over an average duration of 218.8 days (Namerow et al. 2003). Eleven patients (73%) were judged to be responders based on the CGI-I, with improvement in repetitive behaviors in 10 patients (66%) and in irritability in 7 patients (47%). Of the responders, 9 of 10 reportedly had not responded to other SSRIs. Two of 5 patients experiencing adverse effects discontinued treatment. Side effects included headaches, sedation, agitation, and lip dyskinesias.

A 12-week, double-blind, placebo-controlled study of citalopram (mean dosage = 16.5±6.5 mg/day) for repetitive behavior was conducted in 149 children and adolescents (mean age = 9.4 years, range = 5–17 years) with PDDs (King et al. 2009). In contrast to the positive preliminary findings of the retrospective studies, this large-scale controlled study found citalopram to be ineffective for repetitive behaviors. In addition, citalopram was more likely to be associated with adverse effects, including increased energy level, impulsiveness, hyperactivity, decreased concentration, stereotypy, and insomnia, among others.

Escitalopram

Escitalopram, the S-enantiomer of citalopram, is approved for major depressive disorder in adolescents, ages 12–17 years. A 10-week, open-label study of escitalopram (mean dosage = 11.1 mg/day) in 28 children and adolescents (mean age = 10.4 years) with PDDs found that 17 (61%) were treatment responders, with response defined as a 50% reduction on the parent-rated ABC Irritability subscale (Owley et al. 2005). A wide variety of dose response was noted, with some patients unable to tolerate the drug at 10 mg/day, and others showing positive response at the lowest dosage, 2.5 mg/day.

Mirtazapine

Mirtazapine, a drug with both serotonergic and noradrenergic properties, was evaluated in an open-label trial in patients with PDDs (Posey et al. 2001). Twenty-six individuals with PDDs were treated with mirtazapine (7.5–45 mg/day) over a mean duration of 150 days. Nine patients (35%) were considered treatment responders, as measured by the CGI-I, with reduced aggression, self-injury, irritability, hyperactivity, anxiety, insomnia, and depression. No effect on social relatedness or communication impairment was noted. Adverse effects were considered mild and included increased appetite, irritability, and sedation. A retrospective study investigated the effectiveness of mirtazapine (mean dosage = 21.6 mg/day, range = 15–30 mg/day) for inappropriate sexual behavior (e.g., excessive masturbation) in 10 youths, ages 5–16 years, with autism (Coskun et al. 2009). Eight of 10 patients were deemed *much* or *very much improved* on the CGI-I in regard to symptoms of excessive masturbation. Increased appetite, weight gain, and sedation were among the most frequently reported adverse effects.

Venlafaxine

The antidepressant venlafaxine is a dual serotonin and norepinephrine reuptake inhibitor. Low-dose venlafaxine (18.75 mg/day) was associated with decreased hyperactivity and irritability in two adolescents and one young adult with autism over 6 months of treatment (Carminati et al. 2006). A retrospective review of 10 children, adolescents, and young adults with PDDs treated with venlafaxine (6.25–50 mg/day) found that 6 patients (60%) were responders, as defined by the CGI-I (Hollander et al. 2000). The medication was reportedly well tolerated, and improvement was noted in repetitive behaviors, socialization, communication, and inattention. One case report noted increased aggressive behavior when venlafaxine (37.5 mg increased to 75 mg/day) was added to the treatment regimen of an adolescent female with autism who was taking a stable dose of olanzapine (10 mg/day) (Marshall et al. 2003).

Buspirone

Buspirone is a serotonin 5-HT_{1A} receptor partial agonist. Several case reports and small open-label studies have reported on the effectiveness of buspirone in patients with autism. Larger open-label studies have generated conflicting results. An open-label study of buspirone (30–60 mg/day for 28–413 days) found the drug to be ineffective in treating target symptoms, including aggression and self-injury, in 26 adults with mental retardation, which included nine patients with PDDs (King and Davanzo 1996). In another open-label study, 22 children and adolescents with PDDs were treated with buspirone (15–45 mg/day) for 6–8 weeks (Buitelaar et al. 1998). Nine patients (41%) showed significant improvement as measured by the CGI-I, addressing target symptoms of anxiety and irritability. During a continuation phase for treatment responders, one child developed an orofacial-lingual dyskinesia after 10 months of treatment; the dyskinesia remitted after drug discontinuation. No controlled studies of buspirone in patients with PDDs have been reported.

Alpha$_2$-Adrenergic Agonists

Clonidine

Clonidine is an α_2-adrenergic agonist, an extended-release formulation (clonidine ER) of which has FDA approval for attention-deficit/hyperactivity disorder (ADHD) in youth ages 6–17 years. Clonidine has been evaluated in two small controlled trials involving patients with autism. A double-blind, placebo-controlled, crossover trial (6-week treatment periods) of clonidine (4–10 μg/kg/day) was conducted in eight boys with autism (mean age = 8.1 years) who demonstrated symptoms of inattention, impulsivity, and hyperactivity (Jaselskis et al. 1992). The drug was associated with decreased hyperactivity and irritability on teacher and parent ratings, but no treatment-associated differences were found on clinician ratings. Adverse effects of clonidine included hypotension, sedation, and irritability. Transdermal clonidine (5 μg/kg/day) was evaluated in a double-blind, placebo-controlled, crossover study (4-week treatment phases) involving nine males, ages 5–33 years, with autism (Fankhauser et al. 1992). Significant improvement in hyperactivity and anxiety was recorded. The most commonly reported adverse effects were sedation and fatigue.

Guanfacine

Guanfacine is an α_2-adrenergic agonist, an extended-release formulation (guanfacine XR) of which has FDA approval for ADHD in youth ages 6–17 years. Preliminary research suggested that guanfacine may be well tolerated and beneficial for symptoms of hyperactivity in children and adolescents with PDDs (Posey et al. 2004b). A prospective, open-label trial of guanfacine was conducted in 25 youths (mean age=9 years, range=5–14 years) with PDDs and hyperactivity who had previously not responded to methylphenidate (Scahill et al. 2006). In this study, 48% of the subjects demonstrated improvement in hyperactivity at total daily doses of 1–3 mg. Decreased frustration tolerance and tearfulness led to study discontinuation in three participants. A small double-blind, placebo-controlled trial of guanfacine was completed in 11 children with hyperactivity and intellectual disability and/or a PDD (Handen et al. 2008). Forty-five percent of study participants had a significant reduction of hyperactivity. The most common adverse effects included increased irritability and drowsiness. To date, one case report of guanfacine XR in patients with PDDs has been published (Blankenship et al. 2011). The authors found improvement in inattention, hyperactivity, and impulsivity in two patients (4 and 9 years of age) at total daily dosages of 2–3 mg. Adverse effects included sedation and reduced blood pressure.

Psychostimulants

Psychostimulants are considered first-line agents for the treatment of hyperactivity and inattention in patients diagnosed with ADHD (Greenhill et al. 2002b). Whereas some preliminary research concluded that stimulants were generally ineffective and associated with adverse effects in patients with PDDs (Aman 1982; Campbell 1975; Stigler et al. 2004a), other trials have suggested that stimulants may be effective in this population. Methylphenidate has FDA approval for treating ADHD in children and adolescents ages 6–17 years. A double-blind, crossover study (2-week treatment phases) of methylphenidate (10 or 20 mg bid) was conducted in 10 children with autism, ages 7–11 years (Quintana et al. 1995). Overall, a modest benefit of methylphenidate treatment over placebo was found. Adverse effects included insomnia, irritability, and decreased appetite. Another double-blind, placebo-controlled, crossover study of methylphenidate (0.3 and 0.6 mg/kg/day) found a 50% reduction on the Conners Hyperactivity Index in 8 (62%) of 13 children with autism, ages 5–11 years (Handen et al. 2000). Adverse effects, more common at the 0.6-mg/kg/day dosage, included social withdrawal and irritability.

The RUPP Autism Network completed the largest controlled trial of a psychostimulant in patients with PDDs to date (Research Units on Pediatric Psychopharmacology Autism Network 2005a). This study involved 72 youths, ages 5–14 years, with target symptoms of moderate-to-severe hyperactivity. Subjects entered a 1-week test-dose phase in which placebo and three doses (low, medium, high) of methylphenidate were administered. The 66 subjects who tolerated the test-dose phase received 1 week each of placebo and of methylphenidate at three different dosages in random order during a 4-week, double-blind, crossover phase. Those who responded to methylphenidate then entered an 8-week open-label phase. Overall, 35 (49%) of 72 enrolled subjects responded to methylphenidate. Discontinuation of study medication due to adverse effects occurred in 13 (18%) of 72 subjects. These results are consistent with the findings of a smaller study of methylphenidate in 13 youths with PDDs (Di Martino et al. 2004). In the latter study, within 1 hour of a single test dose (0.4 mg/kg), 5 individuals developed increased hyperactivity, stereotypy, dysphoria, or tics, and were unable to tolerate the drug. Six of the remaining 8 subjects responded to the drug, resulting in an overall response rate of 46%.

In contrast to these findings, data from the National Institute of Mental Health (NIMH) Multimodal Treatment of ADHD (MTA) study showed that 69% of subjects responded to methylphenidate treatment, with only 1.4% discontinuing due to adverse effects (Greenhill et al. 2002a). Methylphenidate is less effective and associated with more frequent adverse effects in youth with PDDs and ADHD than in typically developing children with ADHD.

Atomoxetine

The selective norepinephrine reuptake inhibitor atomoxetine is approved for the treatment of children and adolescents, ages 6–17 years, with ADHD. Results of two open-label studies suggest that the drug may decrease symptoms of motor hyperactivity and inattention in higher-functioning children and adolescents with PDDs (Posey et al. 2005; Troost et al. 2006). In the study by Posey et al. (2005), 16 children and adolescents, ages 6–14 years, with PDDs received atomoxetine at a mean dosage of 1.2 mg/kg/day. Twelve (75%) of 16 subjects were deemed responders. The drug was well tolerated, aside from two subjects who discontinued atomoxetine due to irritability. A 10-week, open-label study of atomoxetine (mean dosage 1.2 mg/kg/day) was completed in 12 youths with PDDs (Troost et al. 2006). Although drug treatment led to a 44% reduction in ADHD symptoms, 5 subjects (42%) discontinued the study due to adverse effects such as irritability, nausea, and anxiety. A placebo-controlled, crossover pilot study of atomoxetine was conducted in 16 youths with PDDs and hyperactivity, ages 5–15 years. Nine (56%) of 16 subjects responded to atomoxetine, demonstrating a significant reduction in symptoms of hyperactivity. One subject was rehospitalized for recurrent irritability on the drug. Upper gastrointestinal symptoms and fatigue were frequently reported adverse effects.

Beta-Adrenergic Antagonists

β-Adrenergic blockers are drugs that block norepinephrine receptors, thus limiting norepinephrine neurotransmission. Eight hospitalized adults with autism were described as having improvement in speech and socialization after open-label treatment with propranolol or nadolol (mean dosage = 225 mg/day over 14.2 months) (Ratey et al. 1987). All patients showed a marked decrease in aggression. Six patients (75%) showed improved social skills, and 4 (50%) developed improved speech during treatment. Seven of the patients were taking concomitant antipsychotics during this trial, with five able to decrease and one able to discontinue treatment during the trial. The authors felt that the improvement noted was due to decreased hyperarousal.

Mood Stabilizers

Valproic Acid

The mood stabilizer and antiepileptic drug valproic acid (divalproex sodium) has been investigated in open-label and double-blind, placebo-controlled studies in individuals with autism (Hellings et al. 2005; Hollander et al. 2001, 2006, 2010).

An 8-week, double-blind, placebo-controlled study of valproic acid (mean blood level = 77.8 µg/mL at 8 weeks) was conducted in 30 subjects, ages 6–20 years, with PDDs and significant aggressive behavior (Hellings et al. 2005). In this trial, treatment was not associated with significant improvement in irritability as measured by the ABC or by global symptoms as measured by the CGI-I. One subject developed a rash, which remitted after drug discontinuation, and two subjects developed elevated serum ammonia while taking valproic acid. In an 8-week, double-blind, placebo-controlled trial of valproic acid in 13 patients with autism and interfering repetitive behavior, treatment was associated with a significant reduction in repetitive phenomena as measured by the Children's Yale-Brown Obsessive Compulsive Scale (Hollander et al. 2006). Overall, the drug was well tolerated. A 12-week, double-blind, placebo-controlled study of valproic acid was completed in 27 youth, ages 5–15 years, with PDDs and irritability (Hollander et al. 2010). The authors reported that 62.5% of subjects in the valproic acid group, versus 9% in the placebo group, responded to treatment (mean blood level = 89.8 µg/mL [responders]; 64.3 µg/mL [nonresponders]). Irritability, insomnia, headache, and weight gain were among the adverse effects reported.

Lithium

Lithium has FDA approval for bipolar disorder in youth ages 12–17 years. Three case reports have described the use of the mood stabilizer lithium in patients with PDDs. Two reports have noted reduced manic-like symptoms in individuals with autism and a family history of bipolar disorder (Kerbeshian et al. 1987; Steingard and Biederman 1987). A single report of lithium augmentation of fluvoxamine treatment in an adult with autism noted improvement in symptoms of aggression and irritability after 2 weeks of treatment, as measured by the CGI-I (Epperson et al. 1994).

Lamotrigine

Lamotrigine is an anticonvulsant and mood stabilizer that attenuates some forms of glutamate release via inhibition of sodium, calcium, and potassium channels. The use of lamotrigine (mean dosage = 4.5 mg/kg/day) over a mean duration of 14 months was described in 13 children, ages 3–13 years, with autism and intractable epilepsy (Uvebrant and Bauziene 1994). Eight subjects (62%) showed a decrease in autistic symptoms. Adverse effects included sleep disturbance and rash. In a 4-week, double-blind, placebo-controlled trial of lamotrigine (5 mg/kg/day) in 14 children with autism, ages 3–11 years, Belsito et al. (2001) reported no treatment-associated effect as measured by the ABC, Childhood Autism Rating Scale, and Pre-Linguistic Autism Diagnostic Observation Scale. Insomnia and hyperactivity were the most common side effects reported.

Levetiracetam

Levetiracetam is an anticonvulsant with inhibitory and neuroprotective properties. A 10-week, double-blind, placebo-controlled trial of levetiracetam (mean dosage = 862.5 mg/day, range = 500–1,250 mg/day) was conducted in 20 subjects with autism, ages 5–17 years (Wasserman et al. 2006). No significant difference was found between levetiracetam and placebo on global measures of autism or on measures of irritability, affective instability, and repetitive behavior. Overall, the drug was well tolerated, with mild agitation, aggression, and hyperactivity among the adverse effects reported.

Cholinesterase Inhibitors

Donepezil

The cholinesterase inhibitor donepezil has been evaluated in two open-label reports in patients with PDDs. Improved speech was noted in 25 boys (mean age = 6.6 years) taking donepezil (2.5 or 5 mg/day) over 12 weeks of open-label treatment (Chez et al. 2000). No improvements in social relatedness were noted. Adverse effects included aggression, irritability, sedation, and sleep disturbance. In a retrospective review of open-label donepezil add-on treatment (mean dosage = 9.4 ±1.8 mg/day), Hardan and Handen (2002) reported that four (50%) of eight individuals with autism, ages 7–19 years, who were taking other psychotropic medications responded positively to treatment as measured by the CGI-I. In addition, scores decreased on the Hyperactivity and Irritability subscales of the ABC. In this review, donepezil was generally well tolerated, with one patient developing nausea and vomiting and one patient reporting mild irritability. Handen et al. (2011) investigated the efficacy and tolerability of donepezil on executive functioning in 34 patients with PDDs, ages 8–17 years. The study involved a 10-week, double-blind, placebo-controlled trial of donepezil (5 and 10 mg/day), followed by a 10-week, open-label trial for placebo nonresponders. No significant differences were found between donepezil and placebo on measures of executive functioning. Mild adverse effects associated with the drug included diarrhea, headache, and fatigue.

Rivastigmine

The cholinesterase inhibitor rivastigmine was evaluated in one 12-week, open-label trial in 32 patients with autism (Chez et al. 2004). Treatment-associated improvement was noted in expressive speech and overall autistic behavior using standardized measures.

Galantamine

Galantamine is a cholinesterase inhibitor and nicotinic receptor modulator. A 12-week, open-label trial of galantamine (mean dosage = 18.4 mg/day, range = 12–24 mg/day) was conducted in 13 youths with autism, ages 4–17 years (Nicolson et al. 2006). The drug was well tolerated and considered beneficial for reducing symptoms of aggression, behavioral dyscontrol, and inattention.

Glutamatergic Agents

Amantadine

Amantadine, a compound used to treat influenza, herpes zoster, and Parkinson disease, has known noncompetitive N-methyl-D-aspartate (NMDA) antagonist activity (Kornhuber et al. 1994). In a 4-week, double-blind, placebo-controlled trial in 39 youths with autism, ages 5–19 years, amantadine (final dosage = 5 mg/kg/day) was associated with improved clinician ratings in the domains of hyperactivity and inappropriate speech on the Aberrant Behavior Checklist—Community version (King et al. 2001). No significant treatment-associated improvements were noted on parent ratings. The drug was reportedly well tolerated.

Memantine

Memantine is an uncompetitive NMDA antagonist used in the treatment of Alzheimer disease. The use of memantine (mean dosage = 12.7 mg/day, range = 2.5–30 mg/day) was described in 151 children and adolescents, ages 2–26 years (mean age = 9.3 years), with PDDs over 21 months of treatment (Chez et al. 2007). Although standardized assessments were not used, improvement was shown in language function, social behavior, and (to a lesser degree) stereotypies. Adverse effects included worsened behavior, which occurred in 22 (15%) of the patients. A retrospective study of memantine (mean dosage = 10.1 mg/day, range = 2.5–20 mg/day) found improvement in social withdrawal and inattention in 11 (61%) of 18 patients with PDDs (mean age = 11.4 years, range = 6–15 years) (Erickson et al. 2007). Four subjects discontinued the study, with increased irritability, increased seizure frequency, and excessive sedation among the adverse effects reported. Owley et al. (2006) conducted an 8-week, open-label study of memantine (mean dosage = 0.4 mg/kg/day) in 14 subjects with PDDs, ages 3–12 years (mean age = 7.8 years). Although only 4 (28%) of 14 subjects demonstrated "minimal" improvement on the CGI-I, improvement was noted in memory, social withdrawal, hyperactivity, and irritability. Adverse effects included hyperactivity, which led to drug discontinuation in two subjects.

D-Cycloserine

D-Cycloserine is an antibiotic traditionally used to treat tuberculosis. Additionally, the drug is an NMDA partial agonist that has been shown to reduce the negative symptoms associated with schizophrenia (Goff et al. 1999). In the only published trial to date of D-cycloserine in PDDs, 10 drug-free patients with autism (mean age = 10±7.7 years) participated in an 8-week trial that began with a 2-week placebo lead-in phase, followed by 2 weeks at each of three dosages: 0.7, 1.4, 2.8 mg/kg/day (Posey et al. 2004a). D-Cycloserine was associated with improvement on the CGI-I and the Social Withdrawal subscale of the ABC. Four patients (40%) were considered responders based on CGI-I ratings of *much improved*. Two patients (20%) had to drop out of the study due to development of a transient motor tic and increased echolalia, respectively.

Naltrexone

The opiate receptor antagonist naltrexone has been evaluated in four controlled studies in patients with autism. This research was stimulated by findings of elevated endorphin levels in the blood (Weizman et al. 1984) and cerebrospinal fluid (Gillberg et al. 1985; Ross et al. 1987) of individuals with autism. Although initial reports were promising, subsequent larger, double-blind, placebo-controlled studies have not demonstrated significant efficacy regarding core or associated symptoms of autism (Campbell et al. 1993; Feldman et al. 1999; Leboyer et al. 1992; Willemsen-Swinkels et al. 1995). Overall, the majority of the evidence points toward naltrexone as ineffective in improving autistic symptoms or self-injurious behavior, and as modestly effective in the treatment of hyperactivity.

Secretin

The gastrointestinal peptide secretin stimulates secretion of water and bicarbonate from the pancreas and supports the activity of cholecystokinin, which, in turn, further activates pancreatic secretion. Extensive study of this compound in autism occurred after an initial report of open-label treatment in three patients who experienced improvement in maladaptive behavior and core autistic symptoms (Horvath et al. 1998). After initial reports of secretin's success were described in the mainstream media, its use spread to the point that more than 500,000 doses had been administered to patients with autism by the year 1999 (Kaminska et al. 2002). Fifteen double-blind, placebo-controlled trials have evaluated the use of secretin in patients with autism, and none of the reports concluded that the drug was effective (Sturmey 2005). These reports included single-dose and multiple-dose trials of human or porcine secretin. Although secretin represents one of the most studied compounds in patients with PDDs, no evidence exists to support its use in this diagnostic group.

Safety Issues

In this portion of the chapter, we focus on adverse effects reported for selected classes of medications that are used in PDDs. The section is not meant to be an extensive review of all adverse effects for all drugs previously discussed, but rather to highlight major adverse effects of several commonly used classes of drugs that should be brought to the reader's attention. When selecting a medication, the clinician must educate the patient and caregivers regarding its potential adverse effects.

Atypical Antipsychotics

The use of atypical antipsychotics is associated with a risk of several adverse events that warrant monitoring. Although the atypical antipsychotics purportedly have a decreased risk of EPS and TD in comparison with the typical agents, these events have been reported in individuals with PDDs taking these drugs (Correll et al. 2011; Malone et al. 2002; Zuddas et al. 2000). Hyperprolactinemia is another potential adverse effect that may occur during treatment with an atypical antipsychotic. Studies measuring prolactin levels found treatment with risperidone and paliperidone to be associated with significant elevation in prolactin levels in patients with PDDs, despite the fact that no participants showed clinical signs of hyperprolactinemia (Gagliano et al. 2004; Masi et al. 2001b, 2003; Stigler et al. 2012). Chronic hyperprolactinemia can lead to disordered growth, sexual dysfunction, and osteoporosis (Saito et al. 2004).

In children and adolescents, olanzapine is associated with a considerable risk of weight gain, whereas quetiapine, risperidone, aripiprazole, and paliperidone are associated with a moderate risk (De Hert et al. 2011; Stigler et al. 2012). In contrast, published data in youth suggest that ziprasidone may be associated with a decreased risk of weight gain. The association between weight gain and atypical antipsychotic use in patients with PDDs is of significant concern. Evidence has implicated this class of drugs in the onset or exacerbation of diabetes and hyperlipidemia (De Hert et al. 2011; Stigler et al. 2004b). Regular monitoring of patient weight, as well as fasting glucose and lipids, is highly recommended. In addition, selection of a particular antipsychotic may warrant monitoring of liver functions, blood count, and electrocardiogram (ECG).

Selective Serotonin Reuptake Inhibitors

In 2004, the FDA required SSRI manufacturers to include a black box warning describing the potential for increased suicidality in children and adolescents taking these drugs, especially during the first few months of treatment. With this risk in mind, regular assessment for suicidality must be part of the treatment plan for patients with PDDs taking any of these drugs. In addition, prepubertal patients with PDDs taking SSRIs may be at increased risk of behavioral activation and irritability during SSRI treatment (McDougle et al. 2000). Therefore, clinicians should start by prescribing low dosages of SSRIs for patients and slowly titrate toward an effective dosage.

Psychostimulants

As described earlier, psychostimulants may be less well tolerated in youth with PDDs than in typically developing children with ADHD (Research Units on Pediatric Psychopharmacology Autism Network 2005a). Adverse effects that warrant close monitoring include increased irritability, agitation, hyperactivity, decreased appetite, weight loss, insomnia, exacerbation/development of tics, and psychosis (rarely). In addition, this drug class may rarely be associated with cardiovascular adverse events, with persons who have preexisting heart conditions at higher risk. A baseline medical history and physical examination are recommended to identify at-risk individuals with structural cardiac abnormalities or other cardiovascular symptoms (Correll et al. 2011).

Alpha$_2$-Adrenergic Agonists

α_2-Adrenergic agonists are typically well tolerated, aside from possible adverse effects of sedation and hypotension. Depressive symptoms may worsen or be induced as well. A baseline ECG prior to beginning this class of drugs is recommended whenever possible, particularly in persons with a significant history of cardiovascular problems.

Atomoxetine

In 2005, the FDA required manufacturers of atomoxetine to include a black box warning regarding potential increased suicidal ideation in children and adolescents treated with this drug. Because of this risk, regular assessment for suicidality in patients taking atomoxetine is warranted. In addition, rare cases of hepatic dysfunction associated with atomoxetine warrant ongoing assessment for signs and symptoms of liver failure in patients with PDDs taking this drug (Formanek 2005).

Mood Stabilizers

Among the anticonvulsants, valproic acid is frequently used to treat persons with PDDs. Drug levels should be monitored on a regular basis to ensure that levels remain in the therapeutic range. Patients should be regularly assessed for symptoms of valproic acid toxicity, including nausea, vomiting, ataxia, tremor, dizziness, headache, confusion, and somnolence. Hepatotoxicity is a possible serious adverse effect associated with the drug, warranting periodic liver function tests (Dreifuss et al. 1987). Pancreatitis is another rare but potentially life-threatening complication. In addition, because of the risk of thrombocytopenia, a blood count including platelets should be obtained in all patients receiving this drug.

Risks from taking another mood stabilizer, lithium, include impaired renal and thyroid function, thus warranting regular monitoring (Scahill et al. 2001). In addition, baseline ECGs are recommended. Lithium levels must be monitored on a regular basis during treatment. Toxic levels of lithium are often close to the therapeutic range (0.6–1.2 µg/mL), thus making it essential to monitor for signs and symptoms of lithium toxicity during treatment. Signs of toxicity include lethargy, nausea, vomiting, diarrhea, tremor, weakness, and seizures.

Practical Management Strategies

A multimodal approach to the management of autism and related disorders is essential. This approach often incorporates speech therapy, occupational therapy, physical therapy, educational interventions, and social skills training. Ongoing collaboration with the youth's educational team at school can ease transitions, decrease adverse behaviors, and optimize learning in the classroom setting. In addition, behavior therapy may be of particular importance in that it may decrease the need for pharmacotherapy in patients with PPDs. Even with the use of such interventions, however, medication is often required to decrease the maladaptive behaviors commonly observed in youth with PDDs.

The pharmacotherapy of PDDs is based on a target symptom approach (Figure 7–1). As described in this chapter, a variety of medications may impact specific target symptom domains in this population. The algorithm provides an overview of drug treatment strategies for three symptom domains commonly encountered in PDDs: irritability (tantrums, aggression, self-injury), motor hyperactivity and inattention, and interfering repetitive phenomena.

Children presenting with mild symptoms of irritability may derive benefit from an initial trial of an α_2-adrenergic agonist. The emergence of more severe symptoms often requires treatment with an atypical antipsychotic. From a clinical standpoint, mood stabilizers may also be efficacious, primarily in postpubertal individuals.

Symptoms of hyperactivity and inattention are also frequently observed in children with PDDs. Emerging evidence suggests that α_2-adrenergic agonists, as well as atomoxetine and stimulants, may be effective in this population. However, it is important to weigh the risks and benefits involved with the use of these drugs. Given that the α_2-adrenergic agonist guanfacine is generally well tolerated, a trial of this drug is generally recommended prior to trials of either stimulants or atomoxetine.

Research has demonstrated that the majority of children with interfering repetitive phenomena do not benefit from treatment with SSRIs. Because of potential activation that may be associated with this drug class in prepubertal individuals, use of low dosages and a slow titration schedule are recommended. In general, the atypical antipsychotics should be considered for treatment-resistant symptoms of hyperactivity and inattention, as well as for interfering repetitive behaviors.

Conclusions

Research into pharmacotherapy for PDDs will continue to explore the efficacy and tolerability of currently available drugs, as well as the use of novel agents, to address specific interfering target symptoms. Larger-scale controlled studies are needed to further inform the effectiveness of glutamatergic agents for core social impairment. In addition, the pharmacological management of comorbid mood and anxiety symptoms remains understudied in this diagnostic group. Although youth with PDDs often present with interfering symptoms in several domains, research to date has focused on the use of one drug to treat a specific group of symptoms. Studies of coactive pharmacological treatment strategies targeting more than one symptom domain are needed to better understand the effectiveness, tolerability, and safety of using more than one agent concurrently in the treatment of PDDs.

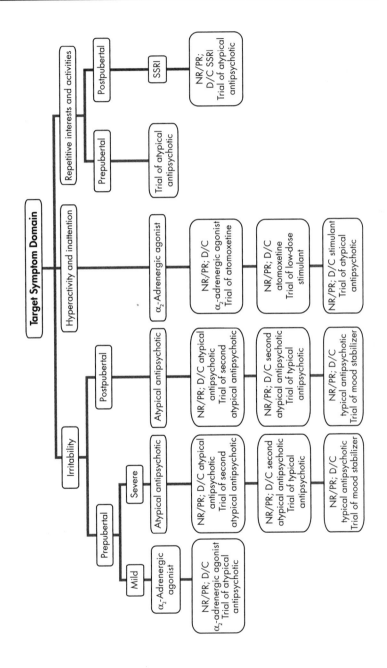

Figure 7–1. A target symptom approach to the pharmacotherapy of pervasive developmental disorders *(opposite page).*

This algorithm provides an overview of drug treatment strategies for three symptom domains commonly encountered in PDDs: aggression and self-injury, motor hyperactivity and inattention, and interfering repetitive phenomena. It is recommended that behavior therapy also be considered at each treatment juncture.

D/C = discontinue; NR/PR = nonresponse/partial response; SSRI = selective serotonin reuptake inhibitor.

Clinical Pearls

- Use a multimodal therapeutic approach to the management of PDDs.
- Prescribe medication to reduce maladaptive behaviors, allowing youth with PDDs to maximize benefit from therapy and educational services.
- Base pharmacotherapy of PDDs on a target symptom approach. Three major target symptom domains in PDDs are irritability (tantrums, aggression, self-injury), hyperactivity/inattention, and repetitive interests/activities.
- Try prescribing an α_2-adrenergic agonist for youth with mild aggression or self-injury, or an atypical antipsychotic for individuals with more severe symptoms.
- Consider risperidone and aripiprazole for the treatment of irritability in youth with autism.
- Keep in mind that prepubertal patients with PDDs may be at increased risk of behavioral activation and irritability during SSRI treatment for interfering repetitive phenomena.
- Remember that stimulants appear less well tolerated by youth with PDDs than by typically developing children with ADHD.
- Consider a trial of guanfacine prior to atomoxetine or a stimulant for symptoms of hyperactivity and inattention in PDDs.

References

Aman MG: Stimulant drug effects in developmental disorders and hyperactivity: toward a resolution of disparate findings. J Autism Dev Disord 12:385–398, 1982

American Psychiatric Association: Diagnostic and Statistical Manual of Mental Disorders, 3rd Edition. Washington, DC, American Psychiatric Association, 1980

American Psychiatric Association: Diagnostic and Statistical Manual of Mental Disorders, 4th Edition, Text Revision. Washington, DC, American Psychiatric Association, 2000

Anderson GM, Freedman DX, Cohen DJ, et al: Whole blood serotonin in autistic and normal subjects. J Child Psychol Psychiatry 28:885–900, 1987

Anderson LT, Campbell M, Adams P, et al: The effects of haloperidol on discrimination learning and behavioral symptoms in autistic children. J Autism Dev Disord 19:227–239, 1989

Arnt J, Skarsfeldt M: Do novel antipsychotics have similar pharmacological characteristics? A review of the evidence. Neuropsychopharmacology 18:63–101, 1998

Autism Speaks: Autism Speaks announces results reported for the Study of Fluoxetine in Autism (SOFIA): first industry-sponsored trial for the Autism Clinical Trials Network (ACTN). February 2009. Available at: www.autismspeaks.org/press/as_announces_sofia_results.php. Accessed May 15, 2012.

Baldessarini RJ, Frankenburg FR: Clozapine: a novel antipsychotic agent. N Engl J Med 14:746–754, 1991

Beherec L, Lambrey S, Quilici G, et al: Retrospective review of clozapine in the treatment of patients with autism spectrum disorder and severe disruptive behaviors. J Clin Psychopharmacol 31:341–344, 2011

Belsito KM, Law PA, Kirk KS, et al: Lamotrigine therapy for autistic disorder: a randomized, double-blind, placebo-controlled trial. J Autism Dev Disord 31:175–181, 2001

Blankenship K, Erickson CA, Stigler KA, et al: Guanfacine extended release in two patients with pervasive developmental disorders. J Child Adolesc Psychopharmacol 21:287–290, 2011

Brodkin ES, McDougle CJ, Naylor ST, et al: Clomipramine in adults with pervasive developmental disorders: a prospective open-label investigation. J Child Adolesc Psychopharmacol 7:109–121, 1997

Buchsbaum MS, Hollander E, Haznedar MM, et al: Effect of fluoxetine on regional cerebral metabolism in autistic spectrum disorders: a pilot study. Int J Neuropsychopharmacol 4:119–125, 2001

Buitelaar JK, van der Gaag RJ, van der Hoeven J: Buspirone in the management of anxiety and irritability in children with pervasive developmental disorders: results of an open-label trial. J Clin Psychiatry 59:56–59, 1998

Burris KD, Molski TF, Xu C, et al: Aripiprazole, a novel antipsychotic, is a high-affinity partial agonist at human dopamine D_2 receptors. J Pharmacol Exp Ther 302:381–389, 2002

Bymaster FP, Hemrick-Luecke SK, Perry KW, et al: Neurochemical evidence for antagonism by olanzapine of dopamine, serotonin, alpha 1-adrenergic and muscarinic receptors in vivo in rats. Psychopharmacology 124:87–94, 1996

Campbell M: Pharmacotherapy in early infantile autism. Biol Psychiatry 10:399–423, 1975

Campbell M, Anderson LT, Meier M, et al: A comparison of haloperidol and behavior therapy and their interaction in autistic children. J Am Acad Child Psychiatry 17:640–655, 1978

Campbell M, Anderson LT, Small AM, et al: Naltrexone in autistic children: behavioral symptoms and attentional learning. J Am Acad Child Adolesc Psychiatry 32:1283–1291, 1993

Campbell M, Armenteros JL, Malone PR, et al: Neuroleptic-related dyskinesias in autistic children: a prospective, longitudinal study. J Am Acad Child Adolesc Psychiatry 36:835–843, 1997

Carminati GG, Deriaz N, Bertschy G: Low-dose venlafaxine in three adolescents and young adults with autistic disorder improves self-injurious behavior and attention deficit/hyperactivity disorder (ADHD)–like symptoms. Prog Neuropsychopharmacol Biol Psychiatry 30:312–315, 2006

Chen NC, Bedair HS, McKay B, et al: Clozapine in the treatment of aggression in an adolescent with autistic disorder. J Clin Psychiatry 62:479–480, 2001

Chez MG, Nowinski CV, Buchanan CP, et al: Donepezil (Aricept) use in children with autistic spectrum disorders. Ann Neurol 48:541, 2000

Chez MG, Aimonovitch M, Buchanan T, et al: Treating autistic spectrum disorders in children: utility of the cholinesterase inhibitor rivastigmine tartrate. J Child Neurol 19:165–169, 2004

Chez MG, Burton Q, Dowling T, et al: Memantine as adjunctive therapy in children diagnosed with autism spectrum disorders: an observation of initial clinical response and maintenance tolerability. J Child Neurol 22:574–579, 2007

Cohen IL, Campbell M, Posner D, et al: Behavioral effects of haloperidol in young autistic children. J Am Acad Child Adolesc Psychiatry 19:665–677, 1980

Conroy J, Meally E, Kearney G, et al: Serotonin transporter gene and autism: a haplotype analysis in an Irish autistic population. Mol Psychiatry 9:587–593, 2004

Correll CU, Kratochvil CJ, March JS: Developments in pediatric psychopharmacology: focus on stimulants, antidepressants, and antipsychotics. J Clin Psychiatry 72:655–670, 2011

Corson AH, Barkenbus JE, Posey DJ, et al: A retrospective analysis of quetiapine in the treatment of pervasive developmental disorders. J Clin Psychiatry 65:1531–1536, 2004

Coskun M, Karakoc S, Kircelli F, et al: Effectiveness of mirtazapine in the treatment of inappropriate sexual behaviors in individuals with autistic disorder. J Child Adolesc Psychopharmacol 19:203–206, 2009

Couturier JL, Nicolson R: A retrospective assessment of citalopram in children and adolescents with pervasive developmental disorders. J Child Adolesc Psychopharmacol 12:243–248, 2002

Davanzo PA, Belin TR, Widawski MH, et al: Paroxetine treatment of aggression and self-injury in persons with mental retardation. Am J Ment Retard 102:427–437, 1998

De Hert M, Dobbelaere M, Sheridan EM, et al: Metabolic and endocrine adverse effects of second-generation antipsychotics in children and adolescents: a systematic review of randomized, placebo controlled trials and guidelines for clinical practice. Eur Psychiatry 26:144–158, 2011

DeLong GR, Ritch CR, Burch S: Fluoxetine response in children with autistic spectrum disorders: correlation with familial major affective disorder and intellectual achievement. Dev Med Child Neurol 44:652–659, 2002

Di Martino A, Melis G, Cianchetti C, et al: Methylphenidate for pervasive developmental disorders: safety and efficacy of acute single dose test and ongoing therapy: an open-pilot study. J Child Adolesc Psychopharmacol 14:207–218, 2004

Dreifuss FE, Santilli N, Langer DH, et al: Valproic acid hepatic fatalities: a retrospective review. Neurology 37:379–385, 1987

Epperson CN, McDougle CJ, Anand A: Lithium augmentation of fluvoxamine in autistic disorder: a case report. J Child Adolesc Psychopharmacol 4:201–207, 1994

Erickson CA, Posey DJ, Stigler KA, et al: A retrospective study of memantine in children and adolescents with pervasive developmental disorders. Psychopharmacology 191:141–147, 2007

Fankhauser MP, Karumanchi VC, German ML, et al: A double-blind, placebo-controlled study of the efficacy of transdermal clonidine in autism. J Clin Psychiatry 53:77–82, 1992

Fatemi SH, Realmuto GM, Khan L, et al: Fluoxetine in treatment of adolescent patients with autism: a longitudinal open-label trial. J Autism Dev Disord 28:303–307, 1998

Feldman HM, Koman BK, Gonzaga AM: Naltrexone and communication skills in young children with autism. J Am Acad Child Adolesc Psychiatry 38:587–593, 1999

Findling RL, Maxwell K, Wiznitzer M: An open clinical trial of risperidone monotherapy in young children with autistic disorder. Psychopharmacol Bull 33:155–159, 1997

Findling RL, McNamara NK, Gracious BL, et al: Quetiapine in nine youths with autistic disorder. J Child Adolesc Psychopharmacol 14:287–294, 2004

Formanek R: New warning about ADHD drug. FDA Consum 39:3, 2005

Gagliano A, Germano E, Pustorino G, et al: Risperidone treatment of children with autistic disorder: effectiveness, tolerability, and pharmacokinetic implications. J Child Adolesc Psychopharmacol 14:39–47, 2004

Gillberg C, Terenius L, Lonnerholm G: Endorphin activity in childhood psychosis. Arch Gen Psychiatry 42:780–783, 1985

Gobbi G, Pulvirenti L: Long-term treatment with clozapine in an adult with autistic disorder accompanied by aggressive behavior. J Psych Neurol 26:340–341, 2001

Goff DC, Tsai G, Levitt J, et al: A placebo-controlled trial of D-cycloserine added to conventional neuroleptics in patients with schizophrenia. Arch Gen Psychiatry 56:21–27, 1999

Gordon CT, State RC, Nelson JE, et al: A double-blind comparison of clomipramine, desipramine, and placebo in the treatment of autistic disorder. Arch Gen Psychiatry 50:441–447, 1993

Greenhill L, Beyer DH, Finkleson J, et al: Guidelines and algorithms for the use of methylphenidate in children with attention-deficit/hyperactivity disorder. J Atten Disord 6 (suppl):S89–S100, 2002a

Greenhill LL, Pliszka S, Dulcan MK, et al; American Academy of Child and Adolescent Psychiatry. Practice parameter for the use of stimulant medications in the treatment of children, adolescents, and adults. J Am Acad Child Adolesc Psychiatry 41:26S–49S, 2002b

Greist JH, Jefferson JW, Kobak KA, et al: Efficacy and tolerability of serotonin transport inhibitors in obsessive-compulsive disorder. Arch Gen Psychiatry 52:53–60, 1995

Handen BL, Johnson CR, Lubetsky M: Efficacy of methylphenidate among children with autism and symptoms of attention-deficit hyperactivity disorder. J Autism Dev Disord 30:245–255, 2000

Handen BL, Sahl R, Hardan AY: Guanfacine in children with autism and/or intellectual disabilities. J Dev Behav Pediatr 29:303–308, 2008

Handen BL, Johnson CR, McAuliffe-Bellin S, et al: Safety and efficacy of donepezil in children and adolescents with autism: neuropsychological measures. J Child Adolesc Psychopharmacol 21:43–50, 2011

Hardan AY, Handen BL: A retrospective open trial of adjunctive donepezil in children and adolescents with autistic disorder. J Child Adolesc Psychopharmacol 12:237–241, 2002

Hellings JA, Weckbaugh M, Nickel EJ, et al: A double-blind, placebo controlled study of valproate for aggression in youth with pervasive developmental disorder. J Child Adolesc Psychopharmacol 15:682–692, 2005

Hollander E, Kaplan A, Cartwright C, et al: Venlafaxine in children, adolescents and young adults with autism spectrum disorders: an open retrospective clinical report. J Child Neurol 15:132–135, 2000

Hollander E, Dolgoff-Kaspar R, Cartwright C, et al: An open trial of divalproex sodium in autism spectrum disorders. J Clin Psychiatry 62:530–534, 2001

Hollander E, Wasserman S, Swanson EN, et al: A double-blind placebo-controlled pilot study of olanzapine in childhood/adolescent pervasive developmental disorder. J Child Adolesc Psychopharmacol 14:287–294, 2004

Hollander E, Phillips A, Chaplin W, et al: A placebo controlled crossover trial of liquid fluoxetine on repetitive behaviors in childhood and adolescent autism. Neuropsychopharmacology 30:582–589, 2005

Hollander E, Soorya L, Wasserman S, et al: Divalproex sodium vs. placebo in the treatment of repetitive behaviours in autism spectrum disorder. Int J Neuropsychopharmacol 9:209–213, 2006

Hollander E, Chaplin W, Soorya L, et al: Divalproex sodium vs. placebo for the treatment of irritability in children and adolescents with autism spectrum disorders. Neuropsychopharmacology 35:990–998, 2010

Horvath K, Stefanatos G, Sokolaki KN, et al: Improved social and language skills after secretin administration in patients with autism spectrum disorders. J Assoc Acad Minor Phys 9:9–15, 1998

Jaselskis CA, Cook EH Jr, Fletcher KE, et al: Clonidine treatment of hyperactive and impulsive children with autistic disorder. J Clin Psychopharmacol 12:322–327, 1992

Kaminska B, Czaja M, Kozielska E, et al: Use of secretin in the treatment of childhood autism. Med Sci Monit 8:RA22–RA26, 2002

Kanner L: Autistic disturbances of affective contact. Nerv Child 2:217–250, 1943

Kerbeshian J, Burd L, Fisher W: Lithium carbonate in the treatment of two patients with infantile autism and atypical bipolar symptomatology. J Clin Psychopharmacol 7:401–405, 1987

King BH, Davanzo P: Buspirone treatment of aggression and self-injury in autistic and nonautistic persons with severe mental retardation. Dev Brain Dysfunc 9:22–31, 1996

King BH, Wright DM, Handen BL, et al: Double-blind, placebo-controlled study of amantadine hydrochloride in the treatment of children with autistic disorder. J Am Acad Child Adolesc Psychiatry 40:658–665, 2001

King BH, Hollander E, Sikich L, et al: Lack of efficacy of citalopram in children with autism spectrum disorders and high levels of repetitive behavior. Arch Gen Psychiatry 66:583–590, 2009

Kornhuber J, Weller M, Schoppmeyer K, et al: Amantadine and memantine are NMDA receptor antagonists with neuroprotective properties. J Neurol Transm Suppl 43:91–104, 1994

Lambrey S, Falissard B, Martin-Barrero M, et al: Effectiveness of clozapine for the treatment of aggression in an adolescent with autistic disorder. J Child Adolesc Psychopharmacol 20:79–80, 2010

Leboyer M, Bouvard MP, Launey JM, et al: Brief report: a double-blind study of naltrexone in infantile autism. J Autism Dev Disord 22:309–319, 1992

Leboyer M, Philippe A, Bouvard M, et al: Whole blood serotonin and plasma beta-endorphin in autistic probands and their first-degree relatives. Biol Psychiatry 45:158–163, 1999

Leysen JE, Gommeren W, Eens A, et al: Biochemical profile of risperidone, a new antipsychotic. J Pharmacol Exp Ther 247:661–670, 1988

Malone RP, Cater J, Sheikh RM, et al: Olanzapine versus haloperidol in children with autistic disorder: an open pilot study. J Am Acad Child Adolesc Psychiatry 40:887–894, 2001

Malone RP, Maislin G, Choudhury MS, et al: Risperidone treatment in children and adolescents with autism: short- and long-term safety and effectiveness. J Am Acad Child Adolesc Psychiatry 41:140–147, 2002

Malone RP, Delaney MA, Hyman SB, et al: Ziprasidone in adolescents with autism: an open-label pilot study. J Child Adolesc Psychopharmacol 17:779–790, 2007

Marcus RN, Owen R, Kamen L, et al: A placebo-controlled, fixed-dose study of aripiprazole in children and adolescents with irritability associated with autistic disorder. J Am Acad Child Adolesc Psychiatry 48:1110–1119, 2009

Marcus RN, Owen R, Manos G, et al: Aripiprazole in the treatment of irritability in pediatric patients (aged 6–17 years) with autistic disorder: results from a 52-week, open-label study. J Child Adolesc Psychopharmacol 21:229–236, 2011a

Marcus RN, Owen R, Manos G, et al: Safety and tolerability of aripiprazole for irritability in pediatric patients with autistic disorder: a 52-week, open-label, multi-center study. J Clin Psychiatry 72:1270–1276, 2011b

Marshall BL, Napolitano DA, McAdam DB, et al: Venlafaxine and increased aggression in a female with autism. J Am Acad Child Adolesc Psychiatry 42:383–384, 2003

Martin A, Koenig K, Scahill L, et al: Open-label quetiapine in treatment of children and adolescents with autistic disorder. J Child Adolesc Psychopharmacol 9:99–107, 1999

Martin A, Koenig K, Anderson GM, et al: Low-dose fluvoxamine treatment of children and adolescents with pervasive developmental disorder: a prospective, open-label study. J Autism Dev Disord 33:77–85, 2003

Masi G, Cosenza A, Mucci M, et al: Open trial of risperidone in 24 young children with pervasive developmental disorders. J Am Acad Child Adolesc Psychiatry 40:1206–1214, 2001a

Masi G, Cosenza A, Mucci M: Prolactin levels in young children with pervasive developmental disorders. J Child Adolesc Psychopharmacol 11:389–394, 2001b

Masi G, Cosenza A, Mucci M, et al: A 3-year naturalistic study of 53 preschool children with pervasive developmental disorders treated with risperidone. J Clin Psychiatry 64:1039–1047, 2003

McDougle CJ, Naylor ST, Cohen DJ, et al: A double-blind, placebo-controlled study of fluvoxamine in adults with autistic disorder. Arch Gen Psychiatry 53:1001–1008, 1996a

McDougle CJ, Naylor ST, Cohen DJ, et al: Effects of tryptophan depletion in drug-free adults with autism. Arch Gen Psychiatry 53:993–1000, 1996b

McDougle CJ, Holmes JP, Bronson MR, et al: Risperidone treatment of children and adolescents with pervasive developmental disorders: a prospective, open-label study. J Am Acad Child Adolesc Psychiatry 36:685–693, 1997

McDougle CJ, Brodkin ES, Naylor ST, et al: Sertraline in adults with pervasive developmental disorder: a prospective open-label investigation. J Clin Psychopharmacol 18:62–66, 1998a

McDougle CJ, Holmes JP, Carlson DC, et al: A double-blind, placebo-controlled study of risperidone in adults with autistic disorder and other pervasive developmental disorders. Arch Gen Psychiatry 55:633–41, 1998b

McDougle CJ, Kresch LE, Posey DJ: Repetitive thoughts and behavior in pervasive developmental disorders: treatment with serotonin reuptake inhibitors. J Autism Dev Disord 30:425–433, 2000

McDougle CJ, Kem DL, Posey DJ: Case series: use of ziprasidone for maladaptive symptoms in youth with autism. J Am Acad Child Adolesc Psychiatry 41:921–927, 2002

McDougle CJ, Scahill L, Aman MG, et al: Risperidone for the core symptom domains of autism: results from the RUPP Autism Network Study. Am J Psychiatry 162:1142–1148, 2005

Namerow LB, Thomas P, Bostic JQ, et al: Use of citalopram in pervasive developmental disorder. J Dev Behav Pediatr 24:104–108, 2003

Nicolson R, Awad G, Sloman L: An open trial of risperidone in young autistic children. J Am Acad Child Adolesc Psychiatry 37:372–376, 1998

Nicolson R, Craven-Thuss B, Smith J: A prospective, open-label trial of galantamine in autistic disorder. J Child Adolesc Psychopharmacol 16:621–629, 2006

Owen R, Sikich L, Marcus RN, et al: Aripiprazole in the treatment of irritability in children and adolescents with autistic disorder. Pediatrics 124:1533–1540, 2009

Owley T, Walton L, Salt J, et al: An open-label trial of escitalopram in pervasive developmental disorders. J Am Acad Child Adolesc Psychiatry 44:343–348, 2005

Owley T, Salt J, Guter S, et al: A prospective, open-label trial of memantine in the treatment of cognitive, behavioral, and memory dysfunction in pervasive developmental disorders. J Child Adolesc Psychopharmacol 16:517–524, 2006

Posey DJ, Litwiller M, Koburn A, et al: Paroxetine in autism. J Am Acad Child Adolesc Psychiatry 38:111–112, 1999

Posey DJ, Guenin KD, Kohn AE, et al: A naturalistic open-label study of mirtazapine in autistic and other pervasive developmental disorders. J Child Adolesc Psychopharmacol 11:267–277, 2001

Posey DJ, Kem DL, Swiezy NB, et al: A pilot study of D-cycloserine in subjects with autistic disorder. Am J Psychiatry 161:2115–2117, 2004a

Posey DJ, Puntney JI, Sasher TM, et al: Guanfacine treatment of hyperactivity and inattention in pervasive developmental disorders: a retrospective analysis of 80 cases. J Child Adolesc Psychopharmacol 14:233–241, 2004b

Posey DJ, Wiegand RE, Wilkerson J, et al: A prospective, open-label study of atomoxetine for ADHD symptoms associated with higher-functioning pervasive developmental disorders. Neuropsychopharmacology 31:S156, 2005

Potenza MN, Holmes JP, Kanes SJ, et al: Olanzapine treatment of children, adolescents, and adults with pervasive developmental disorders: an open-label pilot study. J Clin Psychopharmacol 19:37–44, 1999

Quintana H, Birmaher B, Stedge D, et al: Use of methylphenidate in the treatment of children with autistic disorder. J Autism Dev Disord 25:283–294, 1995

Ratey JJ, Bemporad J, Sorgi J, et al: Brief report: open trial effects of beta-blockers on speech and social behaviors in 8 autistic adults. J Autism Dev Disord 17:439–446, 1987

Remington G, Sloman L, Konstantareas M, et al: Clomipramine versus haloperidol in the treatment of autistic disorder: a double-blind, placebo-controlled, crossover study. J Clin Psychopharmacol 21:440–444, 2001

Research Units on Pediatric Psychopharmacology Autism Network: Risperidone in children with autism and serious behavioral problems. N Engl J Med 347:314–321, 2002

Research Units on Pediatric Psychopharmacology Autism Network: Randomized, controlled, crossover trial of methylphenidate in pervasive developmental disorders with hyperactivity. Arch Gen Psychiatry 62:1266–1274, 2005a

Research Units on Pediatric Psychopharmacology Autism Network. Risperidone treatment of autistic disorder: longer-term benefits and blinded discontinuation after 6 months. Am J Psychiatry 162:1361–1369, 2005b

Ross DL, Klykylo WM, Hitzemann R: Reduction of elevated CSF beta-endorphin by fenfluramine in infantile autism. Pediatr Neurol 3:83–86, 1987

Saito E, Correll C, Gallelli K, et al: A prospective study of hyperprolactinemia in children and adolescents treated with atypical antipsychotic agents. J Child Adolesc Psychopharmacol 14:350–358, 2004

Scahill L, Farkas L, Hamrin V: Lithium in children and adolescents. J Child Adolesc Psychiatr Nurs 14:89–93, 2001

Scahill L, Aman MG, McDougle CJ, et al: A prospective open trial of guanfacine in children with pervasive developmental disorders. J Child Adolesc Psychopharmacol 16:589–598, 2006

Schain RJ, Freedman DX: Studies on 5-hydroxyindole metabolism in autistic and other mentally retarded children. J Pediatr 58:315–320, 1961

Shea S, Turgay A, Carroll A, et al: Risperidone in the treatment of disruptive behavioral symptoms in children with autistic and other pervasive developmental disorders. Pediatrics 114:634–641, 2004

Snead RW, Boon F, Presberg J: Paroxetine for self-injurious behavior. J Am Acad Child Adolesc Psychiatry 33:909–910, 1994

Steingard R, Biederman J: Lithium responsive manic-like symptoms in two individuals with autism and mental retardation. J Am Acad Child Adolesc Psychiatry 26:932–935, 1987

Steingard RJ, Zimnitsky B, DeMaso DR, et al: Sertraline treatment of transition-associated anxiety and agitation in children with autistic disorder. J Child Adolesc Psychopharmacol 7:9–15, 1997

Stigler KA, Desmond LA, Posey DJ, et al: A naturalistic retrospective analysis of psychostimulants in pervasive developmental disorders. J Child Adolesc Psychopharmacol 14:49–56, 2004a

Stigler KA, Potenza MN, Posey DJ, et al: Weight gain associated with atypical antipsychotic use in children and adolescents: prevalence, clinical relevance, and management. Paediatr Drugs 6:33–44, 2004b

Stigler KA, Diener JT, Kohn AE, et al: Aripiprazole in pervasive developmental disorder not otherwise specified and Asperger's disorder: a 14-week, prospective, open-label study. J Child Adolesc Psychopharmacol 19:265–274, 2009

Stigler KA, Mullett JE, Erickson CA, et al: Paliperidone for irritability in adolescents and young adults with autistic disorder. Psychopharmacology (Berl) May 3, 2012 [Epub ahead of print]

Sturmey P: Secretin is an ineffective treatment for pervasive developmental disabilities: a review of 15 double-blind randomized controlled trials. Res Dev Disabil 26:87–97, 2005

Sugie Y, Sugie H, Fukuda T, et al: Clinical efficacy of fluvoxamine and functional polymorphism in a serotonin transporter gene. J Autism Dev Disord 35:377–385, 2005

Tandon R, Harrigan E, Zorn SH: Ziprasidone: a novel antipsychotic with unique pharmacology and therapeutic potential. J Serotonin Res 4:159–177, 1997

Troost PW, Steenbuis MP, Tuynman-Qua HG, et al: Atomoxetine for attention-deficit/ hyperactivity disorder symptoms in children with pervasive developmental disorders: a pilot study. J Child Adolesc Psychopharmacol 16:611–619, 2006

Uvebrant P, Bauziene R: Intractable epilepsy in children: the efficacy of lamotrigine treatment, including non-seizure related benefits. Neuropediatrics 25:284–288, 1994

Wasserman S, Iyengar R, Chaplin WF, et al: Levetiracetam versus placebo in childhood and adolescent autism: a double-blind placebo-controlled study. Int Clin Psychopharmacol 21:363–367, 2006

Weizman R, Weizman A, Thano S, et al: Humoral-endorphin blood levels in autistic, schizophrenic and healthy subjects. Psychopharmacology (Berl) 82:368–370, 1984

Willemsen-Swinkels SHN, Buitelaar JK, Nijhof GJ, et al: Failure of naltrexone hydrochloride to reduce self-injurious and autistic behavior in mentally retarded adults: double-blind placebo-controlled studies. Arch Gen Psychiatry 52:766–773, 1995

Zuddas A, Ledda MG, Fratta A, et al: Clinical effects of clozapine on autistic disorder. Am J Psychiatry 153:738, 1996

Zuddas A, Dimartino A, Muglia P, et al: Long-term risperidone for pervasive developmental disorder: efficacy, tolerability, and discontinuation. J Child Adolesc Psychopharmacol 10:79–90, 2000

8

Tic Disorders

Lawrence Scahill, M.S.N., Ph.D.
Aysegul Selcen Guler, M.D.

Tic disorders, including Tourette syndrome (TS), are movement disorders that begin in childhood and are defined by the presence of enduring motor tics, phonic tics, or both. The tics of TS show an extraordinary range from mild to severe across patients and a fluctuating course within patients (Lin et

This work was supported by National Institute of Mental Health Grants U10MH66764, MH069874, MH083707, and MH080965 to Dr. Scahill and MH070802 to the Tourette Syndrome Association, and a separate grant from the Tourette Syndrome Association to Dr. Scahill.

This work was also supported by National Institute of Mental Health Grants U10MH066764 and R03MH67845-01A1 to Dr. Scahill and National Institute of Nursing Research Grants R15NR007637-01 and M01RR00125 (Yale University).

The authors acknowledge the assistance of Caitlin Tillberg in the preparation of this manuscript.

al. 2002; Roessner et al. 2011). In addition to association with tics, TS is frequently connected with hyperactivity, impulsiveness, distractibility, obsessive-compulsive symptoms, and anxiety (Jankovic 2009). Therefore, the assessment and treatment of children and adolescents with TS correctly include consideration of these multiple sources of impairment. Indeed, although the referral question may be about tics, the presence of attention-deficit/hyperactivity disorder (ADHD), obsessive-compulsive disorder (OCD), or another anxiety disorder may be more pressing than the tic symptoms. In assessment and treatment planning, the clinician must take into account, in addition to the sources of impairment, the domains of functioning that may be adversely affected. For example, TS or an associated condition may contribute to maladaptive, even volatile, family interactions, may interfere with educational progress, and may contribute to unstable peer relationships.

In this chapter, we review the diagnosis and treatment of children with tic disorders. Because of the common co-occurrence of OCD and ADHD in individuals with tic disorders, we also examine the treatment of these disorders in this population. The primary focus of the review is on pharmacological treatments, but emerging findings in behavioral intervention are also examined. Although there is growing interest in deep brain stimulation and repetitive transcranial magnetic stimulation (rTMS), these approaches are not included in this review (for a review of recent developments in surgical approaches to the treatment of refractory TS, see Mink 2009). rTMS, which uses a noninvasive magnetic coil to generate a current into the cortex, has only been studied in small trials (Orth et al. 2005). Before addressing the issues of diagnosis and treatment, we provide a brief review of the epidemiology of tic disorders to underscore their public health importance.

Epidemiology

Transient tics are relatively common in school-age children, affecting 6%–12% (Scahill et al., in press). Tic disorders are defined in DSM-IV-TR (American Psychiatric Association 2000) by the duration and types of tics present. DSM-IV-TR also stipulates that the tics must begin before age 18 years. In practice, however, tics usually begin in early school age, between ages 5 and 7 years.

Historically, TS has been considered a rare and uniformly severe condition. However, prior estimates of prevalence were typically based on counts of clinically ascertained cases. This method resulted in a systematic undercount because it failed to include cases that had not come to clinical attention—perhaps milder cases or cases with poor access to care. To correct this problem, recent studies have surveyed community samples. Not surprisingly, this strategy has resulted in higher estimates of prevalence. Recent studies have also relied on detailed parent interviews and, in some instances, direct observation of the child to confirm the presence of tics. This approach also promotes the identification of milder cases. Furthermore, the recognition of milder cases has encouraged the view that tic disorders, including TS, reside on a continuum from mild to severe. Finally, as in other areas of psychiatry, the introduction of DSM-III (American Psychiatric Association 1980) specified and broadened the diagnostic criteria. For example, in the Isle of Wight study, Rutter et al. (1970) evaluated a sample of 3,000 children ages 10–12 years; in that sample, 4.4% of the children were identified as having tics, but no cases of TS were identified. By contrast, using DSM-III-R (American Psychiatric Association 1987) criteria, Costello et al. (1996) reported a prevalence of 4.2% for all tic disorders combined (transient tic disorder, chronic tic disorder, and TS) in a similar age group of children in the Great Smoky Mountains Study. The differences in diagnostic classification across these two studies appear to be due to differences in definitions rather than true differences in prevalence of tic disorders.

Over the past decade, there have been 10 community surveys on the prevalence of tic disorders in children (Scahill et al., in press). The prevalence of TS has been estimated from a lower bound of 2.6 per 1,000 to an upper bound of 38 per 1,000. This level of imprecision is not ideal for judging public health importance and service need. In a recent critical review of the literature, Scahill et al. (in press) proposed a narrower range of 3–8 cases per 1,000 for TS. Indeed, five studies reported 4–6 cases per 1,000.

The Centers for Disease Control and Prevention (2009) conducted a national telephone survey of nearly 64,000 households with children ages 6–17 years. Parents were asked about the child's health history (e.g., diabetes, asthma, seizures), psychiatric conditions (e.g., TS, ADHD, depression, autism), and health care utilization. A lifetime diagnosis of TS was reported in 3 children per 1,000, for an estimated total count of 148,000 cases nationwide, with a male-to-female ratio of 3:1. This estimate, which is low compared with the 4–6 per 1,000 estimated by Scahill et al. (in press), suggests that some cases go undetected. Because most cases were described as mild according to the parents, missing mild cases is not likely to provide a complete explanation. The report noted a rate of 3.9 per 1,000 in non-Hispanic white children compared with 1.6 per 1,000 for Hispanic and 1.5 per 1,000 for black children, suggesting that race and ethnicity may affect rates of identified cases. Sixty-four percent of the children with TS also had a diagnosis of ADHD; 43% had a history of disruptive behavior, and 40% had a history of anxiety problems.

Diagnosis and Assessment

The assessment of a child suspected of having TS begins with a review of tic symptoms and exploration of associated problems, particularly inattention, impulsiveness and hyperactivity, and obsessive-compulsive symptoms. The review of tic symptoms includes the age at onset and course of symptoms, current severity of motor and phonic tics, presence of premonitory sensations and capacity for tic suppression, overall burden caused by the tics, and treatment approaches implemented to date. Tics tend to be rapid movements or brief vocalizations that are performed in a stereotyped manner. Tics also tend to occur in bouts—brief or extended clusters of tics, followed by a period of relative quiescence. In mild cases, the bouts of tics are brief, with relatively long tic-free periods (an hour to several hours), and may go unnoticed by casual observers. By contrast, individuals with moderate or marked severity may have bouts of forceful tics consisting of multiple movements and vocalization with only brief tic-free periods. Frequent and forceful movements or vocalizations may be easily noticeable across settings and may interfere with everyday activities.

Many patients with TS describe a warning or urge prior to the performance of a tic. This may be described as a vague feeling of tension or a physical feeling occurring in a specific body region. In fact, the body region involved may be the same muscle group inherent in tic expression (Leckman et al. 1993; Woods et al. 2005). Patients with TS also describe an ability to suppress their tics—at least momentarily. The relationship between premonitory sensations and tic suppression is intriguing, though not completely understood. First, young children, ages 7–10 years, may not spontaneously report either of these phenomena. However, by age 10 years, most children with TS describe both the warning before some of their tics and at least a fleeting capacity to suppress tics. Second, children and adults often report that the act of suppressing tics intensifies the urge to perform the tic. This accentuation pushes the tic urge to a crescendo and ultimately makes the tic irresistible (Leckman et al. 1993). Third, although many patients describe the capacity to suppress tics, at least momentarily, few can describe how this is accomplished. Data from functional magnetic resonance imaging (fMRI) suggest that compared with control subjects, patients with TS experience dysregulation of the motor circuit with a lesser capacity to exert "top-down" control. Tic suppression may reflect additional effort to exert voluntary control of dysregulated subcortical output (Wang et al. 2011). Fourth, the effort to suppress tics may reflect the child's gradual awareness that the tics can have social consequences. In other words, as children with TS begin to understand that the tics can have social consequences, they increase their vigilance about the tics and recruit conscious effort to suppress them. The increased vigilance may promote the evolution of premonitory sensations as the child becomes more aware of the earliest signs of tic behavior. This conceptualization has not been specifically tested and remains speculative.

The differential diagnosis of TS and tic disorders is based on the type of tics present (motor or vocal) and the duration of symptoms (American Psychiatric Association 2000). Transient tic disorder is defined by the presence of motor or vocal tics for less than a year. The diagnosis of chronic tic disorder is made when the child has motor or vocal tics (but not both) for longer than a year. TS is defined by the presence of both motor and phonic tics for more than a year. Diagnosis of TS does not require that both motor and phonic tics be present at the same time but does require that both are present during the course of illness. Other key elements in the diagnosis include onset before age 18 years and exclusion of other causes for the tics, such as medication or another medical condition. For example, a child who only showed tics while being treated with a psychostimulant would not be diagnosed with TS. Although the diagnosis of TS is based on history, the diagnosis of TS is more convincing when the tics are actually observed by an experienced clinician.

Although no laboratory tests confirm the diagnosis of TS, selected laboratory tests can help to rule out rare medical problems such as neuroacanthocytosis, Huntington disease, and Wilson disease (Jankovic and Kurlan 2011; Scahill et al. 2006).

The physical and neurological examinations of most children with TS are unremarkable. An abnormal physical examination or positive neurological findings may signal the need for further evaluation in search of other conditions. For example, repetitive eye blinking with momentary loss of conscious awareness may prompt referral for an electroencephalogram (EEG). Referrals for a neurology consultation or an EEG are usually not necessary. Differences in brain volumes on magnetic resonance imaging (MRI), such as larger volumes in prefrontal regions and smaller caudate volumes, have been observed in research studies comparing TS patients with healthy control subjects (Peterson et al. 2001, 2003). In addition, although findings are not consistent across studies, an increased number of dopamine receptors and enhanced dopamine innervation in patients with TS compared with healthy controls have been demonstrated in several functional neuroimaging studies (see Frey and Albin 2006). Computed tomography, MRI, positron emission tomography, and single-photon emission computed tomography are not part of the routine diagnostic evaluation of TS at the present time.

Developmental history and medical history may be informative in the differential diagnosis of TS. A history of social disability, language delay, and stereotypic hand flapping in a child may point to an autism spectrum disorder rather than TS. A thorough evaluation of how the symptoms affect family, interpersonal relationships, and school performance is essential for treatment planning through the identification of priorities for intervention. Similarly, a review of family history for tics, ADHD, and obsessive-compulsive symptoms is warranted as an aid to making the diagnosis and as part of family education. For example, a family in which a newly diagnosed child's paternal uncle has severe TS may need to be reassured that most cases are mild to moderate and that it is unlikely that their child will be as severely affected as the uncle.

Several tic symptom checklists and clinician interviews are available for the assessment of tic severity. Two commonly used instruments are the Tic Symptom Self Report (TSSR) (Allen et al. 2005; Scahill et al. 2003b) and the Yale Global Tic Severity Scale (YGTSS) (Leckman et al. 1989). The TSSR can be used as a self-report for children over age 10 years, although some orientation for the child may be needed on first administration. It can also be completed by parents or teachers to gather information across settings. The reliability of the TSSR has not been formally studied, but the TSSR performed similarly to the YGTSS as a change measure in two placebo-controlled trials (Allen et al. 2005; Scahill et al. 2003b).

The TSSR contains 20 items for motor tics and 20 items for phonic tics. Each item is rated 0–3 for frequency and intensity. The primary advantage of the TSSR is its ease of completion and scoring. The YGTSS is a clinician-rated instrument that surveys the number, frequency, intensity, complexity, and interference of motor tics and phonic tics separately. The examiner reviews a checklist of motor and phonic tics over the past week and then rates each dimension from 0 to 5. Thus, across the five dimensions, the total motor tic score can range from 0 to 25; likewise, the phonic tic score can range from 0 to 25. The Total Tic score (combined total of motor and phonic tic scores, ranging from 0 to 50) is commonly used as an outcome measure in treatment studies (see next section, "Treatment of Tics in Children With Tourette Syndrome"). The YGTSS also has an overall Impairment score ranging from 0 to 50, with a higher score reflecting greater impairment. This scale is meant to capture the patient's impairment and distress due to tics. Although the correlation of the Impairment score and the Total Tic score is statistically significant in group analysis, some patients may show high degrees of impairment in the presence of mild tics. Other patients may show the opposite pattern: high tic severity with lower impairment. The YGTSS has well-established reliability and validity. One of the strengths of the YGTSS is that it allows the rater to incorporate reports of multiple informants (e.g., parent and child) and observations during the interview into the scoring. For example, when asking about the forcefulness of tics, the rater can ask the child and parent to contrast the average tic intensity over the past week to the observed intensity during the interview.

Treatment of Tics in Children With Tourette Syndrome

The first-line treatment for tics in children with TS is *education*, especially the following points:

1. TS is not a progressive condition.
2. In most cases, the tics are mild to moderate in severity.

3. Treating tics may not improve symptoms of ADHD or disruptive behavior.
4. Tics have a fluctuating course, even when a child is taking a tic-suppressing medication.
5. Most children with TS will show a decline in tics by early adulthood (Bloch et al. 2006).

Understandably, parents and children may overfocus on the child's tics. The clinician's role is to help refocus the parents on the child's most pressing problems and to keep the parents mindful of the child's overall development. All of these educational needs may extend to teachers and other school personnel.

Antipsychotics

Early randomized trials demonstrated that the potent dopamine D_2 receptor antagonists haloperidol and pimozide are superior to placebo for suppressing tics (Ross and Moldofsky 1978; Shapiro and Shapiro 1984). Two randomized controlled trials (RCTs) compared pimozide with haloperidol; one study found better results with haloperidol (Shapiro et al. 1989), whereas no difference was found in the other (Sallee et al. 1997). However, the trial by Sallee et al. (1997) indicated that pimozide was better tolerated than haloperidol at equivalent dosages. Compared with current practice, the early studies used high dosages of these drugs (up to 20 mg/day for haloperidol and up to 48 mg/day for pimozide). In contemporary clinical practice, the trend is clearly toward the use of lower dosages, such as 1–4 mg/day for haloperidol and 2–6 mg/day for pimozide (Roessner et al. 2011; Scahill et al. 2006). Fluphenazine, a phenothiazine antipsychotic with dopamine D_1- and D_2-blocking properties, is used in clinical practice, although it has not been well studied. In an open-label trial with subjects that included children and adults, at dosages ranging from 2 to 15 mg/day given in two divided doses, fluphenazine was effective in 17 of 21 patients. A majority of the subjects with previous experience with haloperidol preferred fluphenazine (Goetz et al. 1984).

The atypical antipsychotics available in the United States include risperidone, olanzapine, ziprasidone, quetiapine, paliperidone, asenapine, and clozapine, which have serotonin-blocking effects and variable D_2-blocking properties (Table 8–1). Aripiprazole is a partial dopamine agonist that is believed to act as an antagonist in hyperdopaminergic state. Clozapine, which has low affinity for D_2 receptors, was no better than placebo for the treatment of tics (Caine et al. 1979). Considered in light of the effectiveness of haloperidol and pimozide, the failure of clozapine suggests that D_2 blockade is an important mechanism in tic suppression. To date, the best-studied atypical antipsychotic is risperidone, which is a relatively potent D_2 receptor blocker. It was superior to placebo for tic reduction in two trials (Dion et al. 2002; Scahill et al. 2003b) and equally as effective as pimozide (Bruggeman et al. 2001; Gilbert et al. 2004) and clonidine (Gaffney et al. 2002). Two open-label trials of olanzapine in a total of 30 adult patients offer some encouraging results for the treatment of tics (Budman et al. 2001; Stamenkovic et al. 2000). Ziprasidone was well tolerated and superior to placebo in a randomized trial of 28 children with TS (Sallee et al. 2000). To date, only small case series are available for quetiapine (Mukaddes and Abali 2003) and aripiprazole (Lyon et al. 2009).

The appeal of the atypical antipsychotic drugs is their demonstrated lower probability for neurological side effects such as dystonia, dyskinesia, tremor, and parkinsonism. There is also a presumption that the atypical antipsychotics are less likely to cause tardive dyskinesia in the long term. After more than a decade of experience with the newer antipsychotics, they indeed appear to have a lower likelihood of neurological side effects in the short term. The relative risk of tardive dyskinesia also appears to be lower, but more person-years of exposure may be needed to confirm this assumption.

Although the neurological side-effect burden appears to be lower with the atypical antipsychotics, other adverse effects have emerged in recent years. Chief among the emerging concerns are increased appetite, weight gain, and the potential for metabolic abnormalities (Meyer and Koro 2004). Based on reports from non-TS clinical populations, clozapine appears to be associated with the highest risk of weight gain, followed in order by olanzapine, quetiapine, risperidone, and ziprasidone (Allison and Casey 2001). Other adverse events reported in children and adolescents include social phobia, constipation, drooling, sedation, and cognitive blunting (Aman et al. 2005; Scahill et al. 2003b).

Clinical concerns have also been raised about alterations in cardiac conduction times, such as QTc prolongation. This issue is not new, given that similar concerns have been expressed about pimozide for several years. Although the occurrence of prolonged QTc is presumed to be rare in the dosage ranges used

Table 8–1. Dosing guidelines for antipsychotic drugs used in the treatment of children with tics of moderate or greater severity

Medication[a]	Starting dose (mg)	Usual dosage range (mg/day)	Placebo-controlled trial?
Haloperidol	0.25–0.5	1–4	Yes[b]
Pimozide	0.5–1.0	2–6	Yes[b]
Fluphenazine	0.5–1.0	1.5–10	No
Risperidone	0.25–0.5	1–3	Yes[b]
Ziprasidone	5–10	10–80	Yes[c]
Olanzapine	2.5–5.0	2.5–12.5	No
Quetiapine	25–50	75–150	No
Aripiprazole	2.5–5.0	5–10	No
Asenapine	No reports in TS		No
Paliperidone	No reports in TS		No

[a]Clozapine is not listed because of its complexity of use and failure to show efficacy.
[b]Superior to placebo in more than one study.
[c]Superior to placebo in one study.

in the treatment of tics, an electrocardiogram (ECG) is recommended before starting treatment with pimozide, during the dose adjustment phase, and annually during ongoing treatment (Scahill et al. 2006). Pimozide also appears to be vulnerable to interaction with drugs such as clarithromycin that inhibit cytochrome P450 (CYP) 3A4 (Desta et al. 1999). Of the atypical antipsychotics, ziprasidone appears to increase the QTc to a mild degree. In a series of 20 children with various psychiatric conditions, a modest increase in QTc occurred during treatment with ziprasidone (Blair et al. 2005). Unlike pimozide, however, ziprasidone does not appear to be vulnerable to drug-drug interaction because it does not rely on a single hepatic pathway. Following a delay in U.S. Food and Drug Administration (FDA) approval for the treatment of adults with schizophrenia, ziprasidone is now approved with no specific warnings regarding cardiac monitoring; however, the package insert mentions that ziprasidone is contraindicated in patients with a known history of QTc prolongation. Until more data are available to inform practice, guidelines similar to those used for pimozide have been recommended (Scahill et al. 2006). Antipsychotics that have been studied in RCTs are listed in Table 8–2.

Table 8–2.   Randomized placebo-controlled trials with $N>20$ focused on tic reduction using YGTSS Total Tic score[a]

Study	Drug	N	Duration (weeks)	Treatment effect[b]	Active>placebo?	Dropouts
Gilbert et al. 2000[c]	Pergolide	24	6	4.1	Not reported	5
Sallee et al. 2000	Ziprasidone	28	8	6.9	Yes	2
Cummings et al. 2002	Guanfacine	24	4	5.6	No	Not reported
Scahill et al. 2003b	Risperidone	34	8	6.0	Yes	2
Gilbert et al. 2003	Pergolide	51	8	3.9	No	6
Hoekstra et al. 2004	IVIG	30	14	3.7	No	2
Nicolson et al. 2005[d]	Metoclopramide	28	8	5.9	Yes	4
Toren et al. 2005	Ondansetron	30	3	2.0	No	3
Jankovic et al. 2010	Topiramate	29	10	8.5	Yes	16

Note.   IVIG=intravenous immunoglobulin; YGTSS=Yale Global Tic Severity Scale.
[a]Several other trials (e.g., atomoxetine, guanfacine, selegiline) evaluated tic outcomes on the YGTSS but were primarily focused on attention-deficit/hyperactivity disorder.
[b]Change in active drug – change in placebo.
[c]Includes only the first arm of the crossover trial. Did not include efficacy for the first arm.
[d]Four subjects dropped out; three additional subjects were excluded for protocol violations. Trials with mecamylamine, botulinum toxin, and tetrahydrocannabinol were not included in the table. Trials did not use YGTSS Total Tic score. Levetiracetam was not included because report did not include results for the first arm of the crossover trial.

Nonantipsychotic Medications

Over the past decade, various nonantipsychotic medications have been tried for the treatment of tics, including baclofen, botulinum toxin, guanfacine, intravenous immunoglobulin (IVIG), levetiracetam, mecamylamine, metoclopramide, nicotine, ondansetron, pergolide, tetrabenazine, tetrahydrocannabinol (THC), and topiramate. Most have not been well studied; those that have been studied in RCTs with more than 20 subjects with tics are listed in Table 8–2.

Levetiracetam has been examined in open trials and two RCTs (Awaad et al. 2005). One RCT compared active levetiracetam with placebo ($N=22$) (Smith-Hicks et al. 2007); the other ($N=12$) compared it with clonidine (Hedderick et al. 2009). Both trials used a crossover design and did not provide interpretable information on the first arm of the trial, thereby making it difficult to compare the results with other trials. Nonetheless, the results of these two trials do not support the use of levetiracetam in children with TS.

Müller-Vahl et al. (2003) conducted a double-blind trial of THC in 24 adults with TS. Seven subjects were not included in the analysis. Using the Global score of the YGTSS (Total Tic score plus Impairment score), the authors found no difference between active THC and placebo after 6 weeks of treatment.

The injection of botulinum toxin is now a standard treatment for dystonia. Following encouraging results in three open studies on TS (Jankovic 1994; Kwak et al. 2000), Marras et al. (2001) conducted a placebo-controlled trial of botulinum toxin in TS. The authors reported about a 40% difference between active drug and placebo. Treatment with botulinum toxin involves direct injection into the selected muscle of the motor tic or the laryngeal folds, in the case of vocal tic (Porta et al. 2004). In open-label studies, the botulinum toxin injections appeared to reduce the premonitory sensations as well as the tic at the injection site. Adverse effects include transient soreness at the injection site, weakness of the injected muscle, and loss of voice volume if the vocal cords are the target of treatment. Because benefit is generally confined to the injected muscle group, botulinum toxin should only be considered in cases with a prominent and interfering tic. The dose and frequency of repeat injections have not been standardized. More study is needed to answer these critical issues.

Ondansetron is a selective serotonin 5-HT$_3$ receptor antagonist that was developed as an antiemetic. A placebo-controlled trial provided encouraging though inconclusive results (Toren et al. 2005). In this study, 30 subjects were randomly assigned to receive ondansetron 24 mg/day (8 mg tid) or placebo for the 3-week trial. On one measure of tic severity, there was a significant difference between active drug and placebo. On the more frequently used YGTSS Total Tic score, there was no difference between drug and placebo. In addition to the small sample size, two limitations qualify these findings: First, the duration of trial was only 3 weeks, which may not have been long enough to detect a treatment effect. Second, there was a significant difference in the YGTSS scores at baseline across treatment groups. Ondansetron was well tolerated, and only one of 15 subjects randomly assigned to receive active drug withdrew because of an adverse effect. This subject reported gastrointestinal complaints. Although ondansetron is now available as a generic in the United States, it has the drawback of high cost. Because it is generally not used for open-ended treatment, insurance companies may balk at its use for TS.

Topiramate is an anticonvulsant that is also used to treat migraine. The mechanism of action is not completely understood, but it appears to enhance γ-aminobutyric acid (GABA)–mediated inhibition at GABA$_A$ receptors. It may also have glutamate-blocking properties. An open trial provided initial encouragement for the treatment of tics (Abuzzahab and Brown 2001). Jankovic et al. (2010) enrolled 29 subjects in a 10-week, placebo-controlled trial. Topiramate was started at 25 mg and increased slowly in 25-mg increments to an average dosage of 118 mg/day. The medication is typically administered on a twice-daily schedule. As shown in Table 8–2, the treatment effect on the YGTSS Total Tic score is the largest over any other listed medication, including risperidone (the only studied medication showing superiority to placebo in more than one trial [Dion et al. 2002; Scahill et al. 2003b]). However, the attrition rate in the topiramate trial was considerably larger than in the other trials presented in Table 8–2. The statistical analysis followed the *intent to treat* convention with last observation carried forward. Attrition was greater in the placebo group, suggesting that higher YGTSS scores were carried forward to endpoint in the placebo group. Thus, although these results are encouraging, the relatively large treatment effect of topiramate may be misleading.

Recent reports on the risk of birth defects following fetal exposure to topiramate and the risk, albeit apparently low, of metabolic acidosis warrant discussion of the risk-benefit ratio of this drug in TS. A survey of some 800,000 live births in Denmark over a 12-year period identified 1,532 infants exposed to newer anticonvulsants, including topiramate (Mølgaard-Nielsen and Hviid 2011). The authors reported a slight but not significant increase in the risk of birth defects in infants given topiramate (4.6%) compared with unexposed infants (2.4%). Topiramate is a carbonic anhydrase inhibitor, resulting in lower serum bicarbonate. A significant drop in bicarbonate can cause metabolic acidosis (Mirza et al. 2011). Serum bicarbonate levels of less than 20 mmol/L are considered abnormal and warrant periodic checking. In a sample of 55 adults treated with topiramate for seizures (mean dosage = 300 mg/day; mean duration = 1,490 days), Mirza et al. (2011) reported that 29% of these subjects had low serum bicarbonate levels. Although neither daily dose nor duration of treatment predicted low bicarbonate levels, test results from this study suggest renal tubular acidosis. Indeed, the investigators observed an association between the occurrence of acidosis and a specific carbonic anhydrase isoform in the renal tubule. Renal tubular acidosis may also play a role in the development of kidney stones. In the trial by Jankovic et al. (2010), one subject taking topiramate had a kidney stone during the trial.

Behavioral Treatments

Beginning with the observation that haloperidol could reduce the severity of tics in TS, researchers have been attempting to find medications that are effective and tolerable in this population. As suggested by the results presented in Table 8–2, however, the empirical support for any medication is limited. This state of affairs has prompted renewed interest in behavioral interventions for tics. Two recent federally funded multisite trials provide solid empirical support for a behavioral intervention built on habit reversal training. The first trial included 126 children ages 9–17 who were randomly assigned to a comprehensive behavioral intervention for tics (CBIT) or supportive psychotherapy for 10 weeks. Outcomes were assessed by a rater who was blind to treatment assignment. After 10 weeks of treatment, the CBIT group showed a decrease from 24.7±6.23 to 17.1±7.83 on the YGTSS Total Tic score, compared with 24.6±5.95 at baseline to 21.1±7.69 at endpoint for the control group (treatment effect 4.1) (Piacentini et al. 2010). In the second trial, 122 subjects ages 16–65 years were evaluated in a trial with the same design. In the adult study, the CBIT group showed a decrease from 24.0±6.5 to 17.8±7.3 on the YGTSS Total Tic score compared with 21.8±6.6 at baseline to 19.3±7.4 at endpoint for the control group (treatment effect 3.7) (Wilhelm et al. 2012). To date, these trials are the largest RCTs focused on tics in patients with TS. The results raise important questions about the decision to use medication for treating tics in patients with TS. This is especially true for pediatric populations, in whom the treatment effect is similar to that of the drug studies presented in Table 8–2.

Future Directions

Increasingly, medications selected for treatment development should be and likely will be based on clues from the underlying neurobiology of TS. A recent postmortem study reported significantly fewer inhibitory neurons in the globus pallidus of individuals with TS than in normal control subjects (Kataoka et al. 2010). This finding is consistent with a body of evidence of reduced inhibitory control at the level of the globus pallidus in patients with TS. The implications for drug treatment are not yet clear.

Genetic analysis in a high-density family with TS found an association between a mutation in the histamine synthetic pathway and TS (Ercan-Sencicek et al. 2010). Individuals in the family with a mutation that conferred decreased activity of histidine decarboxylase, the enzyme that converts histidine to histamine, were affected with TS. Family members without this mutation were unaffected. Histamine in the CNS appears to have a regulatory control on other neurotransmitters such as dopamine. This finding suggests that lower levels of histamine may play a role in the pathophysiology of TS.

Four histamine receptor subtypes have been identified: H_1, H_2, H_3, and H_4. Of particular interest is the H_3 receptor, which is an autoreceptor that is central to the regulation of histamine and perhaps downstream effects as well (Benarroch 2010). Based on these findings, drugs that modulate central histamine function are of interest for the treatment of TS. No H_3 compounds are on the market at present, but several are in development for various indications (Gemkow et al. 2009).

Conclusions: Pharmacotherapy for Tics

For children and adolescents with mild tics, medications aimed at reducing tics may not be necessary. For children who have tics that are frequent and forceful, and that interfere with activities of daily living, medication is likely to be indicated. The goal of medication treatment should be to reduce, not eliminate, the tics. The antipsychotic medications haloperidol, pimozide, risperidone, ziprasidone, and fluphenazine appear to be the most effective. Although it is considered effective, haloperidol has fallen out of use because of concerns about short- and long-term adverse effects. Pimozide is effective and generally well tolerated at low dosages, but requires cardiac monitoring and is vulnerable to drug-drug interaction. Risperidone is the best studied of the newer atypical antipsychotics, and is superior to placebo. Despite a lower risk of neurological side effects with risperidone, weight gain is an important clinical concern. Ziprasidone also appears to be effective, but supportive data are limited to one pilot trial. Botulinum toxin may be considered in patients with a single interfering tic. However, treatment guidelines on dose and frequency of injection remain somewhat uncertain. For tics of moderate severity, but not for tics of greater severity, guanfacine or clonidine may also be considered as first-line treatments, given the favorable safety margin of these medications. CBIT requires availability of trained therapists, but it does appear to be a viable alternative to medication for tic reduction.

Treatment of Obsessive-Compulsive Disorder in Children With Tourette Syndrome

Diagnosis and Assessment

OCD is characterized by recurrent, unwanted worries; thoughts or impulses (obsessions) that are difficult to dislodge; and/or repetitive behaviors that the person feels driven to perform (compulsions). Many patients report that attempts to resist the performance of compulsions increases anxiety as well as the urge to perform the compulsion. According to DSM-IV-TR, the obsessions or compulsions must expend at least an hour per day and be the source of distress or impairment. Adolescents and adults with OCD acknowledge that their obsessions or compulsions are excessive. This realization may not be present in younger children.

The lifetime prevalence of OCD is estimated to be 2%–3% in adults (Karno et al. 1988), with similar estimates in adolescents (Valleni-Basile et al. 1994). The prevalence in preadolescents, however, appears to be lower, with estimates in the range of 2/1,000 in children under age 13 years (Costello et al. 1996).

Common obsessions in children and adolescents include contamination worries, fears about harm coming to self or family members, worry about acting on unwanted aggressive impulses, and concern about order and symmetry (Scahill et al. 2003a). Although many children and adolescents report that their obsessions come "out of the blue," careful discussion usually reveals that the obsessive worries occur in specific events and situations. Common compulsions include hand washing, cleaning rituals, repetitive requests for reassurance about disease or harm, arranging objects in patterns, checking, counting, and repeating routine activities (e.g., opening and closing a door, going back and forth across a doorway). In many cases, a close relationship exists between the obsession and the repetitive behavior, as exemplified by fears of contamination and hand washing. By contrast, other patients state that a ritual is done to achieve a sense of completion. In either model, the ritual is associated with at least a temporary relief in anxiety, which reinforces the compulsive habit.

In the assessment of children with tic disorders and OCD, it may be difficult to distinguish between tics and compulsive behaviors. For example, some children may describe a recurring concern that "something bad will happen" if a specific touching ritual is not completed. Another child may perform a similar-appearing ritual but will describe a need or an urge to carry out the behavior in response to an urge that is not related to a fear. This description often sounds similar to satisfying the premonitory sensations preceding tic. Children with these behaviors, who are driven by a sensation or urge, will often describe a need to "get it right" or achieve a sense of completion. In milder cases, the ritual achieves its aim quickly and the child moves on without much notice. In more severe cases, the child gets caught in multiple repetitions, seemingly unable to achieve a sense of completion. Still other children may describe experiences that contain a mixture of "just right" elements and harm reduction. In a series of 80 children and adolescents, we observed differences in the OCD symptom picture according to the presence or absence of chronic tics (Scahill et al. 2003a). Children with OCD without tics tend to perform rituals to prevent harm. By contrast, children with chronic tics and OCD appear to carry out repetitive behaviors to achieve a sense of completion rather than harm reduction. These findings suggest that assessment should consider the events and situations that are associated with the ritualized behaviors and what seems to drive the repetitive behavior—harm reduction or a sense of the need to achieve completion.

Another type of repetitive urge and behavioral sequence warrants mention. Some children describe an intense urge to touch potentially harmful objects such as a flame, the tip of a knife, or a hot stove. These urges and the actions that may follow are probably best viewed as impulsive behaviors rather than compulsive behaviors and do not arise from self-injurious intent. Children may be reluctant to describe these urges, but upon careful inquiry, they may admit to feeling some relief to learn that others have had such experiences.

Several clinician ratings, self-reports, and parent reports have been developed for assessing obsessive-compulsive symptoms in children with TS. A commonly used clinician rating is the Children's Yale-Brown Obsessive Compulsive Scale (CY-BOCS) (Scahill et al. 1997), which was derived from the original adult instrument, the Yale-Brown Obsessive Compulsive Scale (Y-BOCS; Goodman et al. 1989). The CY-BOCS rates time spent, interference, distress, level of resistance and degree of control over the obsessions and compulsions. The CY-BOCS interview may also assist with charting the phenomenology of the obsessive-compulsive symptoms.

Pharmacotherapy of Obsessive-Compulsive Disorder in Tourette Syndrome

Ironically, most randomized controlled trials of serotonin reuptake inhibitors (SRIs) in children and adolescents with OCD have excluded subjects with TS. In addition, some evidence in children and adults suggests that tic-related OCD may be a distinct subtype of OCD (Leckman et al. 1995; Scahill et al. 2003a). Thus, it is not at all clear that SRIs will be effective in children and adolescents with tic-related OCD.

Before treatment with an SRI is initiated for repetitive behavior in a child with TS, a careful inventory of the repetitive behaviors, including the differentiation of rituals from tics, as well as documentation of the impairment, is warranted. As in the treatment of children with OCD who do not have TS, the medication should be started at a low dosage, and the dosage should be increased slowly, with attention to therapeutic and adverse effects. Children treated with clomipramine need an ECG to assess heart rate and QTc interval prior to starting treatment, during dose adjustment, and when the maintenance dosage is achieved, as well as annually thereafter. Parents need to be educated about the potential for drug interaction and encouraged to call before starting any concomitant treatment while the patient is taking clomipramine. (For a more detailed description of OCD treatment, see Chapter 4, "Anxiety Disorders.")

Treatment of ADHD in Children With Tourette Syndrome

Diagnosis and Assessment

ADHD is characterized by the early-childhood onset of an enduring pattern of inattention and/or hyperactivity and impulsive behavior (American Psychiatric Association 2000). Establishing the diagnosis of ADHD to measure symptom severity in children and adolescents requires information from parents, teachers, and the child. The use of multiple informants is necessary to show that the behavioral pattern is consistent across settings. Clinic observation is also important, but some children are able to maintain behavioral control during a clinic visit. ADHD affects 2%–10% of school-age children, depending on the definition and sampling methods used (Polanczyk et al. 2007). ADHD affects up to two-thirds of children from TS clinical samples (Centers for Disease Control and Prevention 2009). The presence of ADHD is associated with substantial impairment unrelated to the severity of the tics (Sukhodolsky et al. 2003). Because the symptoms of ADHD, such as impulsiveness, overactivity, disruptiveness, and distractibility, are likely to interfere with family life, peer relationships, and academic progress, aggressive treatment of ADHD in children with TS is warranted.

A practical method of collecting information from multiple informants across settings and measuring change with treatment is through the use of parent and teacher rating scales. The parent and teacher questionnaires developed by Conners (Goyette et al. 1978); the ADHD Rating Scale (DuPaul et al. 1998); and the Swanson, Nolan, and Pelham Version IV (SNAP-IV) rating scale (Swanson et al. 1999) are examples of reliable and valid behavior scales. Each of these scales is scored from 0 (*symptoms not present*) to 3 (*severe*). The

ADHD Rating Scale and the SNAP-IV have one-to-one correspondence to DSM-IV (American Psychiatric Association 1994) symptoms of ADHD. Both scales have also been shown to be sensitive to change with treatment (Michelson et al. 2001; MTA Cooperative Group 1999; Scahill et al. 2001). Based on clinical and population data on the SNAP-IV and the ADHD Rating Scale, an average per item score of 2.0 on these scales is predictive of ADHD. Despite their practical value, these scales cannot be relied upon as the only means of making the diagnosis.

Medications for ADHD

Stimulants

Stimulants are the first-line agents for the treatment of ADHD (MTA Cooperative Group 1999; see Chapter 2, "Attention-Deficit/Hyperactivity Disorder," in this volume). Due to lack of efficacy or adverse effects, stimulants fail in 10%–20% of children with ADHD (Elia et al. 1991; MTA Cooperative Group 1999). Case reports over the past three decades suggest that stimulants may induce the emergence of tics or an increase in preexisting tics in children with ADHD (Erenberg et al. 1985; Golden 1974; Lipkin et al. 1994; Lowe et al. 1982; Riddle et al. 1995; Varley et al. 2001). Two placebo-controlled trials that *excluded* children with tic disorders (Barkley et al. 1992; Borcherding et al. 1990) also reported the emergence of tics in a small percentage of children treated with stimulants.

This body of evidence has had an enormous impact on clinical practice until relatively recently. Three short-term, placebo-controlled studies in children with ADHD and tic disorders reported no significant increase in tics among subjects treated with stimulants compared with those given placebo (Castellanos et al. 1997; Gadow et al. 1995; Tourette Syndrome Study Group 2002). Two naturalistic studies also provide information on the longer-term effects of stimulants in children with TS (Gadow et al. 1999; Law and Schachar 1999). Although most children in these longer-term studies did not show an increase in tics, acute exacerbations did occur in a few children, resulting in discontinuation of the stimulant or addition of a tic-suppressing medication. Taken together, these findings suggest that stimulants should be considered in the treatment of children with ADHD and tics. (For a detailed review on the use of stimulants in children with TS, see Bloch et al. 2009.)

In the 16-week Treatment of ADHD in Children With Tic Disorders (TACT) trial conducted by the Tourette Syndrome Study Group (2002), 136 children with ADHD and a tic disorder were randomly assigned to placebo, clonidine alone, methylphenidate alone, or clonidine plus methylphenidate. Although the effect was modest, tics declined in all active treatment groups. Monotherapy with clonidine or methylphenidate was effective in reducing teacher-rated ADHD symptoms, but the magnitude was small (38% and 36%, respectively, with no correction for placebo) compared with the level of improvement documented for methylphenidate in the multisite Multimodal Treatment of ADHD (MTA) study (56% for the medication-only group) (MTA Cooperative Group 1999). By contrast, subjects randomly assigned to clonidine plus methylphenidate showed a 57% improvement on ADHD outcomes. Compared with dosages given in the MTA study, the dosage of methylphenidate in the TACT study was relatively low (25.7 mg in two divided doses compared with a range of 31–38 mg in three divided doses in the MTA study). The more conservative approach in the TACT study may explain the lower level of improvement observed in the methylphenidate group. The level of improvement for monotherapy with clonidine in this study is consistent with the results of another study using the same design in children with ADHD uncomplicated by tic disorders (Palumbo et al. 2008). Taken together, the results of the TACT trial indicate that methylphenidate can be used safely in children with TS. Given the conservative dosing for methylphenidate in the TACT study, clinicians may decide against the more aggressive approach described in the MTA study. Although the more conservative approach may be associated with a lower magnitude of effect, it may also be associated with a lower likelihood of adverse effects, including tics. For example, in the TACT trial, approximately one-quarter of the subjects in the methylphenidate-only group showed an increase in tics, which was only slightly higher than the rate observed in the placebo group.

Nonstimulants

Various nonstimulant medications have been used in the treatment of children with ADHD, including the selective noradrenergic reuptake inhibitors atomoxetine and desipramine, the novel antidepressant bupropion, α_2-adrenergic agonists, modafinil, and selegiline, as well as clonidine and guanfacine. Table 8–3 shows the starting dose and usual maintenance dosage of nonstimulant medications that have been evaluated in the treatment of ADHD. In this section, we examine the nonstimulants listed in the table that have been evaluated in children with ADHD and a chronic tic disorder (see Chapter 2, "Attention-Deficit/Hyperactivity Disorder," for descriptions of other nonstimulants used in the treatment of ADHD).

Three nonstimulant drugs are now approved by the FDA for the treatment of children with ADHD: extended-release guanfacine, extended-release clonidine, and atomoxetine. Atomoxetine has been shown to be safe and effective in several RCTs in children and adolescents (Kelsey et al. 2004; Michelson et al. 2001, 2002). A large-scale trial conducted by Newcorn et al. (2008) compared atomoxetine ($n = 222$), osmotic-release methylphenidate ($n = 220$), and placebo ($n = 74$). The 516 subjects (ages 6–16 years) were randomly assigned to one of these three groups for 6 weeks. The rate of positive response was significantly higher for both active treatment groups compared with placebo and higher for methylphenidate compared with atomoxetine.

An 18-week, placebo-controlled study by Allen et al. (2005) evaluated the efficacy and safety of atomoxetine in 148 children (mean age = 11.2 years) with ADHD and a chronic tic disorder. Atomoxetine resulted in a 28% improvement on a clinician-rated measure of ADHD symptoms compared with 14% for placebo. This level of improvement in ADHD symptoms is similar to but slightly lower than that seen with guanfacine, clonidine, and desipramine in this population. At endpoint there was no difference in tic severity across the atomoxetine and placebo groups, suggesting that atomoxetine neither improves nor worsens tics. The adverse effects in this study were also similar to reports on atomoxetine in children with ADHD. Nausea, vomiting, decreased appetite, and weight loss were significantly more frequent in the atomoxetine group than the placebo group. Insomnia, which has been reported in other pediatric ADHD studies, was no different from placebo in this study.

The tricyclic antidepressant desipramine has been used in the treatment of ADHD for over two decades. Placebo-controlled trials in the 1980s and 1990s showed that it was effective for the treatment of ADHD in children without co-occurring tic disorders (Biederman et al. 1989) and in children with ADHD and tic disorders (Singer et al. 1995). Spencer et al. (2002) conducted a 6-week, placebo-controlled study in 41 children with ADHD and a chronic tic disorder. At total daily doses averaging 3.4 mg/kg given in two divided doses,

Table 8–3.   Dosing guidelines for nonstimulant medications used in the treatment of children with tics and attention-deficit/hyperactivity disorder (ADHD)

Medication[a]	Starting dose (mg)	Usual dosage range (mg/day)	Placebo-controlled trial?	
			ADHD[b]	ADHD + tics[c]
Atomoxetine	18–25	36–100	Yes	Yes
Bupropion	25–50	75–150	Yes	No
Clonidine	0.025–0.05	0.2–0.3	Yes	Yes
Clonidine ER	0.1	0.2–0.3	Yes	No
Guanfacine	0.25–0.5	2–3	No	Yes
Guanfacine ER	1	2–4	Yes	No
Modafinil	50–100	200–400	Yes	No
Pindolol	5–10	15–40	Yes	No
Selegiline	5	5–10	No	Yes

Note.   ER = extended release.
[a]Desipramine is not listed, having fallen out of use due to concerns about QTc prolongation.
[b]Children with ADHD without a tic disorder.
[c]Children with ADHD plus a chronic tic disorder.

desipramine was superior to placebo on an ADHD symptom rating scale. The desipramine group improved by 42%, compared with little change in the placebo group. Tics improved by 30% on average in the desipramine group, compared with no change in the placebo group. Adverse effects included decreased appetite, insomnia, and dry mouth. The investigators detected a significant increase in pulse and blood pressure in the desipramine group, but no abnormalities on ECG. Despite these overall positive results, desipramine is falling out of use because of concerns about prolonged cardiac conduction times and reports of sudden death.

Selegiline is a selective monoamine oxidase inhibitor that directly enhances dopamine function in the brain. In addition, it is metabolized to an amphetamine compound in the brain, which may further enhance central catecholamine function. To date, there are two controlled studies of selegiline in children with ADHD. In the first study, Mohammadi et al. (2004) compared selegiline with methylphenidate in a double-blind, randomized trial involving 40 children with ADHD without co-occurring tics. The subjects were ages 6–15 years. After 60 days of treatment at a maximum total daily dose of 40 mg of methylphenidate or 10 mg of selegiline (both dispensed in two divided doses), there was a 54% decrease in the teacher rating for those taking methylphenidate and a 50% improvement for those taking selegiline. Results on parent ratings were slightly more favorable for both medications than were teacher ratings. Headache and decreased appetite were more frequent in the methylphenidate group; otherwise, both medications were well tolerated.

In the other study, Feigin et al. (1996) studied selegiline in 24 children with TS and ADHD using a double-blind, crossover design. Subjects were randomly assigned to receive either selegiline followed by placebo, or placebo followed by selegiline. Despite the 6-week washout between phases, the study design poses serious problems to the interpretation of the results. First, over one-third of the sample dropped out of the study. Second, there was a clear order effect, in that the subjects who received selegiline first showed benefit compared with placebo. By contrast, the subjects who received selegiline second actually showed a mean worsening of ADHD symptoms. Overall, selegiline was no better than placebo. However, a secondary analysis showed a significant effect for selegiline in the first phase. There was no apparent impact of selegiline on tics. Selegiline appears to be well tolerated. At low dosages, there are no dietary restrictions with selegiline, and drug interaction is not a major concern. However, given the inconsistent results to date, more study is needed to demonstrate its efficacy for ADHD symptoms.

The α_2-adrenergic agonists clonidine and guanfacine are also used to treat children with ADHD and co-occurring tic disorders. Indeed, this class of medications is perhaps the most commonly used for the treatment of tics and ADHD in tic disorder clinics (Freeman et al. 2000). Although some evidence suggests that clonidine and guanfacine can reduce tics (Leckman et al. 1991; Scahill et al. 2001), these drugs are more often used in the treatment of ADHD in children who also have a tic disorder. The use of clonidine in children with tic disorders has been evaluated in a number of small studies (e.g., Hunt et al. 1985). The randomized, placebo-controlled trial of desipramine by Singer et al. (1995) involving 34 children also included a clonidine arm in the crossover design. In that study, clonidine was deemed no better than placebo.

As noted earlier, the Tourette Syndrome Study Group (2002) conducted a multisite, randomized trial with four groups: clonidine alone, methylphenidate alone, clonidine plus methylphenidate, and placebo. The clonidine-alone group showed a 40% improvement on the 10-item Conners Abbreviated Symptom Questionnaire—Teacher compared with 38% for the methylphenidate group and 59% for combined treatment. The combined treatment with clonidine and methylphenidate also attenuated side effects associated with each monotherapy. For example, sedation was less of a problem with the combined treatment than with clonidine only, and insomnia was less of a problem with combined treatment than with methylphenidate only.

Adverse effects of clonidine include sedation, dry mouth, headache, irritability, and mid-sleep awakening. Blood pressure and pulse should be measured at baseline and monitored during dose adjustment, although blood pressure is generally not a problem with clonidine. Nonetheless, patients and families should be educated about the potential for rebound increases in blood pressure, tics, and anxiety with abrupt discontinuation (Leckman et al. 1986).

An extended-release formulation of clonidine was approved by the FDA for the treatment of ADHD in late 2010. This product comes in 0.1-mg and 0.2-mg tablets. As with many other extended-release compounds, this product cannot be crushed or cut in half. The manufacturer recommends that this formulation should be given on a twice-daily schedule (morning and night). The product is approved as monotherapy for ADHD or for use in combination with a stimulant at dosages ranging from 0.2 to 0.4 mg/day in divided doses. Results of two clinical trials are summarized on the FDA Web site (www.accessdata.fda.gov/drugsatfda_docs/label/2010/022331s001s002lbl. pdf). Common adverse effects included sedation, fatigue, sleep disturbance, and irritability. Hypotension and bradycardia appeared to be dose dependent, with both occurring more often in the 0.4-mg/day dosage level. However, these complaints rarely led to treatment discontinuation.

Guanfacine is another α_2-adrenergic agonist that entered into clinical practice in the mid-1990s. Interest in guanfacine emerged following animal studies showing that it may be more specific in its action (see Arnsten and Li 2005 for a review). Traditionally, the α_2 agonists were presumed to enhance prefrontal function by decreasing the firing of presynaptic noradrenergic receptors in the locus coeruleus. This reduced firing by locus coeruleus neurons regulates norepinephrine function and decreases arousal. It is now clear that guanfacine has direct effects on prefrontal function by mimicking norepinephrine at α_2 receptors in this region. This pharmacological effect appears to explain the improvements in distractibility, impulsiveness, and overactivity (Arnsten and Li 2005). Two placebo-controlled trials of immediate-release guanfacine in TS populations have been reported (Cummings et al. 2002; Scahill et al. 2001). Guanfacine was associated with a 30% decrease in tics from baseline in both studies. However, these results are difficult to interpret because tic severity at baseline was mild in both of these trials. Whether guanfacine would be effective for the treatment of moderate-to-severe tics remains unanswered.

In a randomized, placebo-controlled trial, Scahill et al. (2001) evaluated 34 children, ages 7–14 years, with ADHD and a chronic tic disorder. After 8 weeks of treatment with dosages ranging from 1.5 to 3.0 mg/day given in three divided doses, the guanfacine group showed 37% improvement on the teacher-rated ADHD Rating Scale, compared with 8% for the placebo group. Sedation led to discontinuation by only one subject. Other adverse effects included a slight drop in mean blood pressure and pulse and mid-sleep awakening in a few subjects. The thrice-daily dosing may have been protective against hypotensive effects by minimizing the fluctuation of the medication level across the day. For example, in a case series of 200 children from a TS clinic who were treated with guanfacine, four subjects had syncopal episodes (King et al. 2006). In this case series, guanfacine was administered in a single bedtime dose. A review by Scahill et al. (2006) indicated that cardiac monitoring with routine ECGs is not necessary when treating children with clonidine or guanfacine. Clearly, blood pressure and pulse should be monitored during dose adjustment and during the maintenance phase.

An extended-release formulation of guanfacine was approved for the treatment of ADHD in 2009. This approval was supported by two large-scale trials that compared multiple fixed doses of extended-release guanfacine with placebo (Biederman et al. 2008; Sallee et al. 2009b). In the 5-week trial by Biederman et al. (2008), 345 subjects, ages 6–17 years, were randomly assigned to 2-, 3-, or 4-mg doses of extended-release guanfacine or placebo. Subjects assigned to active medication started by taking 1 mg per day. The dose was then increased weekly in 1-mg increments until the randomly assigned dose was achieved. All active doses were superior to placebo. Given the short duration of the trial and the fixed-dose strategy, subjects taking the 3- and 4-mg doses were observed on the assigned dose for only 2–3 weeks, making it difficult to interpret the results. The trial by Sallee et al. (2009b) used a similar design and also provided limited information on the optimal dose. These trials have established the short-term safety and efficacy of extended-release guanfacine in children with ADHD. The optimal dose, however, remains somewhat uncertain. In both trials, the percentage decline in symptom severity was similar across the dose range (e.g., 1–4 mg/day). Examination of the weight-adjusted dose suggests that 0.05–0.08 mg/kg/day can be used as a target dose.

Sallee et al. (2009a) enrolled 259 subjects in a 2-year open-label trial of extended-release guanfacine; 206 of the subjects were given guanfacine monotherapy, and 53 were given guanfacine plus stimulant. The report indicates that approximately half the subjects remained in the study for about 1 year, but less than one-fourth of the subjects (60 of 259) completed the 2-year study. Although the reasons for study exit varied and were not always clear, only 31 subjects (12%) exited because of adverse events. Sedation and fatigue were common complaints, occurring in over half the sample treated with guanfacine monotherapy. Among the 53 subjects (20%) who were given a stimulant, however, sedation or fatigue was reported in 11% of cases. These complaints were more common early in treatment and often resolved with dose adjustment. A meaningful drop in blood pressure (e.g., diastolic reading 50 mmHg or lower for children ages 6–12 years) was observed in about a quarter of the sample. However, syncope was rare, occurring in approximately 2% of the sample. Bradycardia (heart rate of 50 or lower) occurred in 15 subjects. Twenty-one subjects showed a 30- to 60-msec increase in QTc, but no subject exceeded the QTc threshold of 480 msec.

Spencer et al. (2009) added extended-release guanfacine to ongoing treatment with methylphenidate ($n=42$) or amphetamine ($n=33$) in 75 subjects (ages 6–17 years) in a 6-week open-label trial. Subjects were selected because they achieved only a partial response to monotherapy with a stimulant. The added guanfacine dose was started at 1 mg/day, with flexible dosing thereafter, up to 4 mg/day as tolerated. The mean dose of extended-release guanfacine was 3 mg (weight-adjusted 0.07 mg/kg/day) at the end of the 6-week trial. On average, the addition of guanfacine resulted in 50% decline on the ADHD Rating Scale score. The group taking methylphenidate appeared to show greater benefit than the group taking amphetamine. The most common adverse events were sedation and fatigue, which occurred in over half the sample. Five subjects withdrew due to adverse effects; one withdrawal was due to marked fatigue, but the other four were not specified. Measurable decreases in blood pressure occurred in 20 subjects. Of these, 15 events occurred in subjects taking the 4-mg/day dose. No syncope or clinically meaningful changes on measures of cardiac conduction were reported.

Conclusions: Pharmacotherapy of ADHD in Tourette Syndrome

Atomoxetine and the α_2-adrenergic agonists are rational choices for the treatment of ADHD in children with chronic tic disorders, especially if an adequate stimulant trial has been unsuccessful. The α_2 agonists may also be used in combination with stimulants. For patients with prominent tics at baseline or for families who decline treatment with a stimulant, the α_2 agonists may also be a rational alternative.

Theoretical and practical reasons exist for selecting guanfacine over clonidine for treatment of ADHD, but the evidence does not clearly favor one of the α_2 agonists over the other. Extended-release formulations of guanfacine and clonidine have been approved for the treatment of ADHD, and a period of trial and error in the clinic is likely needed, especially given the short duration and fixed-dose designs of these pivotal trials. This approval includes the use of these new formulations in combination with stimulants. Because of their relative safety, the α_2 agonists can also be considered as a first-line treatment for tics independent of ADHD, although the evidence supporting this approach is not strong. The findings with selegiline for the treatment of ADHD in children with TS are inconclusive.

Clinical Pearls

- Advise patients and their families that Tourette syndrome is frequently associated with ADHD, obsessive-compulsive symptoms, and anxiety.
- Consider education to be the first-line treatment for tics in children with Tourette syndrome.
- Remember that pharmacotherapy specifically targeted at reducing tics may not be needed for children and adolescents with mild tics.
- Consider psychostimulants, particularly methylphenidate, as a treatment option for children with ADHD and tics.

- Consider referring patients with tics for behavioral intervention based on habit reversal training.

References

Abuzzahab FS, Brown VL: Control of Tourette's syndrome with topiramate. Am J Psychiatry 158:968, 2001

Allen AJ, Kurlan RM, Gilbert DL, et al: Atomoxetine treatment in children and adolescents with ADHD and comorbid tic disorders. Neurology 65:1941–1949, 2005

Allison DB, Casey DE: Antipsychotic-induced weight gain: a review of the literature. J Clin Psychiatry 62:22–31, 2001

Aman MG, Arnold LE, McDougle CJ, et al: Acute and long-term safety and tolerability of risperidone in children with autism. J Child Adolesc Psychopharmacol 15:869–884, 2005

American Psychiatric Association: Diagnostic and Statistical Manual of Mental Disorders, 3rd Edition. Washington, DC, American Psychiatric Association, 1980

American Psychiatric Association: Diagnostic and Statistical Manual of Mental Disorders, 3rd Edition, Revised. Washington, DC, American Psychiatric Association, 1987

American Psychiatric Association: Diagnostic and Statistical Manual of Mental Disorders, 4th Edition. Washington, DC, American Psychiatric Association, 1994

American Psychiatric Association: Diagnostic and Statistical Manual of Mental Disorders, 4th Edition, Text Revision. Washington, DC, American Psychiatric Association, 2000

Arnsten AF, Li BM: Neurobiology of executive functions: catecholamine influences on prefrontal cortical functions. Biol Psychiatry 57:1377–1384, 2005

Awaad Y, Michon AM, Minarik S: Use of levetiracetam to treat tics in children and adolescents with Tourette's syndrome. Mov Disord 20:714–718, 2005

Barkley RA, McMurray MB, Edelbrock CS, et al: Side effects of methylphenidate in children with attention deficit hyperactivity disorder: a systematic, placebo-controlled evaluation. Pediatrics 86:184–192, 1992

Benarroch EE: Histamine in the CNS: multiple functions and potential neurologic implications. Neurology 75:1472–1479, 2010

Biederman J, Baldessarini RJ, Wright V, et al: A double-blind placebo controlled study of desipramine in the treatment of ADD, I: efficacy. J Am Acad Child Adolesc Psychiatry 28:777–784, 1989

Biederman J, Melmed RD, Patel A, et al: A randomized, double-blind, placebo-controlled study of guanfacine extended release in children and adolescents with attention-deficit/hyperactivity disorder. Pediatrics 121:E73–E84, 2008

Blair J, Scahill L, State M, et al: Electrocardiographic changes in children and adolescents treated with ziprasidone: a prospective study. J Am Acad Child Adolesc Psychiatry 44:73–79, 2005

Bloch MH, Peterson BS, Scahill L, et al: Adulthood outcome of tic and obsessive-compulsive symptom severity in children with Tourette's syndrome. Arch Pediatr Adolesc Med 160:65–69, 2006

Bloch MH, Panza KE, Landeros-Weisenberger A, et al: Meta-analysis: treatment of attention-deficit/hyperactivity disorder in children with comorbid tic disorders. J Am Acad Child Adolesc Psychiatry 48:884–893, 2009

Borcherding BG, Keysor CS, Rapoport JL, et al: Motor/vocal tics and compulsive behaviors on stimulant drugs: is there a common vulnerability? Psychiatry Res 33:83–94, 1990

Bruggeman R, van der Linden C, Buitelaar GS, et al: Risperidone versus pimozide in Tourette's syndrome: a comparative double-blind parallel group study. J Clin Psychiatry 62:50–56, 2001

Budman CL, Gayer A, Lesser M, et al: An open-label study of the treatment efficacy of olanzapine for Tourette's disorder. J Clin Psychiatry 62:290–294, 2001

Caine ED, Polinsky RJ, Kartzinel R, et al: The trial use of clozapine for abnormal involuntary disorders. Am J Psychiatry 136:317–320, 1979

Castellanos FX, Giedd JN, Elia J: Controlled stimulant treatment of ADHD and comorbid Tourette's syndrome: effects of stimulant and dose. J Am Acad Child Adolesc Psychiatry 36:589–596, 1997

Centers for Disease Control and Prevention: Prevalence of diagnosed Tourette syndrome in persons aged 6–17 years—United States, 2007. MMWR Morb Mortal Wkly Rep 58:581–585, 2009

Costello EJ, Angold A, Burns BJ, et al: The Great Smoky Mountains Study of Youth: goals, design, methods, and the prevalence of DSM-III-R disorders. Arch Gen Psychiatry 53:1129–1136, 1996

Cummings DD, Singer HS, Krieger M, et al: Neuropsychiatric effects of guanfacine in children with mild Tourette's syndrome: a pilot study. Clin Neuropharmacol 25:325–332, 2002

Desta Z, Kerbusch T, Flockhart DA: Effect of clarithromycin on the pharmacokinetics and pharmacodynamics of pimozide in healthy poor and extensive metabolizers of cytochrome P450 2D6 (CYP2D6). Clin Pharmacol Ther 65:10–20, 1999

Dion Y, Annable L, Sandor P, et al. Risperidone in the treatment of Tourette's syndrome: a double-blind, placebo-controlled trial. J Clin Psychopharmacol 22:31–39, 2002

DuPaul GJ, Power TJ, McGoey KE, et al: Reliability and validity of parent and teacher ratings of attention-deficit/hyperactivity disorder symptoms. Journal of Psychoeducation Assessment 16:55–68, 1998

Elia J, Borcherding BG, Rapoport JL, et al: Methylphenidate and dextroamphetamine treatments of hyperactivity: are there true non-responders? Psychiatry Res 36:141–155, 1991

Ercan-Sencicek AG, Stillman AA, Ghosh AK, et al: L-histidine decarboxylase and Tourette's syndrome. N Engl J Med 362:1901–1908, 2010

Erenberg G, Cruse RP, Rothner AD: Gilles de la Tourette's syndrome: effects of stimulant drugs. Neurology 35:1346–1348, 1985

Feigin A, Kurlan R, McDermott MP, et al: A controlled trial of deprenyl in children with Tourette's syndrome and attention deficit hyperactivity disorder. Neurology 46:965–968, 1996

Freeman RD, Fast DK, Burd L, et al: An international perspective on Tourette's syndrome: selected findings from 3,500 individuals in 22 countries. Dev Med Child Neurol 42:436–447, 2000

Frey KA, Albin RL: Neuroimaging of Tourette's syndrome. J Child Neurol 21:672–677, 2006

Gadow KD, Sverd J, Sprafkin J, et al: Efficacy of methylphenidate for attention-deficit hyperactivity disorder in children with tic disorder. Arch Gen Psychiatry 52:444–455, 1995

Gadow KD, Sverd J, Sprafkin J, et al: Long-term methylphenidate therapy in children with comorbid attention-deficit hyperactivity disorder and chronic multiple tic disorder. Arch Gen Psychiatry 56:330–336, 1999

Gaffney GR, Perry PJ, Lund BC, et al: Risperidone versus clonidine in the treatment of children and adolescents with Tourette's syndrome. J Am Acad Child Adolesc Psychiatry 41:330–336, 2002

Gemkow MJ, Davenport AJ, Harich S, et al: The histamine H3 receptor as a therapeutic drug target for CNS disorders. Drug Discov Today 14:509–515, 2009

Gilbert DL, Batterson JR, Sethuraman G, et al: Tic reduction with risperidone versus pimozide in a randomized, double-blind, crossover trial. J Am Acad Child Adolesc Psychiatry 43:206–214, 2004

Goetz CG, Tanner CM, Klawans HL: Fluphenazine and multifocal tic disorders. Arch Neurol 41:271–272, 1984

Golden GS: Gilles de la Tourette's syndrome following methylphenidate administration. Dev Med Child Neurol 16:76–78, 1974

Goodman WK, Price LH, Rasmussen SA, et al: The Yale-Brown Obsessive Compulsive Scale, II: validity. Arch Gen Psychiatry 46:1012–1016, 1989

Goyette CH, Conners CK, Ulrich RF: Normative data on revised Conners Parent and Teacher Rating Scales. J Abnorm Child Psychol 6:221–236, 1978

Hedderick EF, Morris CM, Singer HS: Double-blind, crossover study of clonidine and levetiracetam in Tourette syndrome. Pediatr Neurol 40:420–425, 2009

Hoekstra PJ, Minderaa RB, Kallenberg CG: Lack of effect of intravenous immunoglobulins on tics: a double-blind placebo-controlled study. J Clin Psychiatry 65:537–542, 2004

Hunt RD, Minderaa RB, Cohen DJ: Clonidine benefits children with attention deficit disorder and hyperactivity: report of a double-blind placebo-crossover therapeutic trial. J Am Acad Child Psychiatry 24:617–629, 1985

Jankovic J: Botulinum toxin in the treatment of dystonic tics. Mov Disord 9:347–349, 1994

Jankovic J: Treatment of hyperkinetic movement disorders. Lancet Neurol 8:844–856, 2009

Jankovic J, Kurlan R: Tourette syndrome: evolving concepts. Mov Disord 26:1149–1156, 2011

Jankovic J, Jimenez-Shahed J, Brown LW: A randomised, double-blind, placebo-controlled study of topiramate in the treatment of Tourette syndrome. J Neurol Neurosurg Psychiatry 81:70–73, 2010

Karno M, Golding JM, Sorenson SB, et al: The epidemiology of obsessive-compulsive disorder in five US communities. Arch Gen Psychiatry 45:1094–1098, 1988

Kataoka Y, Kalanithi PS, Grantz H, et al: Decreased number of parvalbumin and cholinergic interneurons in the striatum of individuals with Tourette syndrome. J Comp Neurol 518:277–291, 2010

Kelsey DK, Sumner CR, Casat CD, et al: Once-daily atomoxetine treatment for children with attention-deficit/hyperactivity disorder, including an assessment of evening and morning behavior: a double-blind, placebo-controlled trial. Pediatrics 114:E1–E8, 2004

King A, Harris P, Fritzell J, et al: Syncope in children with Tourette's syndrome treated with guanfacine. Mov Disord 21:419–420, 2006

Kwak CH, Hanna PA, Jankovic J: Botulinum toxin in the treatment of tics. Arch Neurol 57:1190–1193, 2000

Law SF, Schachar RJ: Do typical clinical doses of methylphenidate cause tics in children treated for attention-deficit hyperactivity disorder? J Am Acad Child Adolesc Psychiatry 38:944–951, 1999

Leckman JF, Ort S, Caruso KA, et al: Rebound phenomena in Tourette's syndrome after abrupt withdrawal of clonidine. Arch Gen Psychiatry 43:1168–1176, 1986

Leckman JF, Riddle MA, Hardin MT, et al: The Yale Global Tic Severity Scale: initial testing of a clinician-rated scale of tic severity. J Am Acad Child Adolesc Psychiatry 28:566–573, 1989

Leckman JF, Hardin MT, Riddle MA, et al: Clonidine treatment of Gilles de la Tourette's syndrome. Arch Gen Psychiatry 48:324–328, 1991

Leckman JF, Walker DE, Cohen DJ: Premonitory urges in Tourette's syndrome. Am J Psychiatry 150:98–102, 1993

Leckman JF, Grice DE, Barr LC, et al: Tic-related vs. non-tic-related obsessive compulsive disorder. Anxiety 1:208–215, 1995

Lin H, Yeh CB, Peterson BS, et al: Assessment of symptom exacerbations in a longitudinal study of children with Tourette's syndrome or obsessive-compulsive disorder. J Am Acad Child Adolesc Psychiatry 41:1070–1077, 2002

Lipkin PH, Goldstein IJ, Adesman AR: Tics and dyskinesias associated with stimulant treatment in attention-deficit hyperactivity disorder. Arch Pediatr Adolesc Med 148:859–861, 1994

Lowe TL, Cohen DJ, Detlor J, et al: Stimulant medications precipitate Tourette's syndrome. JAMA 26:1729–1731, 1982

Lyon GJ, Samar S, Jummani R, et al: Aripiprazole in children and adolescents with Tourette's disorder: an open-label safety and tolerability study. J Child Adolesc Psychopharmacol 19:623–33, 2009

Marras C, Andrews D, Sime E, et al: Botulinum toxin for simple motor tics: a randomized, double-blind, controlled clinical trial. Neurology 56:605–610, 2001

Meyer JM, Koro CE: The effects of antipsychotic therapy on serum lipids: a comprehensive review. Schizophr Res 70:1–17, 2004

Michelson D, Faries D, Wernicke J, et al: Atomoxetine in the treatment of children and adolescents with attention-deficit/hyperactivity disorder: a randomized, placebo-controlled, dose-response study. Pediatrics 108:E83, 2001

Michelson D, Allen AJ, Busner J, et al: Once-daily atomoxetine treatment for children and adolescents with attention deficit hyperactivity disorder: a randomized, placebo-controlled study. Am J Psychiatry 159:1896–1901, 2002

Mink JW: Clinical review of DBS for Tourette syndrome. Front Biosci (Elite Ed) 1:72–76, 2009

Mirza NS, Alfirevic A, Jorgensen A, et al: Metabolic acidosis with topiramate and zonisamide: an assessment of its severity and predictors. Pharmacogenet Genomics 21:297–302, 2011

Mohammadi MR, Ghanizadeh A, Alaghband-Rad J, et al: Selegiline in comparison with methylphenidate in attention deficit hyperactivity disorder children and adolescents in a double-blind, randomized clinical trial. J Child Adolesc Psychopharmacol 14:418–425, 2004

Mølgaard-Nielsen D, Hviid A: Newer-generation antiepileptic drugs and the risk of major birth defects. JAMA 305:1996–2003, 2011

MTA Cooperative Group: A 14-month randomized clinical trial of treatment strategies for attention-deficit/hyperactivity disorder. The MTA Cooperative Group. Multimodal Treatment Study of Children With ADHD. Arch Gen Psychiatry 56:1073–1086, 1999

Mukaddes NM, Abali O: Quetiapine treatment of children and adolescents with Tourette's disorder. J Child Adolesc Psychopharmacol 13:295–299, 2003

Müller-Vahl KR, Schneider U, Prevedel H, et al: Delta 9-tetrahydrocannabinol (THC) is effective in the treatment of tics in Tourette syndrome: a 6-week randomized trial. J Clin Psychiatry 64:459–465, 2003

Newcorn JH, Kratochvil CJ, Allen AJ, et al: Atomoxetine and osmotically released methylphenidate for the treatment of attention deficit hyperactivity disorder: acute comparison and differential response. Am J Psychiatry 165:721–730, 2008

Nicolson R, Craven-Thuss B, Smith J, et al: A randomized, double-blind, placebo-controlled trial of metoclopramide for the treatment of Tourette's disorder. J Am Acad Child Adolesc Psychiatry 44:640–646, 2005

Orth M, Kirby R, Richardson MP, et al: Subthreshold rTMS over pre-motor cortex has no effect on tics in patients with Gilles de la Tourette's syndrome. Clin Neurophysiol 116:764–768, 2005

Palumbo DR, Sallee FR, Pelham WE Jr, et al: Clonidine for attention-deficit/hyperactivity disorder: I. Efficacy and tolerability outcomes. J Am Acad Child Adolesc Psychiatry 47:180–188, 2008

Peterson BS, Staib L, Scahill L, et al: Regional brain and ventricular volumes in Tourette's syndrome. Arch Gen Psychiatry 58:427–440, 2001

Peterson BS, Thomas P, Kane MJ, et al: Basal ganglia volumes in patients with Gilles de la Tourette's syndrome. Arch Gen Psychiatry 60:415–424, 2003

Piacentini J, Woods DW, Scahill L, et al: Behavior therapy for children with Tourette disorder: a randomized controlled trial. JAMA 303:1929–1937, 2010

Polanczyk G, Lima MS, Horta BL, et al: The worldwide prevalence of attention deficit/hyperactivity disorder: a systematic review and meta-regression analyses. Am J Psychiatry 164:942–948, 2007

Porta M, Maggioni G, Ottaviani F, et al: Treatment of phonic tics in patients with Tourette's syndrome using botulinum toxin type A. Neurol Sci 24:420–423, 2004

Riddle MA, Lynch KA, Scahill L, et al: Methylphenidate discontinuation and re-initiation during long-term treatment of children with Tourette's disorder and attention-deficit hyperactivity disorder. J Child Adolesc Psychopharmacol 5:205–214, 1995

Roessner V, Rothenberger A, Rickards H, et al: European clinical guidelines for Tourette Syndrome and other tic disorders. Eur Child Adolesc Psychiatry 20:153–154, 2011

Ross MS, Moldofsky H: A comparison of pimozide and haloperidol in the treatment of Gilles de la Tourette's syndrome. Am J Psychiatry 135:585–587, 1978

Rutter M, Tizard J, Whitmore K: Education, Health, and Behavior. London, Longman, 1970

Sallee FR, Nesbitt L, Jackson C, et al: Relative efficacy of haloperidol and pimozide in children and adolescents with Tourette's disorder. Am J Psychiatry 154:1057–1062, 1997

Sallee FR, Kurlan R, Goetz CG, et al: Ziprasidone treatment of children and adolescents with Tourette's syndrome: a pilot study. J Am Acad Child Adolesc Psychiatry 39:292–299, 2000

Sallee FR, Lyne A, Wigal T, et al: Long-term safety and efficacy of guanfacine extended release in children and adolescents with attention-deficit/hyperactivity disorder. J Child Adolesc Psychopharmacol 19:215–226, 2009a

Sallee FR, McGough J, Wigal T, et al: Guanfacine extended release in children and adolescents with attention deficit-hyperactivity disorder: a placebo controlled trial. J Am Acad Child Adolesc Psychiatry 48:155–165, 2009b

Scahill L, Riddle MA, McSwiggin-Hardin M, et al: Children's Yale-Brown Obsessive Compulsive Scale: reliability and validity. J Am Acad Child Adolesc Psychiatry 36:844–852, 1997

Scahill L, Chappell PB, Kim YS, et al: Guanfacine in the treatment of children with tic disorders and ADHD: a placebo-controlled study. Am J Psychiatry 158:1067–1074, 2001

Scahill L, Kano Y, King RA, et al: Influence of age and tic disorders on obsessive-compulsive disorder in a pediatric sample. J Child Adolesc Psychopharmacol 13(suppl):7–18, 2003a

Scahill L, Leckman JF, Schultz RT, et al: A placebo-controlled trial of risperidone in Tourette's syndrome. Neurology 60:1130–1135, 2003b

Scahill L, Erenberg G, Berlin CM, et al: Contemporary assessment and pharmacotherapy of Tourette's syndrome. NeuroRx 3:192–206, 2006

Scahill L, Specht M, Bradbury K: The Prevalence of TS and Clinical Characteristics in Children: Movement Disorders (in press)

Shapiro AK, Shapiro E: Controlled study of pimozide vs. placebo in Tourette's syndrome. J Am Acad Child Adolesc Psychiatry 23:161–173, 1984

Shapiro E, Shapiro AK, Fulop G, et al: Controlled study of haloperidol, pimozide, and placebo for the treatment of Gilles de la Tourette's syndrome. Arch Gen Psychiatry 46:722–730, 1989

Singer HS, Brown J, Quaskey S, et al: The treatment of attention-deficit hyperactivity disorder in Tourette's syndrome: a double-blind placebo-controlled study with clonidine and desipramine. Pediatrics 95:74–81, 1995

Smith-Hicks CL, Bridges DD, Paynter NP, et al: A double blind randomized placebo control trial of levetiracetam in Tourette syndrome. Mov Disord 22:1764–1770, 2007

Spencer T, Biederman J, Coffey B, et al: A double-blind comparison of desipramine and placebo in children and adolescents with chronic tic disorder and comorbid attention-deficit/hyperactivity disorder. Arch Gen Psychiatry 59:649–656, 2002

Spencer TJ, Greenbaum M, Ginsberg LD, et al: Safety and effectiveness of coadministration of guanfacine extended release and psychostimulants in children and adolescents with attention-deficit/hyperactivity disorder. J Child Adolesc Psychopharmacol 19:501–510, 2009

Stamenkovic M, Schindler SD, Aschauser HN, et al: Effective open-label treatment of Tourette's disorder with olanzapine. Int Clin Psychopharmacol 15:23–28, 2000

Sukhodolsky D, Scahill L, Zhang H, et al: Disruptive behavior in children with Tourette's syndrome: association of ADHD comorbidity, tic severity, and functional impairment. J Am Acad Child Adolesc Psychiatry 42:98–105, 2003

Swanson J, Lerner M, March J, et al: Assessment and intervention for attention-deficit/hyperactivity disorder in the schools: lessons from the MTA study. Pediatr Clin North Am 46:993–1009, 1999

Toren P, Weizman A, Ratner S, et al: Ondansetron treatment in Tourette's disorder: a 3-week, randomized, double-blind, placebo-controlled study. J Clin Psychiatry 66:499–503, 2005

Tourette Syndrome Study Group: Treatment of ADHD in children with tics: a randomized controlled trial. Neurology 58:527–536, 2002

Valleni-Basile LA, Garrison CZ, Jackson KL, et al: Frequency of obsessive-compulsive disorder in a community sample of young adolescents, J Am Acad Child Adolesc Psychiatry 33:782–791, 1994

Varley CK, Vincent J, Varley P, et al: Emergence of tics in children with attention deficit hyperactivity disorder treated with stimulant medications. Compr Psychiatry 42:228–233, 2001

Wang Z, Maia TV, Marsh R, et al: The neural circuits that generate tics in Tourette's syndrome. Am J Psychiatry 168:1326–1337, 2011

Wilhelm S, Peterson AL, Piacentini J, et al: Randomized trial of behavior therapy for adults with Tourette's disorder. Arch Gen Psychiatry 69:795–803, 2012

Woods DW, Piacentini J, Himle MB, et al: Premonitory Urge for Tics Scale (PUTS): initial psychometric results and examination of the premonitory urge phenomenon in youths with tic disorders. J Dev Behav Pediatr 26:397–403, 2005

9

Early Schizophrenia and Psychotic Illnesses

Christopher N. David, B.A.

Nitin Gogtay, M.D.

Judith L. Rapoport, M.D.

By virtually every clinical and neurobiological measure, childhood-onset or very early-onset schizophrenia—defined as the onset of psychotic symptoms before age 13 years—is continuous with the adult disorder. Clinically, childhood-onset schizophrenia (COS) resembles the adult form in its cardinal positive symptoms of hallucinations, delusions, and thought disorder, and the constellation of negative symptoms such as lack of drive and flattened affect. Neurobiologically, it shares many of the same neuroanatomical anomalies, risk genes, and neuropsychological deficits as adult-onset schizophrenia (for a review, see Rapoport et al. 2005b). The disorder is rare, and as is often the case with very early-onset illnesses, psychotic disorders in children are usually more severe than their adult counterparts (Childs and Scriver 1986). COS is thus associated with a particularly severe disruption of cognitive and social development, and the burden to the family can be devastating. The term *early-onset schizophrenia (EOS)* has been used to describe onset before age 18 years (American Academy of Child and Adolescent Psychiatry 2001). Although many studies considered in this chapter include patients with symptom onset during adolescence, we emphasize studies among patients with COS (onset before age 13).

History and Classification of Psychosis in Children

Although the existence of childhood schizophrenia was recognized early in the twentieth century (Kraepelin 1919), the term *psychosis* was used broadly in children, and a spectrum of behavioral disorders and autism were also grouped under the category of childhood schizophrenia (Volkmar 1996). The landmark studies by Kolvin first established the clinical distinction between autism and other psychotic disorders of childhood (Kolvin 1971). Even today, however, high rates of initial misdiagnosis remain due to symptom overlap, particularly for mood disorders, and the presence of relatively fleeting hallucinations and delusions in nonpsychotic pediatric patients, although more recent studies aim to clarify positive phenomena across pediatric populations (Polanczyk et al. 2010). Anxiety and stress are probably the most common causes of hallucinations in preschool children, and the prognosis of these phenomena is usually benign. On the other hand, psychotic phenomena in school-age children are likely to be more persistent and are associated with significantly greater mental illness, particularly within schizophrenia (David and Rapoport 2012; David et al. 2011; Polanczyk et al. 2010). According to data from a large birth cohort, self-reported psychotic symptoms at age 11 predicted a high risk (odds ratio 16.4) of schizophreniform diagnoses by age 26 (Poulton et al. 2000).

A heterogeneous but sizable group of children referred to the National Institute of Mental Health (NIMH) Childhood-Onset Schizophrenia study since 1991 show transient psychotic symptoms and multiple developmental abnormalities that cannot be adequately characterized by existing DSM-IV

(American Psychiatric Association 1994) categories (the diagnosis of psychosis not otherwise specified would probably be made). Therefore, the term *multidimensionally impaired* (MDI) has been used to capture the mix of stress-related transient episodes of psychosis, emotional instability, impaired interpersonal skills, and information-processing deficits exhibited by these children (Frazier et al. 1994; Kumra et al. 1998). Along with children with COS, the children with MDI have been longitudinally followed up and have provided a medication-matched contrast for various clinical and neuroimaging studies. In this chapter, we focus on the rarer form of COS due to the unique psychiatric vantage point provided by this more markedly severe subset of psychosis (Rapoport et al. 2005b).

Epidemiology

Because of the rarity of COS, large-scale epidemiological studies are not feasible. A study of hospital admissions of 312 psychotic youths over a 13-year period in Denmark found only four patients who were younger than age 13 years (Thomsen 1996). Our own experience at the NIMH indicates that most children receiving the diagnosis of schizophrenia do not meet criteria for schizophrenia. After 3,500 screenings, only 250 children have been offered inpatient admission and only 120 patients have received a diagnosis of COS. The next most common diagnosis was mood disorder with psychotic features.

Course and Outcome

Long-term follow-up of EOS cases indicates chronic illness and impairment. Hollis (2000) found that compared with individuals with nonschizophrenic psychoses, a large cohort diagnosed with EOS (mean age at onset = 14 years) had significantly worse outcomes at a mean follow-up of 11 years, as characterized by a chronic illness course and severe impairments in social relationships. An even longer follow-up of 42 years found that earlier age at onset among 44 patients retrospectively meeting diagnostic criteria for COS was associated with a much poorer clinical outcome and high levels of disability (Eggers and Bunk 1997). Greenstein et al. (2006) reported on a prospective follow-up study over a mean of 5 years with 32 children in an NIMH cohort, and noted that despite optimal pharmacotherapy, there was evidence of high levels of disability and residual psychotic symptoms. Data from these various studies suggest a particularly disabling course of illness.

The prognosis of those in the MDI group, on the other hand, is notably improved. A follow-up of 32 MDI patients showed that none developed schizophrenia, but 12 (38%) met the criteria for bipolar I disorder within 2–8 years of follow-up (Gogtay et al. 2007; Nicolson et al. 2001; Stayer et al. 2005).

Rationale for Psychopharmacological Treatment

Patients with EOS typically have a more chronic course of illness, greater cognitive impairment, more negative symptoms, and more severe social consequences than patients with adult-onset schizophrenia (Correll 2010). Although psychosocial interventions are important, the mainstay of treatment is pharmacological treatment, particularly with antipsychotic medication.

Most classifications of antipsychotics divide the medications into typical, or first-generation, antipsychotics and atypical, or second-generation, antipsychotics. The typical antipsychotics are all high-affinity antagonists of dopamine D_2 receptors, a property that remains the most plausible explanation for their therapeutic effects. Dopamine D_2 receptor antagonism also explains, in part, one of the other key features of typical antipsychotics: the high rate of unwanted side effects, particularly extrapyramidal symptoms and tardive dyskinesia (see later section, "Extrapyramidal Side Effects"). Atypical antipsychotics differ pharmacologically from previous antipsychotic agents in their lower affinity for D_2 receptors and greater affinities for other neuroreceptors (Burstein et al. 2005). They are also thought to have lower incidences of extrapyramidal side effects (EPS), tardive dyskinesia, and hyperprolactinemia, although the atypicals vary considerably in their side-effect profiles (Abi-Dargham and Laruelle 2005; Miyamoto et al. 2005; Tajima et al. 2009). In clinical practice, atypical agents have become the treatment of choice for patients with COS. For example, in a review of practices in the United States, the prescription of atypical antipsychotics increased by nearly 500% between 1995 and 2000, and accounted for the majority of antipsychotic prescriptions among children and adolescents (N.C. Patel et al. 2002). Indeed, the ratio of atypical antipsychotics to traditional antipsychotics used is greater for child (2.7:1) and adolescent (3.8:1) patients than for adults (1.6:1) (Sikich et al. 2004).

Pharmacotherapy

In evaluating the efficacy of antipsychotics in patients with COS, we discuss double-blind studies in depth. We include summaries of the larger prospective open trials of atypicals that reflect current practices and share our experience with newer medications. It should be stressed here that antipsychotics have a wide use in childhood disorders and that information about use of both typical and atypical medications is presented throughout this manual.

Typical Antipsychotics

Efficacy of Typical Antipsychotics Versus Placebo in COS

Early studies in EOS addressed the important question of whether antipsychotics have any treatment efficacy through a comparison with placebo (Pool et al. 1976; Spencer et al. 1992) (Table 9–1). In one of the earliest such studies, Pool et al. (1976) conducted a double-blind, placebo-controlled trial comparing haloperidol (mean dosage=9.8 mg/day) with loxapine (mean dosage=87.5 mg/day) and placebo in 75 hospitalized adolescents. All three groups showed significant improvement, as assessed with the Clinical Global Impression (CGI) Scale, although patients rated as severely or very severely ill at baseline showed a trend toward more improvement with the active treatments (88% for loxapine and 72% for haloperidol) than with placebo (38%). This trial had several limitations. First, the criteria for diagnosis of schizophrenia rested on clinical consensus, and it is unclear whether all of these subjects would meet contemporary DSM-IV-TR (American Psychiatric Association 2000) criteria for schizophrenia. The exact age at onset of first symptoms was not given, so not all of the subjects may have had an onset of symptoms by age 13 years, and the degree of prior treatment resistance was also not provided. Despite these caveats, it remains a landmark study establishing the efficacy of typical antipsychotics in COS. Additional trials of typical antipsychotics in EOS are summarized in Table 9–1, alongside the landmark atypical trial of the Treatment of Early Onset Schizophrenia Spectrum Disorders (TEOSS) study (McClellan et al. 2007; Sikich et al. 2008).

Spencer et al. (1992), in a double-blind, placebo-controlled study with a crossover design, randomly assigned 12 children with DSM-III-R (American Psychiatric Association 1987) schizophrenia to receive either haloperidol for 4 weeks followed by placebo for 4 weeks, or placebo for 4 weeks followed by haloperidol for 4 weeks. Most of these subjects likely had at least partially treatment-resistant illness, because most were hospitalized and had prior exposure to psychotropic medications, although exact details of prior antipsychotic response were not given. On the primary outcome measures (CGI) and ratings of positive psychotic symptoms, the haloperidol group alone showed a significant improvement (with a fall from a baseline score of 5.15 to 2.99 in the haloperidol group [$P<0.001$]), with no significant change in the placebo group. The authors note that a relatively small dosage of haloperidol, with a range of 0.5–3.5 mg/day, was optimal.

Comparison of Efficacy of Typical Antipsychotics

Several studies have directly compared the efficacy of two typical antipsychotics in the absence of a placebo wing, including double-blind comparisons of fluphenazine and haloperidol (Engelhardt et al. 1973), thiothixene and thioridazine (Realmuto et al. 1984), and loxapine and haloperidol (Versiani et al. 1977) (see Table 9–1). All studies reported high rates of response (based on the CGI), ranging from 54% to over 90%, and the antipsychotics did not differ significantly from each other on nearly all outcome measures. However, these earlier studies all suffered from the same problem: the criteria used to define schizophrenia were unclear, and change in specific psychotic symptoms was not reported, limiting the applicability to current practice.

Indeed, given current prescribing practices, most comparisons of typical agents are of historical interest. However, the results of the NIMH Clinical Antipsychotic Trials of Intervention Effectiveness (CATIE) project, which demonstrated equal efficacy of the typical perphenazine and four atypical antipsychotics in adults with chronic schizophrenia, may renew interest in the use of typical antipsychotics for psychosis (Lieberman et al. 2005).

Table 9–1. Selected controlled trials of antipsychotics in patients with childhood-onset schizophrenia

Study	Medications	Mean dosage	N	Mean age (years)	Design	Criteria	Response rate
Typical antipsychotics							
Engelhardt et al. 1973	Fluphenazine Haloperidol	10 mg/day 10 mg/day	15 15	10	Randomized, double-blind	CGI *much* or *very much improved*	93% (14/15) 87% (13/15)
Pool et al. 1976	Loxapine Haloperidol Placebo	87.5 mg/day 9.8 mg/day —	26 25 24	15	Randomized, double-blind	CGI *much* or *very much improved*	88% (23/26) 72% (18/25) 38% (9/24)
Versiani et al. 1977	Loxapine Haloperidol	70 mg/day 8 mg/day	25 25	16	Randomized, double-blind	CGI *much* or *very much improved*	64% (16/25) 60% (15/25)
Realmuto et al. 1984	Thiothixene Thioridazine	0.26 mg/kg/day 2.57 mg/kg/day	13 8	15	Randomized, single-blind	CGI *much* or *very much improved*	54% (7/13) 63% (5/8)
Spencer et al. 1992	Haloperidol Placebo	8.8 mg/day —	12 12	9	Randomized, double-blind, crossover	Marked improvement on clinical judgment	75% (9/12) 0% (0/12)
Atypical antipsychotics							
McClellan et al. 2007; Sikich et al. 2008	Olanzapine Risperidone Molindone	2.5–20 mg/day 0.5–6 mg/day 10–140 mg/day (+ 1 mg/day benztropine)	119 (116 treated)	8–19	Randomized, double-blind, parallel-group design at four sites	20% reduction in baseline PANSS scores; marked improvement on CGI as well	34% 46% 50%

Note. CGI=Clinical Global Impression Scale; PANSS=Positive and Negative Syndrome Scale.

Atypical Antipsychotics

Mechanisms of Action

The advent of atypical agents appeared to herald an era of treatment for schizophrenia with the possibility of more efficacious agents and more favorable side-effect profiles (Kane et al. 1988). Several reviews have considered the issue of what makes an atypical agent atypical (e.g., Kapur and Remington 2001). Most agree on a lower risk of EPS and a lack of prolactin level elevation, with some additionally claiming that the atypicals are more effective in ameliorating the negative symptoms of schizophrenia, although this differential effect is likely to be small (with an effect size on the order of 0.1 [Cohen's d]). In terms of pharmacological properties, most atypicals have a higher affinity for serotonin receptors, specifically the 5-HT_{2A} family, and, to a lesser extent, the dopamine D_4 receptor. However, neither property is necessary for atypicality. For example, amisulpride is a relatively pure D_2/D_3 antagonist lacking serotonin receptor antagonism, and several typicals, including haloperidol, have high affinity for D_4 receptors. More recently, it has been proposed that atypical antipsychotics may have a faster rate of dissociation from the D_2 receptor, allowing the drug to be more responsive to endogenous dopamine, thus allowing an antipsychotic effect while avoiding EPS and prolactin elevation. Amato et al. (2011) recently discussed the dynamic dopamine and serotonin responses in both treatment action and failure of such atypicals. Their work highlights specific changes in dopaminergic response and their reversal as a possible fundamental underpinning for the antipsychotic's action and failure, respectively.

Efficacy of Atypical Antipsychotics

Since this book's first edition appeared, olanzapine, risperidone, aripiprazole, and quetiapine have been approved by the U.S. Food and Drug Administration (FDA) for the treatment of children and adolescents ages 13–17 with schizophrenia. In addition, paliperidone has been approved for the treatment of adolescents with schizophrenia as young as age 12. Second-generation antipsychotics, particularly olanzapine, risperidone, and quetiapine, were found to be the most frequently administered medications in a naturalistic longitudinal study of early-onset first psychotic episodes (Castro-Fornieles et al. 2008), and were shown to differ in their side effects but to result in similar clinical improvements. We look at atypicals individually to highlight understandings in their differences and respective strengths.

The peer-reviewed studies discussed in the following subsections complement additional randomized controlled trials (RCTs) sponsored by pharmaceutical and other organizations, all of which provided support for the FDA's approval of olanzapine, risperidone, aripiprazole, and quetiapine for the treatment of children and adolescents ages 13–17 with schizophrenia. As future trials continue to emerge in the literature, the nuances behind the efficacy and advantages of the choice of atypical antipsychotics will become clearer.

Risperidone. A 6-week open-label study of risperidone (mean dosage = 3.14 mg/day) in 11 treatment-naïve adolescents who met DSM-IV criteria for schizophrenia reported significant improvements in ratings on the CGI, Brief Psychiatric Rating Scale (BPRS), and Positive and Negative Syndrome Scale (PANSS) (positive but not negative symptoms) (Zalsman et al. 2003). Another study reported a categorical response rate of 60% (response defined with the CGI) among 10 adolescents (Armenteros et al. 1997). The dosages of risperidone in this study were higher (mean dosage = 6.6 mg/day), perhaps reflecting the inclusion of a large proportion of subjects with a history of treatment resistance.

In one 6-week, randomized, double blind, placebo-controlled study, 160 adolescents with schizophrenia, ages 13–17 years, received placebo; light, but flexible, dosages of risperidone 1–3 mg/day; or risperidone 4–6 mg/day (Haas et al. 2009b). Both risperidone groups were found to have significantly improved PANSS scores compared with the placebo group (P<0.001). Adverse effects were present at higher rates in both risperidone groups (75% and 76%) than in patients given placebo (54%). The higher-dosage group also had increased rates of dizziness, hypertonia, and EPS than the lower-dosage group. Haas et al. also published a study of adolescents with schizophrenia who were randomized 1:1 on risperidone dosages of 1.5–6.0 mg/day (n=125) or 0.15–0.6 mg/day (n=132) (Haas et al. 2009a). The researchers noted that although treatment was well tolerated, patients given the higher dosage had a mean body weight change of 3.2 kg (standard deviation [SD] = 3.49), alongside other treatment-emergent adverse events occurring at a 74% rate, whereas those taking the lower dosage had a mean body weight change of 1.7 kg (SD = 3.29) and a 65% rate of adverse events. In consideration of the low overall EPS and lack of prolactin-related adverse symptoms, the authors suggest that a risk-benefit analysis reasonably supports a 1- to 3-mg/day dosage for adolescents with schizophrenia (Haas et al. 2009b).

Olanzapine. In some of the earliest work in COS at the NIMH, initial study data suggested only modest improvement among subjects receiving open-label olanzapine, with a reported 17% improvement on the BPRS but only a 1% improvement in positive symptoms and no significant change in CGI Improvement scale (CGI-I) scores (Kumra et al. 1998). These modest gains may reflect the treatment-refractory nature of the illnesses in most of the NIMH cohort.

In a group of nine children with treatment-refractory schizophrenia, Mozes et al. (2003) found an overall more impressive response in a 12-week open-label olanzapine study, with significant improvement on all outcome measures. Studies that include a treatment-naïve population or those involving subjects with minimal prior exposure to antipsychotics show more robust effects. For example, among patients in an outpatient study, Findling et al. (2003) found robust responses in both negative and positive symptoms. Similarly, Ross et al. (2003) reported 37% full response and 32% partial response rates for school-age children with schizophrenia given olanzapine. Notably, this significant improvement was observed only at the 1-year mark, and there was evidence of an increasing amelioration of negative symptoms with time, emphasizing the need for such longer-term studies. The more recent literature echoes similar findings, although some researchers recommend considering olanzapine as a second-line agent in EOS due to its heightened risks for significant weight gain and lipid dysregulation (Deniau et al. 2008), which are discussed further in the section "Treatment of Side Effects" later in this chapter.

Shaw et al. (2006) performed an 8-week, double-blind RCT of olanzapine versus clozapine with a 2-year open-label follow-up in a large sample of children, ages 7–16 years, who met unmodified DSM-IV criteria for schizophrenia and were resistant to treatment with at least two antipsychotics. Compared with clozapine (see "Use of Clozapine in Treating COS" later in this chapter), olanzapine demonstrated a less consistent profile of clinical improvement. Although the results do not definitively demonstrate the superiority of clozapine over olanzapine in treatment-refractory COS, the study suggests that in an independent, dichotomous comparison of the two antipsychotics, clozapine has a more favorable clinical response profile and is better balanced against associated adverse events. In another randomized, single-blind, 6-month study conducted in 50 adolescents with early-onset psychosis, no changes were observed in patients' cognitive performance, and there was no evidence of differential efficacy of olanzapine or quetiapine on cognitive improvement (Robles et al. 2011).

Nonetheless, recent work has continued to highlight the complex relationship between olanzapine's potential for clinical response and its adverse side effects. One multisite, international, randomized (2:1), double-blind, controlled trial assessed 117 adolescent patients with schizophrenia receiving flexible dosages of olanzapine, 2.5–20.0 mg/day ($n=72$, mean age = 16.1 years), or placebo ($n=35$, mean age = 16.3 years) for up to 6 weeks (Kryzhanovskaya et al. 2009b). Olanzapine-treated adolescents showed significantly greater improvement in a comprehensive battery of measures: PANSS total ($P=0.005$) and positive scores ($P=0.002$), BPRS total score ($P=0.003$), and CGI Severity of Illness subscale score ($P=0.004$). Patients receiving olanzapine gained more weight (4.3 kg vs. 0.1 kg, $P<0.001$) and had higher prolactin and triglyceride mean levels when compared with patients given placebo (Kryzhanovskaya et al. 2009b).

In a pooled analysis of olanzapine safety in adolescent schizophrenia populations and a comparison of these data with those of adults treated with olanzapine, Kryzhanovskaya et al. (2009a) reviewed the data from the acute phase of multiple olanzapine trials with a mean daily dosage of 10.6 mg/day (exposure = 48,946 patient days). Among the adolescents ($N=454$), 2 (0.4%) attempted suicide and 13 (2.9%) had suicidal ideation. The most common adverse events were increased appetite (17.4%), increased weight (31.7%), and somnolence (19.8%). The adolescents gained significantly more weight than did adults (7.4 kg vs. 3.2 kg, $P<0.001$). Specifically, within the placebo-controlled database, adolescents demonstrated significantly greater increases in prolactin levels (11.4 µg/L, $P<0.001$) from baseline to the study endpoint (47.4% had high levels), and the overall magnitude of prolactin and weight increases was greater in adolescents than in adults (Kryzhanovskaya et al. 2009a).

In a continuation of the TEOSS study (see McClellan et al. 2007 and Sikich et al. 2008 in Table 9–1, and discussion in "Efficacy of Typical Antipsychotics Versus Placebo in COS" above), patients with schizophrenia (ages

8–19 years) who had improved during an 8-week, randomized, double-blind acute trial of olanzapine, risperidone, or molindone (plus benztropine) were eligible to continue taking the same medication for up to 44 additional weeks under double-blind conditions. No particular agent was found to demonstrate superior efficacy; instead, patients taking all three medications exhibited typical weight gain and other metabolic side effects (Findling et al. 2010b; Sikich et al. 2008).

Aripiprazole. Aripiprazole has a unique receptor profile, with partial agonist action at D_2 and 5-HT$_{1A}$ receptors. According to Normala and Hamidin (2009), aripiprazole has unique properties of fewer metabolic complications and EPS than are commonly observed with other atypicals used to treat children and adolescents with EOS.

In past years, a double-blind study comparing aripiprazole with risperidone at the NIMH was stopped early when the first two patients randomly assigned to receive aripiprazole showed precipitous declines in mental state. Given the treatment-resistant nature of the NIMH cohort, this result does not mean the agent would not be of use in a treatment-naïve population, and reports of its usefulness in this population are only beginning to emerge.

After this book's first edition, work emerged on the tolerability of aripiprazole up to the maximum approved adult dosage (30 mg/day) in patients ages 10–17 years. Patients received aripiprazole for up to 12 days by forced titration to achieve dosages of 20, 25, or 30 mg/day (Findling et al. 2008a), and then received the maximum dosage for 14 more days. Aripiprazole proved generally well tolerated; even though all patients experienced at least one adverse side effect, none met criteria for a serious classification. The pharmokinetics of aripiprazole's administration in youth appeared linear across the dosage range and was comparable with previous pharmokinetic observations in adults.

Findling et al. (2008b) enrolled adolescents (ages 13–17 years) with schizophrenia in a 6-week, multicenter, double-blind, randomized controlled trial comparing aripiprazole (10 or 30 mg/day) with placebo. Compared with patients given placebo, those taking either aripiprazole dosage showed statistically significant improvement in PANSS total scores and improvement in PANSS Hostility factor scores. Although the drug was well tolerated overall, extrapyramidal syndromes, somnolence, and tremors emerged at twice the rate for placebo. The authors noted, however, that both the 10-mg/day and the 30-mg/day dosages of aripiprazole proved to have a superior efficacy to placebo in treating acute schizophrenia in this young population. The 30-mg/day dosage showed significant contrasts to placebo by week 3, whereas changes in the 10-mg/day dosage did not appear until week 6 (Findling et al. 2008b).

In light of this research, aripiprazole has been suggested as a possible initial choice for treatment, with a better risk-benefit ratio than risperidone (Goeb et al. 2010), or as an augmentation option with alternative treatments such as repetitive transcranial magnetic stimulation (rTMS) (Normala and Hamidin 2009).

Quetiapine. Quetiapine has a higher affinity for 5-HT_{2A} receptors relative to D_2 receptors and affinity for α_1-adrenergic and dopamine D_1 receptors, but relatively little muscarinic action. Two open-label studies suggest that quetiapine has some efficacy in psychotic disorders in children (McConville et al. 2003; Shaw et al. 2001).

A recent double-blind, randomized, fixed-dose comparison of 200 mg/day versus 400 mg/day of quetiapine in 141 drug-naïve, acutely ill patients (ages 15–25 years) with first-episode psychosis demonstrated both dosages to be safe and well tolerated, although global and social functioning improved more in the 200-mg group than in the 400-mg group (Berger et al. 2008). In addition, the 200-mg group showed improvement on the Scale for the Assessment of Negative Symptoms (SANS) Anhedonia-Asociality subscale, whereas a slight worsening was seen in the 400-mg group. The second phase of the study, a single-blind, naturalistic, flexible-dose, 8-week period, highlighted that regardless of the initial dose, the clinician's ability to flexibly modify the dose resulted in similar quetiapine levels (average=268 mg/day for both high- and low-dosage groups) after 12 weeks. The researchers recommend conservative quetiapine dosing, beginning with 250–300 mg/day, for the new-onset, previously untreated patient.

Ziprasidone and paliperidone. Ziprasidone has a complex pharmacology, acting as an agonist at 5-HT_{1A} receptors and an antagonist at 5-HT_{1D} and 5-HT_{2C} receptors—properties that may confer antidepressant effects. Published studies of the drug's use in patients with COS remain scarce, although efficacy in open-label studies of youth with a variety of disorders has been reported (Barnett 2003). One industry-supported double-blind, placebo-controlled, flexible-dose study failed to show any difference in efficacy between treatment with ziprasidone and placebo in 283 adolescent participants (Findling et al. 2010a).

Paliperidone is now approved for use in patients with schizophrenia as young as age 12, following recent additions of double-blind trials to the literature (Singh et al. 2011).

Amisulpride. Some recent publications have discussed amisulpride as a possible alternative antipsychotic to treat adolescent schizophrenia (Varol Tas and Guvenir 2009), although the drug is not approved in the United States. Despite claims that amisulpride is associated with fewer extrapyramidal symptoms, a few case reports of induced tardive dyskinesia have surfaced in adult as well as adolescent patients. These findings have encouraged other analyses, and some results suggest that a combination of amisulpride and multiple other medications, especially antidepressants, may synergistically raise rates of tardive dyskinesia (Goyal and Sinha 2010). Other work suggests that amisulpride does not provide any efficacy advantage over other atypicals, except a possible reduction in weight gain (Hamann et al. 2003; Martin et al. 2002). Currently, amisulpride's use for greater efficacy in treatment of COS has been found to be limited in scope; with minimal available data in the literature, no definitive conclusions can be drawn about amisulpride (Komossa et al. 2009).

Efficacy of Atypical Antipsychotics Versus Typical Antipsychotics in COS

A direct comparison between two atypical antipsychotics, olanzapine and risperidone, and the most commonly prescribed typical agent, haloperidol, has been made in a double-blind, parallel treatment study (Sikich et al. 2004). The 8-week study included 75 children and adolescents with psychotic symptoms stemming from a wide range of underlying diagnoses. All three treatments were associated with marked and significant reductions in Brief Psychiatric Rating Scale for Children (BPRS-C) total scores, which fell to 50% of the baseline score in the risperidone group, 44% of the baseline score in the olanzapine group, and 67% of the baseline score in the haloperidol group. The categorical response rates, like most outcome measures, did not differ significantly, but there was a trend toward better response rates with the atypicals: 74% (14/19) with risperidone, 88% (14/16) with olanzapine, and 53% (8/15) with haloperidol. However, there are important limitations to the applicability of these findings to COS, because these trials included a diagnostically heterogeneous group, and only half of the subjects had a diagnosis of schizophrenia. A large proportion of the subjects were receiving other psychotropic medications; however, no differences in response rates were found across treatment groups for participants who were treated exclusively with an antipsychotic. The findings of the study are also congruent with an 8-week, open-label, nonrandomized comparison of olanzapine, risperidone, and haloperidol in 43 adolescents with schizophrenia, in which all three agents were found to be equally efficacious (Gothelf et al. 2003).

Since the first edition of this book was published, Kennedy et al. (2007) examined the Cochrane Schizophrenia Group Trials Register in 2006–2007 for antipsychotic effects in COS. Use of typical or atypical antipsychotics emerged as the only significant distinction criterion in treatment groups. Although Kennedy et al. noted that any benefit from atypical use was offset by an increase in adverse effects, Halloran et al. (2010) found that atypical antipsychotics are the common primary treatment choice for children who have severe psychosis or multiple psychiatric diagnoses.

Sikich, McClellan, and their colleagues have presented work from the TEOSS study (McClellan et al. 2007; Sikich et al. 2008), undertaken as a result of the debate regarding the increased efficacy of second-generation atypical antipsychotics. This double-blind multisite trial randomly assigned children with EOS and schizoaffective disorder to risperidone (0.5–6 mg/day), olanzapine (2.5–20 mg/day), or molindone (10–140 mg/day, plus 1 mg/day of benztropine) for 8 weeks. Results from the 116 pediatric patients receiving treatment indicated that no significant difference in response rate was seen among treatment groups (see Table 9–1), although risperidone and olanzapine were implicated in the greatest risk for weight gain, cholesterol, and lipoprotein levels, with olanzapine causing greater changes than risperidone. The patients taking molindone had higher rates of akathisia self-reports.

In follow-up work from the TEOSS study, Findling et al. (2010b) found that patients who demonstrated improvement during the 8-week randomized trial thereafter continued taking the same medication (for up to 44 weeks, still under double-blind conditions). Treatment effects were maintained, but participants had very poor adherence rates (only 12%) by 52 weeks. These data confirmed the authors' earlier suppositions that no one medication had significantly improved efficacy compared with the others, and although the olanzapine and risperidone groups experienced higher weight gain during the acute trial, maintenance treatment showed no significant differences, with increased weight gain and side effects seen across all groups. From these findings, the researchers call into question recent trends of nearly sole use of atypical antipsychotics for schizophrenia treatment in youth, while pointing out the considerable metabolic complications resulting from their administration.

New Considerations in Antipsychotic Administration and Management

Due to an increased risk of relapse following antipsychotic discontinuation, current medical strategies attempt to prevent relapse and maintain efficacy by encouraging continuous medication exposure for steadied maintenance. New arguments, however, have arisen to challenge the long-upheld clinical practice of daily antipsychotic administration (Remington and Kapur 2010). In response, calls for mixed antipsychotic management in such patients have complicated what is still an unclear issue. For example, recent work indicates that adolescents with schizophrenia may benefit from aripiprazole augmentation during clozapine treatment for an overall increase in effectiveness, a strategy that has previously improved CGI ratings (Bachmann et al. 2009). Still, future prospective studies for pediatric and adolescent populations will be needed to better understand clinical effectiveness for such specific combinations.

Age-Specific Pharmacotherapy Considerations

Recent work has identified factors, such as age at onset, diagnosis subtype, premorbid adjustment, and cognitive functioning, that have meaningful impact on treatment response trajectories (Levine and Rabinowitz 2010). Vahia et al. (2010) observed nuances in treatment variations for patients with early- and late-onset schizophrenia. The EOS group differed from the late-onset group on all measures of psychopathology and cognitive functioning; however, despite similarities on measures of depression severity, education, and negative symptoms, early-onset patients included more males, represented more severe generalized psychopathology of positive symptoms, and were observed to require higher antipsychotic dosages. Interestingly, the differences between early- and late-onset subgroups remained significant after adjustments for gender, age, illness duration, and negative symptom severity, thereby highlighting treatment differences influenced by age at onset of psychosis. Similarly, in a Japanese study, Uchida et al. (2008) found age to be a vital factor in determining appropriate antipsychotic dosages for patients with schizophrenia spectrum disorders; dosage increases progressed with patient age through the third decade, then reached a plateau for two decades, before a decrease commenced.

Use of Clozapine in Treating COS

Clozapine has emerged as the gold-standard antipsychotic for treatment-refractory cases of schizophrenia (Kane et al. 1988). Most, but not all, meta-analyses suggest that clozapine is more efficacious than typical and possibly most atypical antipsychotics in the short term (Davis et al. 2003; Geddes et al. 2000; Leucht et al. 2003; Moncrieff 2003). Unfortunately, the benefits of clozapine must be weighed against its severe adverse side effects, particularly agranulocytosis.

The clinical trials of clozapine in COS have all incorporated the criteria of treatment resistance, which is a convention for current routine clinical use. Thus, no data are available on the efficacy of clozapine as a first-line agent in COS (unlike in adult schizophrenia; see Lieberman et al. 2003). With this in mind, a striking result is that all open trials found clear efficacy for clozapine in children who were not helped by other medications. Frazier et al. (1994) found that 9 of 11 adolescents from the NIMH cohort showed greater than a 33% reduction in BPRS ratings, and only one patient showed clinical deterioration. Turetz et al. (1997) demonstrated a similar reduction of approximately 50% on all psychopathology scales in a report of 11 children who had shown no response to neuroleptic agents. The latter authors noted that the response occurred relatively early in treatment, between weeks 2 and 8, and was sustained at a 4-month follow-up.

Clozapine has been compared with both atypical and typical antipsychotics. In the first study, Kumra et al. (1996) compared haloperidol, probably the most widely used typical antipsychotic at the time of the study (1990–1996), with clozapine, randomly assigning 21 children to receive haloperidol or clozapine for 6 weeks. Clozapine was markedly superior on all components of the BPRS and overall ratings of clinical improvement—a striking finding, given the small sample and the severity of illness at baseline. The mean dosage of haloperidol was 16.8 mg/day, which is at the upper end of the contemporary treatment range. Such relatively high dosages have been implicated in an excess of side effects that mimic the negative symptoms of schizophrenia and lead to an underestimation of antipsychotic efficacy (Geddes et al. 2000). However, given the history of previous resistance to antipsychotics among the patients in this study, high dosages would have been expected and were guided by clinical judgment.

We subsequently compared the efficacy and safety of olanzapine, a widely used atypical, with clozapine. In an 8-week, double-blind RCT with a 2-year follow-up, 25 patients with COS were randomly assigned to receive treatment (12 to clozapine and 13 to olanzapine). Using intent-to-treat analyses, we found that clozapine was associated with a significant reduction in all outcome measures, with olanzapine showing a rather less impressive improvement (Figure 9–1).

A direct comparison of treatment efficacy showed that there was generally no significant difference between the groups, but a significant advantage for clozapine did emerge in the alleviation of negative symptoms of schizophrenia (producing a 45% greater reduction in SANS ratings; $P = 0.04$, effect size = 0.89). The size of the differential effect on negative symptoms is therefore large and in marked contrast to studies in adults with schizophrenia, which report no significant difference between olanzapine and clozapine in treating negative symptoms, despite a larger sample size and power to detect smaller effects (Bitter et al. 2004; Tollefson et al. 2001; Volavka et al. 2002). The improvement in negative symptoms is unlikely to have been an epiphenomenon of improvement in mood or EPS, given that there was no correlation between change in these indices and change in negative symptoms.

Data on the effectiveness and tolerability of antipsychotics in the longer term are of importance; however, with some significant exceptions (Findling et al. 2004; Ross et al. 2003), such data are scarce in the pediatric literature. In the NIMH trial, Shaw et al. (2006) found that by the 2-year stage, 15 of the 18 patients were being treated with clozapine, because olanzapine produced moderately sustained treatment response for only 2 patients. The patients receiving clozapine showed modest but no significant improvement in clinical ratings from the end of the double-blind trial to the 2-year assess-

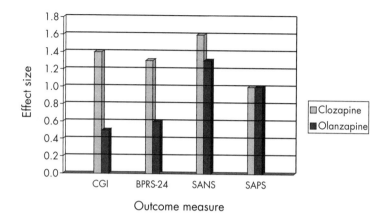

Figure 9–1.   Effect sizes of clozapine and olanzapine in a double-blind trial in 25 patients with childhood-onset schizophrenia. BPRS-24=Brief Psychiatric Rating Scale (24-item); CGI=Clinical Global Impression Scale; SANS=Scale for the Assessment of Negative Symptoms; SAPS=Scale for the Assessment of Positive Symptoms.

ment. Thus, clozapine appears to be generally a highly efficacious choice in a treatment-resistant population.

Considerable interest has been shown in determining what attributes afford clozapine its efficacy. In a study of 54 patients with COS, we found that outcome at 2 years (using the Children's Global Assessment Scale) was associated with a less severe illness at baseline and a greater initial clinical response to clozapine during the first 6 weeks of treatment (Shaw et al. 2006), as has been reported in studies of adults with schizophrenia (Pickar et al. 1994; Sporn et al. 2007). Intriguingly, the ratio of one of the metabolites of clozapine, N-desmethylclozapine (NDMC), to clozapine, was the only variable that was significantly associated with response at 6 weeks. This result replicated a finding in an adult-onset schizophrenia study, which indicated that a greater NDMC-to-clozapine ratio, but not the concentrations of clozapine and NDMC themselves, is associated with better response (Weiner et al. 2004).

Just after publication of the first edition of this book, Findling et al. (2007a) discussed evidence in support of the FDA's eventual allowance for clozapine use in children and adolescents, based on controlled treatment trial data showing clozapine to be more effective for treatment-refractory pediatric patients than at least two typical antipsychotic medications (Kumra et al. 2008c; Shaw and Rapoport 2006). In addition, a 12-week controlled comparison of clozapine versus high-dose olanzapine (up to 30 mg/day) in adolescents with schizophrenia, ages 10–18 years, supported clozapine as the agent of choice (Kumra et al. 2008a). Significantly more clozapine-treated adolescents met response criteria (66%) than olanzapine-treated subjects (33%), and clozapine proved superior in the reduction (from baseline to endpoint of their analysis) of negative symptoms as well as psychosis cluster scores.

The course of COS is difficult, but the high overall response rates found among patients treated with clozapine are encouraging. Although not currently seen consistently in the NIMH COS study, a finding reported by some studies (e.g., Sholevar et al. 2000) is significantly *greater* improvement with clozapine in *younger* subjects. However, even though clozapine is now better established for treatment-resistant schizophrenia, its use in pediatric populations continues to be rare, mainly due to lingering community concern about its potential adverse effects (Gogtay and Rapoport 2008).

Treatment of Comorbid Conditions

Patients with COS have a very high rate of comorbid conditions. Among 76 children from the NIMH cohort, the most frequent comorbid diagnosis at NIMH screening was depression (54%), followed by obsessive-compulsive disorder (21%) and generalized anxiety disorder (15%) (Gochman et al. 2011). A particularly challenging comorbid condition is attention-deficit/hyperactivity disorder (present in 15% of the NIMH sample). Psychiatrists have often been reluctant to treat these symptoms with stimulants for fear of worsening psychosis. However, Tossell et al. (2004) found that five children showed a significant improvement in the Brief Conners Teacher Rating Scale of inattentive symptoms with stimulant treatment following stabilization with an antipsychotic, without any initial worsening of psychosis. This reflects a more general principle of treatment of comorbidity in the psychotic child: The treatment of the coexisting condition should be modeled on the evidence for each disorder and should *follow* the stabilization of psychosis.

Treatment of Side Effects

The available data from short-term studies suggest that youth might be more sensitive than adults to developing antipsychotic-related adverse side effects (e.g., EPS, prolactin elevation, weight gain) (Kumra et al. 2008c). Because the chronic course of COS necessitates long-term treatment, a thorough consideration of side effects and differential profile is vital in the treatment of pediatric and adolescent populations.

Extrapyramidal Side Effects

EPS are among the most troublesome and distressing unwanted sequelae of treatment with antipsychotic drugs. Pathophysiologically, the blockade of nigrostriatal dopaminergic tracts mimics the neurochemical deficits seen in Parkinson disease and exhibits a similar clinical profile. The mechanisms underlying tardive dyskinesias are less clear but may stem from the development of supersensitivity to dopamine resulting from chronic blockade. As mentioned above in "Mechanisms of Action," atypical antipsychotics have a high serotonin-to-dopamine receptor blockade ratio in the brain. The serotonergic blockade leads to increased dopamine release, which may partially offset the postsynaptic dopaminergic blockade, resulting in fewer EPS (Glazer 2000).

Abnormal movements that arise in the first few hours or days of treatment are typically acute dystonic reactions, manifesting as spasms of the orofacial muscles or oculogyric crises with involuntary upward rotation of the eyes. Dyskinetic movements can affect any body part; for example, a patient may experience frequently tongue protrusion and lip smacking, or may experience continuous writhing or athetoid and choreiform movements of the trunk and limbs. *Pseudoparkinsonism* refers to the classic triad of bradykinesia (slowed or reduced voluntary movements), muscular rigidity, and tremor (although the classic pill-rolling tremor is very rare in neuroleptic-induced parkinsonism). *Akathisia* refers to an intensely dysphoric sensation of restlessness associated with an intense need for movement. Several rating scales have been developed to assess abnormal movements, including the Abnormal Involuntary Movement Scale (Guy 1976), the Barnes Akathisia Rating Scale (Barnes 1989), and the Simpson-Angus Rating Scale (Simpson and Angus 1970).

A comparison of rates of EPS in various studies suggests that typical antipsychotics are associated with high levels of EPS (58%–80%) in patients with COS (Table 9–2). These rates are higher than those typically reported in patients with adult-onset schizophrenia (32%–55% [Bobes et al. 2003; Novick et al. 2010]).

By contrast, five open-label studies of olanzapine and quetiapine, involving patients with varying treatment histories and a range of ages at illness onset, found no significant change in ratings of EPS from baseline (Findling et al. 2003; McConville et al. 2003; Mozes et al. 2003; Ross et al. 2003; Shaw et al. 2001). Three open-label studies of risperidone suggest that this atypical is associated with EPS, akathisia, and acute dystonic reactions, especially at higher dosages (Armenteros et al. 1997; Grcevich et al. 1996; Zalsman et al. 2003). One study reported increases in all measures of movement disorders over a 6-week period (Zalsman et al. 2003). Other studies reported a 19% EPS rate and a 40% rate of dystonic reactions (Armenteros et al. 1997; Grcevich et al. 1996). These findings are supported by direct comparisons of typical and atypical antipsychotics. For example, Sikich et al. (2004) found that haloperidol, but not olanzapine or risperidone, was associated with a significant increase in EPS over an 8-week treatment period.

The management of EPS in children follows the principles derived from adult populations. The antipsychotic is reduced to as low a dosage as possible, with awareness that this reduction may be associated with some temporary increase in abnormal movements. Some clinicians also recommend regular "drug holidays" to observe for the development of EPS, although clearly this possibility has to be weighed against the risk of a recurrence of psychosis. Alternatively, the child can be switched to an agent with a lower potential for EPS, such as quetiapine or olanzapine. For pseudoparkinsonism, anticholinergics are frequently used to good effect. For tardive dyskinesia, two controlled studies in adults suggest that clozapine may be the best overall option, given its ability to treat both the psychosis and the movement disorder, although the risks and attendant intensive monitoring make this a less attractive option. Other medications that carry a lower risk of complications can be used in tardive dyskinesia, with vitamin E having the best evidence base in adult efficacy studies (Attard and Taylor 2012; Lieberman et al. 1991).

Akathisia

Akathisia has been described mostly in association with typical neuroleptics, but also with olanzapine and risperidone (at rates of about 13%) and clozapine (about 7%) (Chengappa et al. 1994; Leucht et al. 1999). In the NIMH cohort, two of 40 children treated with clozapine developed akathisia, which was misinterpreted as a worsening of psychotic symptoms in one case and led to a temporary increase in clozapine dosage and a concomitant worsening of symptoms (Gogtay et al. 2002); however, when the diagnosis was made, propranolol was initiated and ameliorated symptoms greatly, allowing continued treatment with clozapine. Other useful agents include benzodiazepines and, perhaps, anticholinergics.

Neuroleptic Malignant Syndrome

Neuroleptic malignant syndrome, a rare but potentially life-threatening complication of antipsychotics, typically arises in the early stages of treatment and has been attributed to the effects of dopamine blockade. The classic signs and symptoms include severe muscle rigidity and/or marked EPS; autonomic instability, including a high or sometimes fluctuating temperature and blood pressure; delirium; and laboratory findings of elevated creatine kinase and leukocytosis. Atypical antipsychotics probably have a lower incidence and produce perhaps a milder form of neuroleptic malignant syndrome (Caroff et al. 2000). However, some dramatic case studies illustrate the potential for the side effect in adolescents who are only briefly exposed to even atypicals (Hanft et al. 2004). Treatment of neuroleptic malignant syndrome relies on prompt transfer to a medical setting, withdrawal of the neuroleptic, intensive supportive care, and possible treatment with dantrolene and bromocriptine. Psychotic exacerbations during this period of abrupt antipsychotic withdrawal have sometimes been treated successfully with electroconvulsive therapy.

Sedation

High rates of fatigue and/or sedation have been consistently reported in association with nearly all antipsychotics in patients with COS. Rates for haloperidol range from a low of 25% in an NIMH double-blind study (Shaw et al. 2006) to 50% and 66% in two earlier trials of the medication (Pool et al. 1976; Spencer et al. 1992). Other typical antipsychotics have been associated with even higher rates of sedation (Pool et al. 1976; Spencer et al. 1992).

Table 9–2. Rates of extrapyramidal side effects (EPS) in controlled studies of antipsychotics in treatment of childhood-onset schizophrenia

Study	Drug	Mean dosage (mg/day)	Measures	Results
Typical antipsychotics				
Engelhardt et al. 1973	Fluphenazine	10.4	Clinical	8/15 EPS, 1/15 acute dystonia, 0/15 akathisia
	Haloperidol	10.4		4/15 EPS, 0/15 acute dystonia, 1/15 akathisia
Pool et al. 1976	Loxapine	87.5	Clinical, muscular rigidity of parkinsonian type	19/26 EPS
	Haloperidol	9.8		18/25 EPS
	Placebo	—		1/24 EPS
Spencer et al. 1992	Haloperidol	8.8	AIMS	3/12 parkinsonian, 2/12 orofacial dyskinesia, 2/12 acute dystonia
	Placebo	—		0/12
Comparisons of typicals and atypicals				
Kumra et al. 1996	Haloperidol	16	AIMS, SAS	No significant increase from baseline
	Clozapine	176		No significant increase from baseline
Sikich et al. 2004	Olanzapine	12.3	AIMS, SAS	No significant increase from baseline, but 56% taking anticholinergics; no acute dystonia; 2/16 akathisia
	Risperidone	4		No significant increase from baseline, but 53% taking anticholinergics; no acute dystonia; no akathisia
	Haloperidol	5		Significant increase from baseline, and significantly greater than with atypicals; 67% taking anticholinergics; 2/15 acute dystonia, 2/15 akathisia

Table 9–2. Rates of extrapyramidal side effects (EPS) in controlled studies of antipsychotics in treatment of childhood-onset schizophrenia *(continued)*

Study	Drug	Mean dosage (mg/day)	Measures	Results
Comparisons of typicals and atypicals *(continued)*				
Gothelf et al. 2003	Olanzapine	12.9	AIMS, UKU	3/19 EPS, 0/19 dystonia, 0/19 akathisia
	Risperidone	3.3		4/17 EPS, 1/17 dystonia, 1/17 akathisia
	Haloperidol	8.3		4/7 EPS, 2/7 dystonia, 3/7 akathisia
Shaw et al. 2006	Olanzapine	18.1	AIMS, BAS, SAS	No significant change from baseline
	Clozapine	327		No significant change from baseline

Note. AIMS=Abnormal Involuntary Movement Scale; BAS=Barnes Akathisia Rating Scale; SAS=Simpson-Angus Rating Scale; UKU=Udvalg for Kliniske Undersøgelser Side Effect Rating Scale.

Atypical agents also seem to produce this unwanted side effect, and rates of over 50% have been reported for ziprasidone and clozapine, with risperidone occupying an intermediate position (31%), and olanzapine (20%) and quetiapine (20%) having lower, but still high, rates (for a review, see Cheng-Shannon et al. 2004). Interestingly, one study linked initial sedation when taking olanzapine with a better clinical response at 8 weeks, suggesting the need for perseverance with fatigue and sedation occurring early in treatment (Sholevar et al. 2000). The management of sedation is empirical and requires rigorous assessment to exclude underlying psychopathology, maintenance treatment with as low a dosage as possible, encouragement of activity scheduling, and constant motivation.

Weight Gain

Weight gain, reported in association with antipsychotics since their initial use, has become a focus of more interest, given the increased awareness of morbidity and mortality accompanying obesity (Deckelbaum and Williams 2001). In their study of 50 children with psychotic symptoms, Sikich et al. (2004) found a weight gain of 7.1 kg over an 8-week period for children being treated with olanzapine—a value greater than the gains of 4.9 kg and 3.5 kg reported for risperidone and haloperidol, respectively. In a double-blind comparison of clozapine and olanzapine, a similar weight gain of just under 4 kg over an 8-week period was associated with both agents, corresponding to an increase of 1.5 units in the body mass index (BMI) (Shaw et al. 2006), with the most extreme weight gains occurring with clozapine. Correll and colleagues reported changes in glucose and lipid metabolism in pediatric populations with significant metabolic adverse events when clozapine treatment was continued long term (Correll 2011; Correll et al. 2009; Kumra et al. 2008a, 2008b).

Among the atypical antipsychotics other than clozapine, open-label studies report greatest weight gain with olanzapine (see Fedorowicz and Fombonne 2005). Findling et al. (2003) reported a gain of approximately 1 kg/week over an 8-week period (Findling et al. 2003), although a longer-term study suggested that after an initial sharp increase, weight plateaus at around 2 months and then remains more stable (Ross et al. 2003). A systematic review of antipsychotic use in children, regardless of diagnoses, found weight gains of 4% with ziprasidone, 7% with clozapine, 17% with risperidone, and 22% with olanzapine and quetiapine (Cheng-Shannon et al. 2004). In another study, a significant link was found between early-onset diagnoses and the subsequent increase in BMI after 6 months of risperidone use (Goeb et al. 2010). We caution that there may be subtle gender and age confounds in such BMI conclusions, because the general dearth of pediatric studies does not allow for definitive conclusions (Goeb et al. 2010). Indeed, observations of body weight over time considered independently do not satisfactorily highlight a critical clinical problem, although consideration of irregular weight increases should continue (Goeb et al. 2010).

Actively avoiding use of atypical antipsychotics solely on the basis of weight gain concerns is hotly debated in recent literature. A recent study in EOS showed that although atypicals caused a significantly larger ($P=0.04$) gain in baseline weight compared with typical antipsychotics, this difference was not seen 6 weeks later (Hrdlicka et al. 2009). The patients gained, on average, 3.6 kg (SD = 2.6) taking risperidone, 4.4 kg (SD = 2.5) taking olanzapine, and 2.1 kg (SD = 4.0) taking clozapine during the 6 weeks of treatment, but no overall weight gain differences were observed between typical and atypical antipsychotics by the end of the study. These results suggest that pediatric populations probably demonstrate much more variable and individual weight responses to atypical exposure than do adult patients. Because medication noncompliance may follow excessive weight gain that results from increasing use of atypicals in pediatric patients, this should be a particular concern for physicians as they consider social withdrawal and stigma consequences (Goeb et al. 2010).

Similar weight gain concerns occur in adult studies, which should further encourage the clinician to explore this side effect holistically. In a recent study of 400 patients recruited in a 52-week Comparison of Atypicals for First Episode Psychosis (CAFE) study, in which olanzapine, quetiapine, and risperidone were evaluated, 31% of patients were overweight and 18% were obese at baseline (J. K. Patel et al. 2009). In addition, 4.3% of patients met criteria for metabolic syndrome. Mechanistically, the relative affinities of the novel antipsychotics for histamine H_1 receptors appear to be the most robust correlate of these clinical findings, although interactions with serotonergic and dopaminergic receptors are also likely to play a role (Wirshing et al. 1999). Elevated levels of leptin, a hormone secreted by adipocytes that partly regulates body weight, are also greater among the antipsychotics most closely linked with weight gain (Herran et al. 2001). The management of this side effect has typically relied on behavioral programs, which unfortunately have mixed evidence of success (Faulkner et al. 2003). Pharmacological interventions are also unproven; some case reports suggest that amantadine, topiramate, and various anorectic agents attenuate antipsychotic-induced weight gain. Metformin has been investigated as a possible effective and safe therapy option to manage weight gain (Klein et al. 2006), although literature on controlled trials remains scare enough to prevent any definitive recommendation for routine clinical use (Canitano 2005; Gracious et al. 2002).

Ultimately, due to short treatment durations, stigma, and methodological challenges, studies focusing on weight gain from antipsychotic treatment remain scarce. The use of antipsychotics seems to be increasing generally, despite adverse side effects. Some literature documents extensive use of expensive atypical antipsychotic medications for off-label purposes, such as sedation, or for other practice patterns; for example, only 15% of one cohort had a diagnosis of schizophrenia (Hartung et al. 2008). Apart from the debate on the generalizability of such atypical pharmacotherapy, we point out that clinicians do seem increasingly more encouraged to pursue such therapies despite the understood metabolic complications. In consideration of the purported unique benefits that these atypicals (e.g., clozapine) may provide in psychiatric populations, particularly in the severe pediatric and treatment-resistant patients, weight gain should be assessed within a risk-benefit ratio specific to the severity of each patient's illness. Clinicians should take into account endocrine changes for youth taking antipsychotics when referencing dosing adjustments based on age, gender, and even growth charts.

Glycemic Control

The link between impaired glycemic control and atypical antipsychotics is well established in both pediatric and adult populations. Sikich et al. (2004) found that olanzapine, but not risperidone or haloperidol, was associated with a trend toward increased fasting blood glucose. Diabetic ketoacidosis, characterized by delirium, dehydration, and hyperventilation, has been reported in adolescents treated with olanzapine (Selva and Scott 2001). In our direct comparison of clozapine and olanzapine (see earlier section, "Use of Clozapine in Treating COS"), we found little evidence for marked hyperglycemia, although comprehensive data were available only for the 8-week phase. The link with impaired glucose control could arise through hyperinsulinemia and the impaired sensitivity to insulin found with use of atypical antipsychotics (Sowell et al. 2002). Additionally, antipsychotics may have direct toxic effects on the pancreas. A final link between antipsychotics and type 2 diabetes mellitus could be through obesity and weight gain associated with both. Despite the lack of a clear association between antipsychotic use and impaired glycemic control in COS, regular blood monitoring seems judicious (Jin et al. 2004).

Hyperlipidemia

Sikich et al. (2004) noted a deleterious increase in low-density lipoprotein and a decrease in high-density lipoprotein in patients randomly assigned to receive olanzapine but not risperidone or haloperidol. In the NIMH cohort, we found high levels of hypercholesterolemia and hypertriglyceridemia in 6 of 15 patients who were followed up for a 2-year period while receiving open-label clozapine (Shaw et al. 2006). Although all cases were detected early and managed through diet and lipid-lowering agents, the high rates underscore the need for regular monitoring for this complication among children maintained on treatment with clozapine and perhaps olanzapine as well (Melkersson et al. 2004).

Hyperprolactinemia

An increase in prolactin secondary to antipsychotics reflects the D_2 receptor blockade in the tuberoinfundibular pathway that releases the tonic inhibition from dopamine upon pituitary lactotropes, leading to increased prolactin (for a review, see Pappagallo and Silva 2004). As a result, elevated prolactin levels are typically produced by the antipsychotics with greatest D_2 affinity (Saito et al. 2004). The sequelae of hyperprolactinemia range from sexual dysfunction, menstrual irregularities, and lactation to decreased bone density and possible cardiovascular disease. Wudarsky et al. (1999) found increased prolactin levels in 36 children with early-onset psychosis after 6 weeks of treatment with either haloperidol or olanzapine but not clozapine. The association may be modulated by gender, because in the NIMH cohort a correlation between olanzapine and prolactin levels was found among girls only (Alfaro et al. 2002). In this study, all but one child remained asymptomatic; the girl with the highest prolactin levels developed transient galactorrhea.

The most effective treatment for symptomatic hyperprolactinemia is either reduction of the dosage of the antipsychotic (Masi et al. 2001) or a switch to an agent possibly less associated with the complication, such as quetiapine (Shaw et al. 2001). Dopamine agonists reinstitute the dopaminergic inhibition of prolactin release, and cabergoline has been used with success in male children with risperidone-induced hyperprolactinemia (Cohen and Biederman 2001), although bromocriptine has a more established role. Whether asymptomatic hyperprolactinemia requires intervention is more controversial, given evidence for the normalization of prolactin levels at 1-year follow-up in disruptive children being treated with risperidone (Findling et al. 2004).

Cardiovascular and Autonomic Side Effects

Several antipsychotics alter repolarization of cardiac muscle, as reflected in a prolonged QT interval. In turn, this change may act as a risk factor for more serious arrhythmias, such as torsades de pointes. In our double-blind study comparing clozapine and olanzapine (see earlier section, "Use of Clozapine in Treating COS"), we found higher rates of supine tachycardia, but no serious arrhythmias, among patients treated with clozapine. However, seven patients in the clozapine wing became hypertensive during the trial, compared with only one patient treated with olanzapine.

Cardiometabolic effects of second-generation antipsychotic medications are of concern to the clinician but have not been sufficiently studied in pediatric and adolescent patients who were previously unexposed to antipsychotic medication. Correll et al. (2009) showed that first-time use of second-generation antipsychotic medications was associated with significant cardiometabolic risk among four common antipsychotic medications despite nominal metabolic variability. Biases regarding baseline weights and race/ethnicity may influence the cardiometabolic risk study (Correll et al. 2009; Mangurian et al. 2010).

Side Effects Particularly Associated With Clozapine

The association between clozapine and neutropenia is well established. In a review of data on more than 1,100 patients treated with clozapine, the risk of agranulocytosis was greater in patients under age 21 than in those ages 21–40 (Alvir et al. 1993). However, Cheng-Shannon et al. (2004) reported two cases of agranulocytosis occurring among 243 children and adolescents treated with clozapine, giving a rate more in line with that seen in the adult population. Due to this connection, clozapine requires intensive blood monitoring. The high rates of neutropenia and agranulocytosis in children are particularly unfortunate given the severity of COS, for which clozapine is often the only effective treatment. As a result, there is considerable interest in developing strategies to maximize the opportunity for children to be treated with clozapine following initial withdrawal due to the development of neutropenia. We have reported on two cases of children, ages 7 and 12 years, diagnosed with very early-onset schizophrenia, who developed neutropenia when initially treated with clozapine (Sporn et al. 2003). In both cases, addition of lithium carbonate was associated with a sustained elevation of the white blood count, allowing a successful rechallenge with clozapine. Clozapine rechallenge should be done with intensive monitoring, which is best performed in highly specialized units.

Epileptiform abnormalities are not uncommon in the electroencephalograms of children and adolescents taking clozapine. Clozapine also has the potential to reduce seizure threshold, and seizures occur in approximately 2% of children taking the medication. Most patients can continue taking clozapine with an adjunctive anticonvulsant, and prophylactic anticonvulsants are justified when patients are given high dosages of clozapine. We recommend gabapentin as an anticonvulsant in clozapine-induced seizures, chosen in view of its relatively benign side-effect profile and its lack of significant drug interactions (Usiskin et al. 2000).

Hypersalivation is a distressingly common side effect of clozapine that has been reported only rarely with use of other antipsychotics. Proposed mechanisms include the action of clozapine at the muscarinic M_4 receptor, blockade of α_2-adrenoceptors, or distortion of the swallowing reflex. Treatment options include chewing gum; reduction in the dosage of clozapine; or treatment with pharmacological agents such as anticholinergics, α_2-adrenergic agonists, and, in extreme cases, botulinum toxin (Kahl et al. 2004). Some studies suggest that the addition of other antipsychotics, such as amisulpride, at low dosages may be efficacious, although a double-blind study found that pirenzepine, one of the most promising agents (based on results of open-label studies), was no more effective than placebo (Bai et al. 2001).

A retrospective study of clinical response, therapeutic dosages, and side effects of long-term clozapine use in Korean children and adolescents with either very early-onset schizophrenia or refractory EOS found significant reductions in hospital days per year in almost all (96.2%) patients receiving clozapine when compared with pretreatment periods (Kim et al. 2008). The researchers noted that clozapine's long-term benefits were also seen in the reduction of hospitalization rates in 14 patients undergoing clozapine treatment for 3 or more years. Neutropenia did develop in 26.9% of patients after 1 year, but contrary to other reports in the literature (Haapasalo-Pesu 2009), none of the patients developed agranulocytosis. Although legitimate concerns for side effects of clozapine continue, clozapine remains a viable and potent option, particularly in younger and treatment-resistant patients (Gogtay and Rapoport 2008).

Early Intervention Studies

A great majority of the existing literature focuses on improving treatment when a patient is already involved with psychiatric services. However, there are several other potential windows for intervention. From earliest childhood, individuals who later develop schizophrenia as adults have subtle motor and cognitive abnormalities, similar to the constellation of deficits found in children at high risk of developing psychosis by virtue of having a parent with schizophrenia (Cornblatt 2002). Many other studies, most notably the large epidemiological study on the course of psychosis (the Age, Beginning, and Course study), have established the existence of a prodromal phase, lasting 2–5 years (Beiser et al. 1993; Hafner et al. 1998). During this time, an individual experiences a marked decline in overall functioning, and mental state is characterized by abnormalities of thought, perception, and action, which appear to be attenuated forms of the positive psychotic symptoms. Nearer the onset of established psychosis, many patients have fully developed positive psychotic symptoms, but these are transient, intermittent, and self-terminating. Finally, several studies have demonstrated that typically a long period of delay occurs between the onset of definite psychotic symptoms and the onset of treatment.

Research into interventions during the period between the development of a DSM-IV-TR psychotic disorder and the beginning of treatment is fueled by evidence that a longer duration of untreated psychosis is linked to poorer clinical outcome in many, but not all, studies (for a review, see Ruhrmann et al. 2005). Additionally, there are concerns that untreated psychosis is not only intensely aversive for the patient but also possibly neurotoxic (Lieberman et al. 1997; Pantelis et al. 2003). The evidence for such secondary prevention is surprisingly scant (e.g., see (Kuipers et al. 2004), given that it forms the current dominant model of health service provision.

Another, more ambitious, strategy attempts to identify people who are prepsychotic or prodromal and intervene during this stage to not only delay but possibly avert an eventual transition to frank psychosis. Considering that the median age at onset of schizophrenia is 19 years, most prodromal subjects are adolescents, making the rise of preventive interventions of particular relevance to the psychiatrist working with children and adolescents.

The feasibility of such preventive intervention relies on the ability to accurately identify subjects who are at high risk of psychosis. The current dominant approach defines patients at ultra-high risk of developing psychosis in the near future, combining the traditional definition of genetic high risk (having a first-degree relative with a psychotic disorder) with early symptomatic and functional changes. McGorry et al. (2003) led the field in developing criteria that suggest ultra-high risk for the development of psychosis. One group at ultra-high risk includes those with trait and state risk factors, meaning those with genetic high risk and/or schizotypal personality disorder, as well as a rapid, recent decline in global function. Other groups at ultra-high risk are those with clusters of attenuated positive symptoms (including unusual thought content/delusional ideation, suspiciousness/persecutory ideas, grandiosity) and brief, limited, or intermittent psychotic symptoms. Overall, approximately 40% of patients meeting these criteria will transition to psychosis (not just schizophrenia) within 12 months, with *psychosis* defined as the presence of positive psychotic symptoms for longer than 1 week (Yung et al. 2003). An alternative approach emphasizes so-called basic symptoms, which are subtle self-experienced neuropsychological deficits, such as thought pressure, perseverative thinking, derealization, and slight perceptual aberrations. In one study using this approach, the Cologne Early Recognition Study, investigators correctly predicted a transition to schizophrenia (not only psychosis) in 78% of cases within 4 years (Klosterkotter et al. 2001), and their work has partly formed the basis of ongoing prevention studies in Germany.

Issues of intervention are contentious. There are at least two ethical and pragmatic objections to using psychotropics during the prodromal phase.

The first is a claim that the evidence base for psychotropic use is scant. This is of particular concern, because even the best current criteria of ultra-high risk are far from perfect, carrying a high rate of false positives, which means that many subjects will be potentially exposed to medications without any clear evidence that they would have developed psychosis if left untreated. The second objection is that taking medication entails contact with psychiatric services and accepting the label of being at risk of developing psychosis, both of which are likely to carry some degree of social stigma.

One of the first studies on early intervention at the prodromal stage was conducted in the United Kingdom (Falloon 1992). In this study, all patients who were prodromal, as defined by DSM-III criteria (American Psychiatric Association 1980), were given psychoeducation, and some patients additionally received low-dose antipsychotics. The study reported a 10-fold decrease in the incidence of schizophrenia in the region compared with a previous period, although the study was uncontrolled and it is unclear which components of the intervention were efficacious.

In the first RCT, McGorry et al. (2003) found that significantly fewer patients who were treated with a mix of low-dose risperidone and psychotherapy progressed to first-episode psychosis by the end of the 6-month trial period compared with a group who received nonspecific "needs-based" interventions (9.7% vs. 35.7%, respectively; $P<0.05$). (This and other RCTs are summarized in Table 9–3.) The significant difference between the groups was not sustained at a 6-month follow-up after the active intervention, however, because of an increase in the number of patients in the specific intervention group who became psychotic. A post hoc analysis suggested that, overall, subjects in the specific-intervention group who received low-dose risperidone had the lowest rates of transition to psychosis, although the numbers were small. Additionally, given the design of the study, it is difficult to determine the specific contribution of risperidone to the findings.

In the Prevention Through Risk Identification, Management, and Education trial comparing olanzapine with placebo, Woods et al. (2003) found that although olanzapine treatment reduced the transition to psychosis rate by 50% (from 35% to 16%), the reduction was not statistically significant. Detailed reporting on the data at 8 weeks after initial randomization suggested that there was more improvement in psychopathology in association with olanzapine treatment, given at a mean dosage of 10 mg over the period

Table 9–3. Randomized trials of interventions for patients at ultra-high risk of developing psychosis

Study	Interventions	N	Outcome measures	Results	Comments
McGorry et al. 2003	NBI vs. SPI (risperidone 1.3 mg/day and CBT)	59	Development of definite psychotic symptoms	10/28 NBI vs. 3/31 SPI developed psychosis at 6 months; difference not sustained at 12 months	Lower rate of development of psychosis in patients who were fully adherent to risperidone (2/14 vs. 7/17)
Woods et al. 2003	Placebo vs. olanzapine	60	Development of psychosis (based on Scale of Prodromal Symptoms)	10/29 placebo vs. 5/31 olanzapine developed psychosis	Significant group difference at 8 weeks using linear mixed-models analyses
Morrison et al. 2004	TAU vs. CT	58	Development of definite psychotic symptoms (based on PANSS)	2/35 CT vs. 4/23 TAU developed psychosis	96% reduction in odds of making a transition to psychosis in CT group[a]

Note.   CBT=cognitive-behavioral therapy; CT=cognitive therapy; NBI=needs-based intervention; PANSS=Positive and Negative Syndrome Scale; SPI=specific preventive intervention; TAU=treatment as usual.
[a]After adjustment for potential moderating variables.

(with a significant interaction of groups with scores on the PANSS and Scale of Prodromal Symptoms in a linear, mixed-model regression). However, there was also marked weight gain in the olanzapine group during this period (mean = 4 kg vs. 0.3 kg in the placebo group; $P<0.001$).

A descriptive, interim analysis of a German intervention trial comparing amisulpride with placebo indicates beneficial effects of amisulpride not only on attenuated positive symptoms but also on negative and depressive symptoms and global functioning (Ruhrmann et al. 2003). Whether these promising initial results will be sustained by future work with additional data is unclear.

The potential use of nonpharmacological interventions alone in prodromal patients has also proved to be a promising avenue. Morrison et al. (2004) found that 5.7% of patients receiving cognitive therapy compared with 17.4% receiving "treatment as usual" developed psychosis over a 1-year period. In addition, cognitive therapy appeared to reduce the intensity of the prodromal symptoms themselves (Morrison et al. 2004).

Moreover, it is not at all clear that antipsychotics are necessarily the only, or the best, pharmacological intervention. In the Hillside Recognition and Prevention Program, adolescents first were identified as being at risk of developing psychosis on the basis of specific combination deficits of neurocognitive deficits and then were treated (Cornblatt 2002). Unlike in other studies, the adolescents did not have to display any attenuated positive symptoms. The 54 adolescents in this group were treated on an unrandomized, open-label basis with either antipsychotics or antidepressants (selective serotonin reuptake inhibitors). Interestingly, the antidepressants, often given in combination with mood stabilizers, were as effective as the antipsychotics in promoting clinical improvement.

A recent review agrees that randomized clinical trials may suggest a possible positive effect upon the completion of treatment (Masi and Liboni 2011). However, without significantly stronger results in the literature, continuing concerns regarding side effects and nonadherence preclude any validation to standardize prodromal intervention in a typical clinical setting (de Koning et al. 2009).

Conclusions

In consideration of the lack of clear treatment guidelines to guide the child psychiatrist through this controversial field, further work to develop understanding of primary and secondary preventions is necessary to move forward. Current reviews have summarized the recent literature advocating for proper pharmacotherapy to greatly increase the efficacy of psychosocial interventions (Masi and Liboni 2011). Low pharmacological effect sizes, remission rates, and frequent adverse side effects, mainly metabolic, highlight the importance of future research incorporating randomized, placebo-controlled studies as well as long-term, naturalistic follow-ups of large patient samples.

Clinical Pearls

- Remember that childhood-onset schizophrenia is similar to the adult form of the disorder but much more rare, usually more severe, and more difficult to treat.
- Consider antipsychotics to be the mainstay of treatment because they are superior to placebo.
- Keep in mind that although older RCTs suggest a trend toward superior efficacy for the atypicals olanzapine and risperidone over haloperidol in the treatment of childhood psychoses, this clinical trend is complicated by recent work with a molindone comparison.
- Consider a trial of clozapine because it remains the antipsychotic with clear, superior efficacy for severe forms of early psychosis, particularly in childhood-onset and treatment-resistant cases.
- Advise patients and their families that all antipsychotics are associated with adverse side effects, including EPS with the typicals and metabolic complications with the newer atypicals.
- Remain aware that it is unclear whether treatment during the prodromal phase immediately preceding the onset of frank psychosis is effective.

References

Abi-Dargham A, Laruelle M: Mechanisms of action of second generation antipsychotic drugs in schizophrenia: insights from brain imaging studies. Eur Psychiatry 20:15–27, 2005

Alfaro CL, Wudarsky M, Nicolson R, et al: Correlation of antipsychotic and prolactin concentrations in children and adolescents acutely treated with haloperidol, clozapine, or olanzapine. J Child Adolesc Psychopharmacol 12:83–91, 2002

Alvir JM, Lieberman JA, Safferman AZ, et al: Clozapine-induced agranulocytosis: incidence and risk factors in the United States. N Engl J Med 329:162–167, 1993

Amato D, Natesan S, Yavich L, et al: Dynamic regulation of dopamine and serotonin responses to salient stimuli during chronic haloperidol treatment. Int J Neuropsychopharmacol 14:1327–1339, 2011

American Academy of Child and Adolescent Psychiatry: Practice parameter for the assessment and treatment of children and adolescents with schizophrenia. J Am Acad Child Adolesc Psychiatry 40 (suppl):4S–23S, 2001

American Psychiatric Association: Diagnostic and Statistical Manual of Mental Disorders, 3rd Edition. Washington, DC, American Psychiatric Association, 1980

American Psychiatric Association: Diagnostic and Statistical Manual of Mental Disorders, 3rd Edition, Revised. Washington, DC, American Psychiatric Association, 1987

American Psychiatric Association: Diagnostic and Statistical Manual of Mental Disorders, 4th Edition. Washington, DC, American Psychiatric Association, 1994

American Psychiatric Association: Diagnostic and Statistical Manual of Mental Disorders, 4th Edition, Text Revision. Washington, DC, American Psychiatric Association, 2000

Armenteros JL, Whitaker AH, Welikson M, et al: Risperidone in adolescents with schizophrenia: an open pilot study. J Am Acad Child Adolesc Psychiatry 36:694–700, 1997

Attard A, Taylor DM: Comparative effectiveness of atypical antipsychotics in schizophrenia: what have real-world trials taught us? CNS Drugs 26:491–508, 2012

Bachmann CJ, Lehr D, Theisen FM, et al: Aripiprazole as an adjunct to clozapine therapy in adolescents with early onset schizophrenia: a retrospective chart review. Pharmacopsychiatry 42:153–157, 2009

Bai YM, Lin CC, Chen JY, et al: Therapeutic effect of pirenzepine for clozapine-induced hypersalivation: a randomized, double-blind, placebo-controlled, cross-over study. J Clin Psychopharmacol 21:608–611, 2001

Barnes TR: A rating scale for drug-induced akathisia. Br J Psychiatry 154:672–676, 1989

Barnett M: Ziprasidone monotherapy in pediatric bipolar disorder. Poster presented at the 156th Annual Meeting of the American Psychiatric Association, San Francisco, CA, May 2003

Beiser M, Erickson D, Fleming JA, et al: Establishing the onset of psychotic illness. Am J Psychiatry 150:1349–1354, 1993

Berger GE, Proffitt TM, McConchie M, et al: Dosing quetiapine in drug-naive first-episode psychosis: a controlled, double-blind, randomized, single-center study investigating efficacy, tolerability, and safety of 200 mg/day vs. 400 mg/day of quetiapine fumarate in 141 patients aged 15 to 25 years. J Clin Psychiatry 69:1702–1714, 2008

Bitter I, Dossenbach MR, Brook S, et al: Olanzapine versus clozapine in treatment-resistant or treatment-intolerant schizophrenia. Prog Neuropsychopharmacol Biol Psychiatry 28:173–180, 2004

Bobes J, Gibert J, Ciudad A, et al: Safety and effectiveness of olanzapine versus conventional antipsychotics in the acute treatment of first-episode schizophrenic inpatients. Prog Neuropsychopharmacol Biol Psychiatry 27:473–481, 2003

Burstein ES, Ma J, Wong S, et al: Intrinsic efficacy of antipsychotics at human D2, D3, and D4 dopamine receptors: identification of the clozapine metabolite N-desmethylclozapine as a D2/D3 partial agonist. J Pharmacol Exp Ther 315:1278–1287, 2005

Canitano R: Clinical experience with topiramate to counteract neuroleptic induced weight gain in 10 individuals with autistic spectrum disorders. Brain Dev 27:228–232, 2005

Caroff SN, Mann SC, Campbell EC, et al: Atypical antipsychotics and neuroleptic malignant syndrome. Psychiatr Ann 30:314–321, 2000

Castro-Fornieles J, Parellada M, Soutullo CA, et al: Antipsychotic treatment in child and adolescent first-episode psychosis: a longitudinal naturalistic approach. J Child Adolesc Psychopharmacol 18:327–336, 2008

Chengappa KN, Shelton MD, Baker RW, et al: The prevalence of akathisia in patients receiving stable doses of clozapine. J Clin Psychiatry 55:142–145, 1994

Cheng-Shannon J, McGough JJ, Pataki C, et al: Second-generation antipsychotic medications in children and adolescents. J Child Adolesc Psychopharmacol 14:372–394, 2004

Childs B, Scriver CR: Age at onset and causes of disease. Perspect Biol Med 29:437–460, 1986

Cohen LG, Biederman J: Treatment of risperidone-induced hyperprolactinemia with a dopamine agonist in children. J Child Adolesc Psychopharmacol 11:435–440, 2001

Cornblatt BA: The New York high risk project to the Hillside Recognition and Prevention (RAP) program. Am J Med Genet 114:956–966, 2002

Correll CU: Symptomatic presentation and initial treatment for schizophrenia in children and adolescents. J Clin Psychiatry 71:E29, 2010

Correll CU: Safety and tolerability of antipsychotic treatment in young patients with schizophrenia. J Clin Psychiatry 72:E26, 2011

Correll CU, Manu P, Olshanskiy V, et al: Cardiometabolic risk of second-generation antipsychotic medications during first-time use in children and adolescents. JAMA 302:1765–1773, 2009

David CN, Rapoport JL: The neurodevelopment of hallucinations, in The Neuroscience of Hallucinations. Edited by Jardris R. New York, Springer, 2012

David CN, Greenstein D, Clasen L, et al: Childhood onset schizophrenia: high rate of visual hallucinations. J Am Acad Child Adolesc Psychiatry 50:681–686.E3, 2011 [Epub]

Davis JM, Chen N, Glick ID: A meta-analysis of the efficacy of second-generation antipsychotics. Arch Gen Psychiatry 60:553–564, 2003

Deckelbaum RJ, Williams CL: Childhood obesity: the health issue. Obes Res 9 (suppl): 239S–243S, 2001

de Koning, MB, Bloemen OJ, van Almsvoort TA, et al: Early intervention in patients at ultra high risk of psychosis: benefits and risks. Acta Psychiatr Scand 119:426–442, 2009

Deniau E, Bonnot O, Cohen D: [Drug treatment of early onset schizophrenia]. Presse Med 37:853–858, 2008

Eggers C, Bunk D: The long-term course of childhood-onset schizophrenia: a 42-year follow-up. Schizophr Bull 23:105–117, 1997

Engelhardt DM, Polizos P, Waizer J, et al: A double-blind comparison of fluphenazine and haloperidol in outpatient schizophrenic children. J Autism Child Schizophr 3:128–137, 1973

Falloon IR: Early intervention for first episodes of schizophrenia: a preliminary exploration. Psychiatry 55:4–15, 1992

Faulkner G, Soundy AA, Lloyd K: Schizophrenia and weight management: a systematic review of interventions to control weight. Acta Psychiatr Scand 108:324–332, 2003

Fedorowicz VJ, Fombonne E: Metabolic side effects of atypical antipsychotics in children: a literature review. Psychopharmacology 19:533–550, 2005

Findling RL, McNamara NK, Youngstrom EA, et al: A prospective, open-label trial of olanzapine in adolescents with schizophrenia. J Am Acad Child Adolesc Psychiatry 42:170–175, 2003

Findling RL, Aman MG, Eerdekens M, et al: Long-term, open-label study of risperidone in children with severe disruptive behaviors and below-average IQ. Am J Psychiatry 161:677–684, 2004

Findling RL, Frazier JA, Gerbino-Rosen G, et al: Is there a role for clozapine in the treatment of children and adolescents? J Am Acad Child Adolesc Psychiatry 46:423–428, 2007a

Findling RL, Reed MD, O'Riordan MA, et al: A 26-week open-label study of quetiapine in children with conduct disorder. J Child Adolesc Psychopharmacol 17:1–9, 2007b

Findling RL, Kauffman RE, Sallee FR, et al: Tolerability and pharmacokinetics of aripiprazole in children and adolescents with psychiatric disorders: an open-label, dose-escalation study. J Clin Psychopharmacol 28:441–446, 2008a

Findling RL, Robb A, Nyilas M, et al: A multiple-center, randomized, double-blind, placebo-controlled study of oral aripiprazole for treatment of adolescents with schizophrenia. Am J Psychiatry 165:1432–1441, 2008b

Findling RL, Cavus I, Pappadopulos E, et al: A placebo-controlled trial to evaluate the efficacy and safety of flexibly dosed oral ziprasidone in adolescent subjects with schizophrenia. Presented at the 2nd Biannual Schizophrenia International Research Conference, Florence, Italy, 2010a

Findling RL, Johnson JL, McClellan J, et al: Double-blind maintenance safety and effectiveness findings from the Treatment of Early Onset Schizophrenia Spectrum (TEOSS) study. J Am Acad Child Adolesc Psychiatry 49:583–594; quiz 632, 2010b

Frazier JA, Gordon CT, McKenna K, et al: An open trial of clozapine in 11 adolescents with childhood-onset schizophrenia. J Am Acad Child Adolesc Psychiatry 33:658–663, 1994

Geddes J, Freemantle N, Harrison P, et al: Atypical antipsychotics in the treatment of schizophrenia: systematic overview and meta-regression analysis. BMJ 321:1371–1376, 2000

Glazer WM: Extrapyramidal side effects, tardive dyskinesia, and the concept of atypicality. J Clin Psychiatry 61 (suppl):16–21, 2000

Gochman P, Miller R, Rapoport JL: Childhood-onset schizophrenia: the challenge of diagnosis. Curr Psychiatry Rep 13:321–322, 2011

Goeb JL, Marco S, Duhamel A, et al: [Metabolic side effects of risperidone in early onset schizophrenia]. Encephale 36:242–252, 2010

Gogtay N, Rapoport J: Clozapine use in children and adolescents. Expert Opin Pharmacother 9:459–465, 2008

Gogtay N, Sporn A, Alfaro CL, et al: Clozapine-induced akathisia in children with schizophrenia. J Child Adolesc Psychopharmacol 12:347–349, 2002

Gogtay N, Ordonez A, Herman DH, et al: Dynamic mapping of cortical development before and after the onset of pediatric bipolar illness. J Child Psychol Psychiatry 48:852–862, 2007

Gothelf D, Apter A, Reidman J, et al: Olanzapine, risperidone and haloperidol in the treatment of adolescent patients with schizophrenia. J Neural Transm 110:545–560, 2003

Goyal N, Sinha VK: Amisulpride-induced tardive dyskinesia in childhood onset schizophrenia. Prog Neuropsychopharmacol Biol Psychiatry 34:728–729, 2010

Gracious BL, Krysiak TE, Youngstrom EA: Amantadine treatment of psychotropic-induced weight gain in children and adolescents: case series. J Child Adolesc Psychopharmacol 12:249–257, 2002

Grcevich SJ, Findling RL, Rowane WA, et al: Risperidone in the treatment of children and adolescents with schizophrenia: a retrospective study. J Child Adolesc Psychopharmacol 6:251–257, 1996

Greenstein D, Lerch J, Shaw P, et al: Childhood onset schizophrenia: cortical brain abnormalities as young adults. J Child Psychol Psychiatry 47:1003–1012, 2006

Guy W: Clinical Global Impressions, in ECDEU Assessment Manual for Psychopharmacology, Revised (NIMH Publ No 76-338). Rockville, MD, National Institute of Mental Health, 1976, pp 218–222

Haapasalo-Pesu KM: [Clozapine in the treatment of under-age schizophrenia]. Duodecim 125:1635–1638, 2009

Haas M, Eerdekens M, Kushner S, et al: Efficacy, safety and tolerability of two dosing regimens in adolescent schizophrenia: double-blind study. Br J Psychiatry 194:158–164, 2009a

Haas M, Unis AS, Armenteros J, et al: A 6-week, randomized, double-blind, placebo-controlled study of the efficacy and safety of risperidone in adolescents with schizophrenia. J Child Adolesc Psychopharmacol 19:611–621, 2009b

Hafner H, Maurer K, Loffler W, et al: The ABC Schizophrenia Study: a preliminary overview of the results. Soc Psychiatry Psychiatr Epidemiol 33:380–386, 1998

Halloran DR, Swindle J, Takemoto SK, et al: Multiple psychiatric diagnoses common in privately insured children on atypical antipsychotics. Clin Pediatr (Phila) 49:485–490, 2010

Hamann J, Kissling W, Leucht S, et al: New generation antipsychotics for first episode schizophrenia. Cochrane Database of Systematic Reviews 2003, Issue 4. Art. No.: CD004410. DOI: 10.1002/14651858.CD004410.

Hanft A, Eggleston CF, Bourgeois JA: Neuroleptic malignant syndrome in an adolescent after brief exposure to olanzapine. J Child Adolesc Psychopharmacol 14:481–487, 2004

Hartung DM, Wisdom JP, Pollack DA, et al: Patterns of atypical antipsychotic subtherapeutic dosing among Oregon Medicaid patients. J Clin Psychiatry 69:1540–1547, 2008

Herran A, Garcia-Unzueta MT, Amado JA, et al: Effects of long-term treatment with antipsychotics on serum leptin levels. Br J Psychiatry 179:59–62, 2001

Hollis C: Adult outcomes of child- and adolescent-onset schizophrenia: diagnostic stability and predictive validity. Am J Psychiatry 157:1652–1659, 2000

Hrdlicka M, Zedkova I, Blatny M, et al: Weight gain associated with atypical and typical antipsychotics during treatment of adolescent schizophrenic psychoses: a retrospective study. Neuro Endocrinol Lett 30:256–261, 2009

Jin H, Meyer JM, Jeste DV: Atypical antipsychotics and glucose dysregulation: a systematic review. Schizophr Res 71:195–212, 2004

Kahl KG, Hagenah J, Zapf S, et al: Botulinum toxin as an effective treatment of clozapine-induced hypersalivation. Psychopharmacology 173:229–230, 2004

Kane J, Honigfeld G, Singer J, et al: Clozapine for the treatment-resistant schizophrenic: a double-blind comparison with chlorpromazine. Arch Gen Psychiatry 45:789–796, 1988

Kapur S, Remington G: Atypical antipsychotics: new directions and new challenges in the treatment of schizophrenia. Annu Rev Med 52:503–517, 2001

Kennedy E, Kumar A, Datta SS: Antipsychotic medication for childhood-onset schizophrenia. Cochrane Database of Systematic Reviews 2007, Issue 3. Art. No.: CD004027. DOI: 10.1002/14651858.CD004027.pub2.

Kim Y, Kim BN, Cho SC, et al: Long-term sustained benefits of clozapine treatment in refractory early onset schizophrenia: a retrospective study in Korean children and adolescents. Hum Psychopharmacol 23:715–722, 2008

Klein DJ, Cottingham EM, Sorter M, et al: A randomized, double-blind, placebo-controlled trial of metformin treatment of weight gain associated with initiation of atypical antipsychotic therapy in children and adolescents. Am J Psychiatry 163:2072–2079, 2006

Klosterkotter J, Hellmich M, Steinmeyer EM, et al: Diagnosing schizophrenia in the initial prodromal phase. Arch Gen Psychiatry 58:158–164, 2001

Kolvin I: Studies in the childhood psychoses, I: diagnostic criteria and classification. Br J Psychiatry 118:381–384, 1971

Komossa K, Rummel-Kluge C, Schmid F, et al: Aripiprazole versus other atypical antipsychotics for schizophrenia. Cochrane Database of Systematic Reviews 2009, Issue 4. Art. No.: CD006569. DOI: 10.1002/14651858.CD006569.pub3.

Kraepelin E: Dementia Praecox and Paraphrenia. Huntington, NY, Robert E Krieger, 1919

Kryzhanovskaya LA, Robertson-Plouch CK, Xu W, et al: The safety of olanzapine in adolescents with schizophrenia or bipolar I disorder: a pooled analysis of 4 clinical trials. J Clin Psychiatry 70:247–258, 2009a

Kryzhanovskaya LA, Schulz SC, McDougle C, et al: Olanzapine versus placebo in adolescents with schizophrenia: a 6-week, randomized, double-blind, placebo-controlled trial. J Am Acad Child Adolesc Psychiatry 48:60–70, 2009b

Kuipers E, Holloway F, Rabe-Hesketh S, et al: An RCT of early intervention in psychosis: Croydon Outreach and Assertive Support Team (COAST). Soc Psychiatry Psychiatr Epidemiol 39:358–363, 2004

Kumra S, Frazier JA, Jacobsen LK, et al: Childhood-onset schizophrenia: a double-blind clozapine-haloperidol comparison. Arch Gen Psychiatry 53:1090–1097, 1996

Kumra S, Jacobsen LK, Lenane M, et al: Childhood-onset schizophrenia: an open-label study of olanzapine in adolescents. J Am Acad Child Adolesc Psychiatry 37:377–385, 1998

Kumra S, Kranzler H, Gerbino-Rosen G, et al: Clozapine and "high-dose" olanzapine in refractory early onset schizophrenia: a 12-week randomized and double-blind comparison. Biol Psychiatry 63:524–529, 2008a

Kumra S, Kranzler H, Gerbino-Rosen G, et al: Clozapine versus "high-dose" olanzapine in refractory early onset schizophrenia: an open-label extension study. J Child Adolesc Psychopharmacol 18:307–316, 2008b

Kumra S, Oberstar JV, Sikich L, et al: Efficacy and tolerability of second-generation antipsychotics in children and adolescents with schizophrenia. Schizophr Bull 34:60–71, 2008c

Leucht S, Pitschel-Walz G, Abraham D, et al: Efficacy and extrapyramidal side-effects of the new antipsychotics olanzapine, quetiapine, risperidone, and sertindole compared to conventional antipsychotics and placebo: a meta-analysis of randomized controlled trials. Schizophr Res 35:51–68, 1999

Leucht S, Wahlbeck K, Hamann J, et al: New generation antipsychotics versus low-potency conventional antipsychotics: a systematic review and meta-analysis. Lancet 361:1581–1589, 2003

Levine SZ, Rabinowitz J: Trajectories and antecedents of treatment response over time in early episode psychosis. Schizophr Bull 36:624–632, 2010

Lieberman JA, Saltz BL, Johns CA, et al: The effects of clozapine on tardive dyskinesia. Br J Psychiatry 158:503–510, 1991

Lieberman JA, Sheitman BB, Kinon BJ: Neurochemical sensitization in the pathophysiology of schizophrenia: deficits and dysfunction in neuronal regulation and plasticity. Neuropsychopharmacology 17:205–229, 1997

Lieberman JA, Phillips M, Gu H, et al: Atypical and conventional antipsychotic drugs in treatment-naive first-episode schizophrenia: a 52-week randomized trial of clozapine vs. chlorpromazine. Neuropsychopharmacology 28:995–1003, 2003

Lieberman JA, Stroup TS, McEvoy JP, et al: Effectiveness of antipsychotic drugs in patients with chronic schizophrenia. N Engl J Med 353:1209–1223, 2005

Mangurian C, Fuentes-Afflick E, Newcomer JW, et al: Risks from antipsychotic medications in children and adolescents. JAMA 303:729–730, 2010

Martin S, Ljo H, Peuskens J, et al: A double-blind, randomised comparative trial of amisulpride versus olanzapine in the treatment of schizophrenia: short-term results at two months. Curr Med Res Opin 18:355–362, 2002

Masi G, Liboni F: Management of schizophrenia in children and adolescents: focus on pharmacotherapy. Drugs 71:179–208, 2011

Masi G, Cosenza A, Mucci M: Prolactin levels in young children with pervasive developmental disorders during risperidone treatment. J Child Adolesc Psychopharmacol 11:389–394, 2001

McClellan J, Sikich L, Findling RL, et al: Treatment of early onset schizophrenia spectrum disorders (TEOSS): rationale, design, and methods. J Am Acad Child Adolesc Psychiatry 46:969–978, 2007

McConville B, Carrero L, Sweitzer D, et al: Long-term safety, tolerability, and clinical efficacy of quetiapine in adolescents: an open-label extension trial. J Child Adolesc Psychopharmacol 13:75–82, 2003

McGorry PD, Yung AR, Phillips LJ: The "close-in" or ultra high-risk model: a safe and effective strategy for research and clinical intervention in prepsychotic mental disorder. Schizophr Bull 29:771–790, 2003

Melkersson KI, Dahl ML, Hulting AL: Guidelines for prevention and treatment of adverse effects of antipsychotic drugs on glucose-insulin homeostasis and lipid metabolism. Psychopharmacology 175:1–6, 2004

Miyamoto S, Duncan GE, Marx CE, et al: Treatments for schizophrenia: a critical review of pharmacology and mechanisms of action of antipsychotic drugs. Mol Psychiatry 10:79–104, 2005

Moncrieff J: Clozapine vs. conventional antipsychotic drugs for treatment-resistant schizophrenia: a re-examination. Br J Psychiatry 183:161–166, 2003

Morrison AP, French P, Walford L, et al: Cognitive therapy for the prevention of psychosis in people at ultra-high risk: randomised controlled trial. Br J Psychiatry 185:291–297, 2004

Mozes T, Greenberg Y, Spivak B, et al: Olanzapine treatment in chronic drug-resistant childhood-onset schizophrenia: an open-label study. J Child Adolesc Psychopharmacol 13:311–317, 2003

Nicolson R, Lenane M, Brookner F, et al: Children and adolescents with psychotic disorder not otherwise specified: a 2- to 8-year follow-up study. Compr Psychiatry 42:319–325, 2001

Normala I, Hamidin A: The use of aripiprazole in early onset schizophrenia: safety and efficacy. Med J Malaysia 64:240–241, 2009

Novick D, Haro JM, Bertsch J, et al: Incidence of extrapyramidal symptoms and tardive dyskinesia in schizophrenia: thirty-six-month results from the European schizophrenia outpatient health outcomes study. J Clin Psychopharmacol 30:531–540, 2010

Pantelis C, Velakoulis D, McGorry PD, et al: Neuroanatomical abnormalities before and after onset of psychosis: a cross-sectional and longitudinal MRI comparison. Lancet 361:281–288, 2003

Pappagallo M, Silva R: The effect of atypical antipsychotic agents on prolactin levels in children and adolescents. J Child Adolesc Psychopharmacol 14:359–371, 2004

Patel JK, Buckley PF, Woolson S, et al: Metabolic profiles of second-generation antipsychotics in early psychosis: findings from the CAFE study. Schizophr Res 111:9–16, 2009

Patel NC, Sanchez RJ, Johnsrud MT, et al: Trends in antipsychotic use in a Texas Medicaid population of children and adolescents: 1996 to 2000. J Child Adolesc Psychopharmacol 12:221–229, 2002

Pickar D, Litman RE, Hong WW, et al: Clinical response to clozapine in patients with schizophrenia. Arch Gen Psychiatry 51:159–160, 1994

Polanczyk G, Moffitt TE, Arseneault L, et al: Etiological and clinical features of childhood psychotic symptoms: results from a birth cohort. Arch Gen Psychiatry 67:328–338, 2010

Pool D, Bloom W, Mielke DH, et al: A controlled evaluation of loxitane in seventy-five adolescent schizophrenic patients. Curr Ther Res Clin Exp 19:99–104, 1976

Poulton R, Caspi A, Moffitt TE, et al: Children's self-reported psychotic symptoms and adult schizophreniform disorder: a 15-year longitudinal study. Arch Gen Psychiatry 57:1053–1058, 2000

Rapoport JL, Addington AM, Frangou S, et al: The neurodevelopmental model of schizophrenia: update 2005. Mol Psychiatry 10:434–449, 2005a

Rapoport JL, Addington A, Frangou S: The neurodevelopmental model of schizophrenia: what can very early onset cases tell us? Curr Psychiatry Rep 7:81–82, 2005b

Realmuto GM, Erickson WD, Yellin AM, et al: Clinical comparison of thiothixene and thioridazine in schizophrenic adolescents. Am J Psychiatry 141:440–442, 1984

Remington G, Kapur S: Antipsychotic dosing: how much but also how often? Schizophr Bull 36:900–903, 2010

Robles O, Zabala A, Bombin I, et al: Cognitive efficacy of quetiapine and olanzapine in early onset first-episode psychosis. Schizophr Bull 37:405–415, 2011

Ross RG, Novins D, Farley GK, et al: A 1-year open-label trial of olanzapine in school-age children with schizophrenia. J Child Adolesc Psychopharmacol 13:301–309, 2003

Ruhrmann S, Schultze-Lutter F, Klosterkotter J: Early detection and intervention in the initial prodromal phase of schizophrenia. Pharmacopsychiatry 36 (suppl): S162–S167, 2003

Ruhrmann S, Schultze-Lutter F, Maier W, et al: Pharmacological intervention in the initial prodromal phase of psychosis. Eur Psychiatry 20:1–6, 2005

Saito E, Correll CU, Gallelli K, et al: A prospective study of hyperprolactinemia in children and adolescents treated with atypical antipsychotic agents. J Child Adolesc Psychopharmacol 14:350–358, 2004

Selva KA, Scott SM: Diabetic ketoacidosis associated with olanzapine in an adolescent patient. J Pediatr 138:936–938, 2001

Shaw JA, Lewis JE, Pascal S, et al: A study of quetiapine: efficacy and tolerability in psychotic adolescents. J Child Adolesc Psychopharmacol 11:415–424, 2001

Shaw P, Rapoport JL: Decision making about children with psychotic symptoms: using the best evidence in choosing a treatment. J Am Acad Child Adolesc Psychiatry 45:1381–1386, 2006

Shaw P, Sporn A, Gogtay N, et al: Childhood-onset schizophrenia: a double-blind, randomized clozapine-olanzapine comparison. Arch Gen Psychiatry 63:721–730, 2006

Sholevar EH, Baron DA, Hardie TL: Treatment of childhood-onset schizophrenia with olanzapine. J Child Adolesc Psychopharmacol 10:69–78, 2000

Sikich L, Hamer RM, Bashford RA, et al: A pilot study of risperidone, olanzapine, and haloperidol in psychotic youth: a double-blind, randomized, 8-week trial. Neuropsychopharmacology 29:133–145, 2004

Sikich L, Frazier JA, McClellan J, et al: Double-blind comparison of first- and second-generation antipsychotics in early onset schizophrenia and schizo-affective disorder: findings from the treatment of early onset schizophrenia spectrum disorders (TEOSS) study. Am J Psychiatry 165:1420–1431, 2008

Simpson GM, Angus JW: A rating scale for extrapyramidal side effects. Acta Psychiatr Scand Suppl 212:11–19, 1970

Singh J, Robb A, Vijapurkar U, et al: A randomized, double-blind study of paliperidone extended-release in treatment of acute schizophrenia in adolescents. Biol Psychiatry 70:1179–1187, 2011

Sowell MO, Mukhopadhyay N, Cavazzoni P, et al: Hyperglycemic clamp assessment of insulin secretory responses in normal subjects treated with olanzapine, risperidone, or placebo. J Clin Endocrinol Metab 87:2918–2923, 2002

Spencer EK, Kafantaris V, Padron-Gayol MV, et al: Haloperidol in schizophrenic children: early findings from a study in progress. Psychopharmacol Bull 28:183–186, 1992

Sporn A, Gogtay N, Ortiz-Aguayo R, et al: Clozapine-induced neutropenia in children: management with lithium carbonate. J Child Adolesc Psychopharmacol 13:401–404, 2003

Sporn A, Gogtay N, Bobb A, et al: Clozapine treatment of childhood-onset schizophrenia: evaluation of efficacy, adverse effects, and long-term outcome. J Am Acad Child Adolesc Psychiatry 46:1349–1356, 2007

Stayer C, Sporn A, Gogtay N, et al: Multidimensionally impaired: the good news. J Child Adolesc Psychopharmacol 15:510–519, 2005

Tajima K, Fernandez H, Lopez-Ibor JL, et al: Schizophrenia treatment. Critical review on the drugs and mechanisms of action of antipsychotics. Actas Esp Psiquiatr 37:330–342, 2009

Thomsen PH: Schizophrenia with childhood and adolescent onset: a nationwide register-based study. Acta Psychiatr Scand 94:187–193, 1996

Tollefson GD, Birkett MA, Kiesler GM, et al: Double-blind comparison of olanzapine versus clozapine in schizophrenic patients clinically eligible for treatment with clozapine. Biol Psychiatry 49:52–63, 2001

Tossell JW, Greenstein DK, Davidson AL, et al: Stimulant drug treatment in childhood-onset schizophrenia with comorbid ADHD: an open-label case series. J Child Adolesc Psychopharmacol 14:448–454, 2004

Turetz M, Mozes T, Toren P, et al: An open trial of clozapine in neuroleptic-resistant childhood-onset schizophrenia. Br J Psychiatry 170:507–510, 1997

Uchida H, Suzuki T, Mamo DC, et al: Effects of age and age of onset on prescribed antipsychotic dose in schizophrenia spectrum disorders: a survey of 1,418 patients in Japan. Am J Geriatr Psychiatry 16:584–593, 2008

Usiskin SI, Nicolson R, Lenane M, et al: Gabapentin prophylaxis of clozapine-induced seizures. Am J Psychiatry 157:482–483, 2000

Vahia IV, Palmer BW, Depp C, et al: Is late-onset schizophrenia a subtype of schizophrenia? Acta Psychiatr Scand 122:414–426, 2010

Varol Tas F, Guvenir T: Amisulpride treatment of adolescent patients with schizophrenia or schizo-affective disorders. Eur Child Adolesc Psychiatry 18:511–513, 2009

Versiani M, Bueno J, Mundim M: A double-blind comparison between loxapine and chlordiazepoxide in the treatment of anxiety. Psychopharmacol Bull 13:22–24, 1977

Volavka J, Czobor P, Sheitman B, et al: Clozapine, olanzapine, risperidone, and haloperidol in the treatment of patients with chronic schizophrenia and schizoaffective disorder. Am J Psychiatry 159:255–262, 2002

Volkmar FR: Childhood and adolescent psychosis: a review of the past 10 years. J Am Acad Child Adolesc Psychiatry 35:843–851, 1996

Weiner DM, Meltzer HY, Veinbergs I, et al: The role of M1 muscarinic receptor agonism of N-desmethylclozapine in the unique clinical effects of clozapine. Psychopharmacology 177:207–216, 2004

Wirshing DA, Wirshing WC, Kysar L, et al: Novel antipsychotics: comparison of weight gain liabilities. J Clin Psychiatry 60:358–363, 1999

Woods SW, Breier A, Zipursky RB, et al: Randomized trial of olanzapine versus placebo in the symptomatic acute treatment of the schizophrenic prodrome. Biol Psychiatry 54:453–464, 2003 [erratum: 54:497, 2003]

Wudarsky M, Nicolson R, Hamburger SD, et al: Elevated prolactin in pediatric patients on typical and atypical antipsychotics. J Child Adolesc Psychopharmacol 9:239–245, 1999

Yung AR, Phillips LJ, Yuen HP, et al: Psychosis prediction: 12-month follow-up of a high-risk ("prodromal") group. Schizophr Res 60:21–32, 2003

Zalsman G, Carmon E, Martin A, et al: Effectiveness, safety, and tolerability of risperidone in adolescents with schizophrenia: an open-label study. J Child Adolesc Psychopharmacol 13:319–327, 2003

Index

*Page numbers printed in **boldface** type refer to tables or figures.*